Instructor's Resource Manual

DAVI-ELLEN CHABNER, BA, MAT

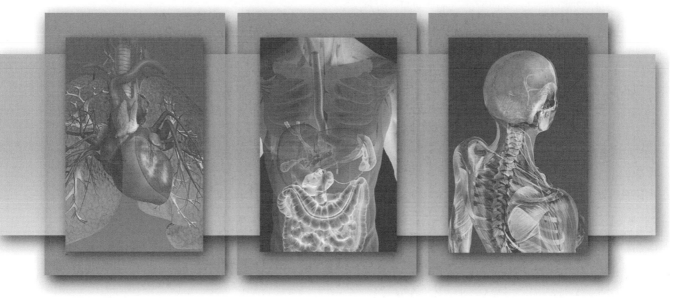

The Language
of Medicine

Eighth Edition

SAUNDERS
ELSEVIER

SAUNDERS
ELSEVIER

11830 Westline Industrial Drive
St. Louis, Missouri 63146

INSTRUCTOR'S RESOURCE MANUAL FOR THE
LANGUAGE OF MEDICINE, EIGHTH EDITION

Notice

Neither the Publisher nor the Author assumes any responsibility for any loss or injury and/or damage to persons or property arising out of or related to any use of the material contained in this book. It is the responsibility of the treating practitioner, relying on independent expertise and knowledge of the patient, to determine the best treatment and method of application for the patient.

The Publisher

ISBN 13: 978-1-4160-3490-2
ISBN 10: 1-4160-3490-0

Executive Editor: Jeanne Wilke
Senior Developmental Editor: Becky Swisher
Publishing Services Manager: Patricia Tannian
Project Manager: John Casey
Senior Designer: Ellen Zanolle

Printed in United States of America

Last digit is the print number: 9 8 7 6 5 4 3 2 1

TABLE OF CONTENTS

Introduction..1

How to Use the Textbook and Instructor's Manual 1

    Proposals for Courses 3

    Classroom Methods 5

    Ancillary Products: Back-of-Book CD, Instant Translator,
    Instructor's Resource Manual 7

Chapter One—Basic Word Structure

    Multiple Choice Quiz...11

    Exercise Quiz 13

    Dictation and Comprehension Quiz 15

    Spelling Quiz 16

    Pronunciation Quiz 17

    Review Sheet Quiz 18

    Crossword Puzzle 19

    Answers to the Quizzes 20

    Answers to Combining Forms and Terminology Sections....................22

Chapter Two—Terms Pertaining to the Body as a Whole

    Multiple Choice Quiz...27

    Exercise Quiz 29

    Dictation and Comprehension Quiz 31

    Spelling Quiz 32

    Pronunciation Quiz 33

    Diagram Quiz...35

    Review Sheet Quiz 36

Crossword Puzzle 38

Answers to the Quizzes 39

Answers to Combining Forms and Terminology Sections.....................................41

Chapter Three—Suffixes

Multiple Choice Quiz..43

Exercise Quiz..45

Dictation and Comprehension Quiz 47

Spelling Quiz..48

Pronunciation Quiz..49

Review Sheet Quiz..50

Crossword Puzzle 51

Answers to the Quizzes 53

Answers to Combining Forms and Terminology Sections.....................................55

Chapter Four—Prefixes

Multiple Choice Quiz..59

Exercise Quiz..61

Dictation and Comprehension Quiz 63

Spelling Quiz..64

Pronunciation Quiz..65

Review Sheet Quiz..66

Crossword Puzzle 67

Answers to the Quizzes 68

Answers to Combining Forms and Terminology Sections.....................................70

Chapter Five—Digestive System

Multiple Choice Quiz..75

Exercise Quiz..77

Dictation and Comprehension Quiz: Vocabulary 80

Dictation and Comprehension Quiz: Pathological Symptoms 81

Dictation and Comprehension Quiz: Pathological Conditions..............................82

Spelling Quiz..83

Pronunciation Quiz..84

Diagram Quiz...85

Vocabulary Quiz...86

Crossword Puzzle 88

Answers to the Quizzes 89

Answers to Combining Forms and Terminology Sections.. 92

Chapter Six—Additional Suffixes and Digestive System Terminology

Multiple Choice Quiz.. 95

Exercise Quiz 97

Dictation and Comprehension Quiz 99

Spelling Quiz 100

Pronunciation Quiz 101

Review Sheet Quiz 102

Crossword Puzzle 104

Practical Applications 105

Answers to the Quizzes 106

Answers to Combining Forms and Terminology Sections.. 109

Chapter Seven—Urinary System

Multiple Choice Quiz.. 113

Exercise Quiz 115

Dictation and Comprehension Quiz 117

Spelling Quiz 118

Pronunciation Quiz 119

Diagram Quiz... 120

Vocabulary Quiz... 121

Review Sheet Quiz 123

Crossword Puzzle 124

Practical Applications... 125

Answers to the Quizzes 126

Answers to Combining Forms and Terminology Sections.. 129

Chapter Eight—Female Reproductive System

Multiple Choice Quiz.. 133

Exercise Quiz 135

Dictation and Comprehension Quiz: Vocabulary and Terminology 138

Dictation and Comprehension Quiz: Pathological Conditions, Clinical
Tests and Procedures 139

Spelling Quiz 141

Pronunciation Quiz 142

Diagram Quiz 143

Vocabulary Quiz 144

Review Sheet Quiz 147

Crossword Puzzle 148

Practical Applications 149

Answers to the Quizzes 151

Answers to Combining Forms and Terminology Sections 154

Chapter Nine—Male Reproductive System

Multiple Choice Quiz 158

Exercise Quiz 160

Dictation and Comprehension Quiz 162

Spelling Quiz 163

Pronunciation Quiz 164

Diagram Quiz 165

Vocabulary Quiz 166

Review Sheet Quiz 168

Crossword Puzzle 169

Practical Applications 170

Answers to the Quizzes 171

Answers to Combining Forms and Terminology Sections 174

Chapter Ten—Nervous System

Multiple Choice Quiz 176

Exercise Quiz 178

Dictation and Comprehension Quiz: Vocabulary and Terminology 181

Dictation and Comprehension Quiz: Pathology 182

Spelling Quiz 183

Pronunciation Quiz 184

Diagram Quiz 185

Vocabulary Quiz 186

Review Sheet Quiz 188

Crossword Puzzle 189

Practical Applications 190

Answers to the Quizzes 191

Answers to Combining Forms and Terminology Sections 194

Chapter Eleven—Cardiovascular System

Multiple Choice Quiz...198

Exercise Quiz...200

Dictation and Comprehension Quiz: Vocabulary and Terminology 203

Dictation and Comprehension Quiz: Pathology...204

Spelling Quiz...205

Pronunciation Quiz...206

Abbreviations Quiz 207

Diagram Quiz...208

Vocabulary Quiz...209

Review Sheet Quiz 211

Crossword Puzzle 212

Practical Applications...213

Answers to the Quizzes 216

Answers to Combining Forms and Terminology Sections...219

Chapter Twelve—Respiratory System

Multiple Choice Quiz...221

Exercise Quiz...223

Dictation and Comprehension Quiz: Vocabulary and Terminology 226

Dictation and Comprehension Quiz: Pathology...227

Spelling Quiz...228

Pronunciation Quiz...229

Abbreviations Quiz 230

Diagram Quiz...231

Vocabulary Quiz...232

Review Sheet Quiz 234

Crossword Puzzle 235

Practical Applications...236

Answers to the Quizzes 238

Answers to Combining Forms and Terminology Sections...241

Chapter Thirteen—Blood System

Multiple Choice Quiz...245

Exercise Quiz...248

Dictation and Comprehension Quiz: Vocabulary 251

Dictation and Comprehension Quiz: Pathology and Tests.......................................252

Spelling Quiz 253

Pronunciation Quiz 254

Diagram Quiz 255

Vocabulary Quiz 256

Review Sheet Quiz 258

Crossword Puzzle 259

Practical Applications 260

Answers to the Quizzes 261

Answers to Combining Forms and Terminology Sections 264

Chapter Fourteen—Lymphatic and Immune Systems

Multiple Choice Quiz 267

Exercise Quiz 269

Dictation and Comprehension Quiz 272

Spelling Quiz 273

Pronunciation Quiz 274

Abbreviations Quiz 275

Diagram Quiz 276

Vocabulary Quiz 277

Review Sheet Quiz 279

Opportunistic Infections Quiz 280

Crossword Puzzle 281

Practical Applications 282

Answers to the Quizzes 283

Answers to Combining Forms and Terminology Sections 286

Chapter Fifteen—Musculoskeletal System

Multiple Choice Quiz 288

Exercise Quiz

    Part I: Bones 290

    Part II: Joints and Muscles 292

Dictation and Comprehension Quiz: Bones 295

Dictation and Comprehension Quiz: Joints and Muscles 296

Spelling Quiz 297

Pronunciation Quiz 298

Abbreviations Quiz 299

Diagram Quiz 300

Vocabulary Quiz 301

Review Sheet Quiz 305

Crossword Puzzle 307

Practical Applications 308

Answers to the Quizzes 309

Answers to Combining Forms and Terminology Sections 313

Chapter Sixteen—Skin

Multiple Choice Quiz 318

Exercise Quiz 320

Dictation and Comprehension Quiz: Vocabulary, Combining Forms, and Suffixes 323

Dictation and Comprehension Quiz: Lesions, Symptoms,
Abnormal Conditions, and Neoplasms 324

Spelling Quiz 326

Pronunciation Quiz 327

Diagram Quiz 328

Vocabulary Quiz 329

Review Sheet Quiz 331

Crossword Puzzle 332

Practical Applications 333

Answers to the Quizzes 334

Answers to Combining Forms and Terminology Sections 337

Chapter Seventeen—Sense Organs: The Eye and The Ear

Multiple Choice Quiz 340

Exercise Quiz

Part I: Eye 342

Part II: Ear 345

Dictation and Comprehension Quiz: Eye 347

Dictation and Comprehension Quiz: Ear 348

Spelling Quiz 349

Pronunciation Quiz 350

Abbreviations Quiz 351

Diagram Quiz

Eye 352

Ear 353

Vocabulary Quiz 354

Review Sheet Quiz 357

Crossword Puzzle 359

Practical Applications 360

Answers to the Quizzes 361

Answers to Combining Forms and Terminology Sections..365

Chapter Eighteen—Endocrine System

Multiple Choice Quiz..368

Exercise Quiz 370

Dictation and Comprehension Quiz: Vocabulary and Terminology 372

Dictation and Comprehension Quiz: Abnormal Conditions, Laboratory Tests, Procedures 373

Spelling Quiz 374

Pronunciation Quiz 375

Abbreviations Quiz 376

Diagram Quiz..377

Vocabulary Quiz..378

Review Sheet Quiz 381

Crossword Puzzle 382

Practical Applications..383

Answers to the Quizzes 384

Answers to Combining Forms and Terminology Sections..387

Chapter Nineteen—Cancer Medicine (Oncology)

Multiple Choice Quiz..391

Exercise Quiz 394

Dictation and Comprehension Quiz 397

Spelling Quiz 398

Pronunciation Quiz 399

Abbreviations Quiz 400

Vocabulary Quiz..401

Review Sheet Quiz 404

Crossword Puzzle 405

Practical Applications..406

Answers to the Quizzes 408

Answers to Combining Forms and Terminology Sections..411

Chapter Twenty—Radiology and Nuclear Medicine

Multiple Choice Quiz 415

Exercise Quiz 417

Dictation and Comprehension Quiz 419

Spelling Quiz 420

Pronunciation Quiz 421

Vocabulary Quiz 422

Review Sheet Quiz 425

Crossword Puzzle 426

Practical Applications 427

Answers to the Quizzes 429

Answers to Combining Forms and Terminology Sections..432

Chapter Twenty-One—Pharmacology

Multiple Choice Quiz 434

Exercise Quiz 436

Dictation and Comprehension Quiz 438

Spelling Quiz 439

Pronunciation Quiz 440

Vocabulary Quiz 441

Review Sheet Quiz 445

Crossword Puzzle 446

Practical Applications 447

Answers to the Quizzes 449

Answers to Combining Forms and Terminology Sections..452

Chapter Twenty-Two—Psychiatry

Multiple Choice Quiz 455

Exercise Quiz 458

Dictation and Comprehension Quiz 461

Spelling Quiz 462

Pronunciation Quiz 463

Vocabulary Quiz 464

Review Sheet Quiz 468

Crossword Puzzle 469

Practical Applications 470

Answers to the Quizzes 471

Answers to Combining Forms and Terminology Sections 474

More Practical Applications 476

Medical Forms 490

Teacher to Teacher 501

Common Usage Terms 510

Medical Terminology Bloopers and Jokes 512

Reference Material 515

Resources 518

INTRODUCTION

How to Use the Textbook and Instructor's Manual

I have prepared this teaching manual for instructors who will be using *The Language of Medicine,* 8th edition, with their medical terminology classes. The manual includes information about the organization of the textbook, sample course plans, classroom methods with practical suggestions for use of the text, quizzes and other materials pertinent to teaching each chapter, description of ancillary products (CD, instant translator, and testbank), examples of practical applications (medical language in context) for use in class, suggestions for classroom activities and methods of other teachers, medical terminology humor, references and resources for supplemental materials, and transparency masters for use with overhead projectors. The organization of the textbook is as follows:

Chapters 1–4

Introductory chapters:

1. Basic Word Structure
2. Terms Pertaining to the Body as a Whole
3. Suffixes
4. Prefixes

These introductory chapters provide a foundation for the study of medical terminology. They teach students to divide words into component parts, recognize basic combining forms, suffixes, and prefixes, and know their meanings. In addition, students gain an understanding of the organization and complexity of the body and become familiar with the location and function of major body organs.

Chapter 1 should be taught first since it is a basic introduction to medical terminology and word analysis. I teach Chapters 2, 3, and 4 in that sequence, but other teachers have commented that they prefer to teach 3 and 4 and then follow with Chapter 2. The text is designed to be flexible so that you can experiment and teach the chapters in your own style.

Each of Chapters 1–4 contains **Word Part/Terminology Lists** (combining forms, suffixes, and prefixes). I use these lists in class to teach the medical terms. For your reference, the meanings of these terms are provided in the Answers to Combining Forms and Terminology sections included in this manual with all the materials for teaching each chapter.

Notice the Practical Applications feature in Chapters 1–4. I find that students enjoy testing their knowledge on these matching activities, and it is a good opportunity to expand their knowledge with related terms and concepts.

Exercises and **Answers** are found at the end of each text chapter. The answers are purposely placed directly after the questions so that students can check their responses easily. The exercises are not designed as tests, but rather as study aids. Students should be reminded to check their answers carefully so that they can benefit from the explanations in the answers sections.

Each chapter also contains a **Pronunciation List**. The Pronunciation List includes terms that are introduced in the chapter. In class, I use the list as an oral exercise and review before the chapter quiz. Students pronounce a term and then give its meaning. At home, students can write the term next to its pronunciation. The more times students write out words and their meanings, the easier it will be for them to learn the material. This is a *workbook* and students should be encouraged to use it in that manner. The CD in the back of the text contains the audio pronunciation of each term on the Pronunciation Lists in every chapter. See page 7, Ancillary Products.

A **Review Sheet** at the end of each chapter lists the combining forms, suffixes, and prefixes used in the chapter. Students in my classes write the meanings of all terms and check their answers with the Glossary of Terms list at the end of the text. I emphasize the *writing* of terms, over and over again, as the key to study. At times, I will use a blank review sheet as a quiz so that students know exactly what they should study. Students may find it helpful to copy these review sheets and complete them multiple times for study.

Chapters 5–18

These chapters explore the terminology of body systems. The format of these chapters follows a specific pattern that you may find useful to follow in teaching:

Introduction: gives an overview of the function of the system.

Anatomy: presents the organs of the system and their locations and functions. Students label simple anatomical diagrams following the directions in the text, and in class, I teach the anatomical terms directly from the diagrams. Students tell me that the **flow diagrams** are especially helpful in study as they review and illustrate the relationship between individual organs within a body system.

Vocabulary: You may use this section as a review of terms previously taught in the anatomy section or as reference for anatomical terms. I ask students to cover the side of the page with the meanings and see if they can explain, in their own words, each term as we examine the list in class.

Combining Forms and Related Terminology: This includes pertinent combining forms and illustrations of their use in medical words. I do this list in class with students by asking them to say the word and give its meaning. I have provided the meanings for your reference in each chapter section of this manual. Students can find meanings for these terms on my web site (http://evolve. elsevier.com/Chabner/language/).

Pathology: These are often more difficult words to divide into parts. As we go over each term in class, I have a student read the paragraph explaining the treatment and etiology of the disease condition so that she or he gains experience in reading terms in a sentence context. This also helps in pronunciation of terms. Often, I will then ask the student to explain the meaning of the sentence in her or his own words. Notice that in order not to overwhelm the student with too much detail, I have put the essential information (meanings of terms) in boldface type. Terms are arranged alphabetically, often anatomically, and by category for easy study and reference.

Clinical Procedures, Laboratory Tests, and Abbreviations: This section, newly organized in this edition for easier study, can be taught in class or used as a reference for students, depending on the amount of time available. Often, clinical procedures are divided into diagnostic and treatment sections.

Practical Applications: These are short examples of how the medical language is used in context. They include actual medical reports, x-ray reports, autopsies, drug descriptions, case studies, and laboratory records. Use these as short exercises in oral reading or as an interesting supplement to the study of the terms in the chapter. Additional Practical Applications are included for every chapter in this manual with questions for material in the text and manual. These questions should help you engage students in dialogue and understanding terms in context. In addition, I have included even more examples of Practical Applications in a separate section of this manual (see

Table of Contents). You can use this and the **Medical Forms** section with your classes as examples of how terms are used in the "real world." I hope that you will communicate any interesting way you use these forms via my e-mail address, MedDavi@aol.com.

Chapters 19–22

These chapters on specialized areas of medicine (Cancer Medicine, Radiology and Nuclear Medicine, Pharmacology, and Psychiatry) continue the basic format of the systems chapters. Many students who do not study these chapters in class find that they can study them on their own and use them as reference for questions that may arise in their work situations.

Glossary and Appendices

The **Glossary** contains a full listing of abbreviations, which should be of practical use, and a Medical Word Parts—English list of all combining forms, suffixes, and prefixes used in the text. An English—Medical Word Parts list follows and includes each English term with its medical counterpart. In this section, I have added when to use a combining form when there are two or more for a particular organ (i.e., nephr/o and ren/o). Again: let me know (MedDavi@aol.com or via the web site) if this helps and communicate your own suggestions as well. There are five **Appendices**. **Appendix I** contains information about forming plurals from singular nouns and gives examples of each. **Appendix II** is a list of commonly encountered abbreviations, acronyms, and symbols. **Appendix III** presents normal laboratory values for blood cells and substances in serum and gives the implications for disease when the values are either too low or too high. **Appendix IV** is an alphabetized list of commonly prescribed drugs and their uses. I hope this will be a useful reference for allied health workers, both on the job and in understanding their own health issues. **Appendix V** is a listing of complementary and alternative medicine terms. You may find creative ways to use this material in teaching as well. The **Index** includes all medical terms defined in the anatomy, vocabulary, pathology, clinical procedures, and laboratory tests sections, with page and illustration references.

Proposals for Courses

The design of *The Language of Medicine* is flexible so that it can be used in courses of varying lengths. An example of a typical two-semester syllabus follows:

Outline for First-Semester Course (16 weeks, 3 hours a week, 48 hours)

Week 1	Basic Word Structure	Chapter 1
Week 2	Terms Pertaining to the Body as a Whole	Chapter 2
Week 3	Suffixes	Chapter 3
Week 4	Prefixes	Chapter 4
Week 5	Digestive System	Chapter 5
Week 6	Additional Suffixes and Digestive System Terminology	Chapter 6
	MIDTERM EXAMINATION	
Week 7	Urinary System	Chapter 7
Week 8	Female Reproductive System	Chapter 8
Week 9	Male Reproductive System	Chapter 9

Week 10	Nervous System	Chapter 10
Week 11	Nervous System	
Week 12	Cardiovascular System	Chapter 11
Week 13	Cardiovascular System	
Week 14	Respiratory System	Chapter 12
Week 15	Respiratory System	
Week 16	Review	
	FINAL EXAMINATION	

Outline for Second-Semester Course (16 weeks, 3 hours a week, 48 hours)

Week 1	Blood System	Chapter 13
Week 2	Lymphatic and Immune Systems	Chapter 14
Week 3	Musculoskeletal System	Chapter 15
Week 4	Musculoskeletal System	
Week 5	Skin	Chapter 16
Week 6	Sense Organs: The Eye and the Ear	Chapter 17
Week 7	Endocrine System	Chapter 18
Week 8	Endocrine System	
	MIDTERM EXAMINATION	
Week 9	Cancer Medicine (Oncology)	Chapter 19
Week 10	Radiology and Nuclear Medicine	Chapter 20
Week 11	Radiology and Nuclear Medicine	
Week 12	Pharmacology	Chapter 21
Week 13	Pharmacology	
Week 14	Psychiatry	Chapter 22
Week 15	Psychiatry	
Week 16	Review	
	FINAL EXAMINATION	

Another example of a course structure was suggested to me by Susan Webb, a medical terminology instructor on Vancouver Island, British Columbia. She teaches a 12-week, 5-hours-a-week (two 2½ hour sessions), 60-hour course. Here is the syllabus for her course:

Week 1	Basic Word Structure	Chapter 1
Week 1	Terms Pertaining to the Body as a Whole	Chapter 2
Week 2	Suffixes	Chapter 3
Week 2	Prefixes	Chapter 4
Week 3	Additional Suffixes and Digestive System Terminology	Chapters 5 and 6
Week 3	Urinary System	Chapter 7

Week 4	Female Reproductive System	Chapter 8
Week 4	Male Reproductive System	Chapter 9
Week 5	Nervous System	Chapter 10
Week 5	Cardiovascular System	Chapter 11
Week 6	Respiratory System	Chapter 12
Week 6	REVIEW	Chapters 1–12
Week 7	Blood System and Review	Chapter 13
Week 7	Lymphatic and Immune Systems	Chapter 14
Week 8	Musculoskeletal System	Chapter 15
Week 8	Skin	Chapter 16
Week 9	Sense Organs: The Eye and the Ear	Chapter 17
Week 9	Endocrine System	Chapter 18
Week 10	Cancer Medicine (Oncology)	Chapter 19
Week 10	Radiology and Nuclear Medicine	Chapter 20
Week 11	Pharmacology	Chapter 21
Week 11	Psychiatry	Chapter 22
Week 12	REVIEW	Chapters 13–22
Week 12	FINAL EXAMINATION	

It may not be possible to cover all the material in your proposed time frame. You must gauge your pace to the ability of the students to absorb the material. My philosophy is to teach less and do it well, rather than rush through the material. You and your students are the best judges of how much of the book you will be able to cover. Students can always study chapters on their own and use as reference the chapters that are not taught.

Classroom Methods

While your teaching style will be characteristically your own, you may find the following ideas helpful:

- Use the method of *inquiry* and *discussion*, in conjunction with lecture. Encourage student participation by asking *why* and *how* questions. The goal is to relate medical terms to the functioning and structure of the body, thereby putting the terms in their proper context. *What* is an erythrocyte? *How* does it function? *What* enables it to carry oxygen? *Why* do body cells need oxygen? *What* is anemia? *Why* is supplemental iron necessary in some forms of the condition?

- Use of inquiry makes you aware of whether your students are "with you." If the class is open to questions and discussion, you will know if the material is being understood. Don't rush through the chapters just to meet a predesignated schedule. The quantity of terms learned should be secondary to a thorough understanding of the meaning of the words.

- Use analogies and examples to illustrate the structure and functioning of parts of the body. For instance, you might compare the pericardium and peritoneum to sheets of polyethylene wrap, enveloping important organs such as the heart and abdominal viscera. Or neutrophils, monocytes, and lymphocytes can be described as the combat forces in your body, fighting against bacterial invasion. The relationship between air sacs (alveoli) and lung capillaries resembles balloons surrounded by fishnetting. Relating the numerous prefixes to familiar words is also helpful. Sub-and exo-, for example, can be associated with words like submarine, subway, exit, and exile. I have included such memory tips in the Answers to Combining Forms and Terminology sections in this manual.

- Give real-life examples of disease processes and procedures. Sometimes, relating the details of an actual medical situation helps fix the concepts and terminology in a student's mind. Personally, I am not shy about telling my classes about my recent colonoscopy or my daughter's experience (I was there, too) of an amniocentesis. You must be careful about getting carried away along this route, so use your and your students' experiences judiciously.

- Use of a medical dictionary and/or dental dictionary is essential. This will enable students to see how many different terms can be made using a single combining form with several different suffixes. Encyclopedic dictionaries give more than simple definitions of terms. They explain disease processes and give information about symptoms and treatments. Students should also be encouraged to use a dictionary when exploring the meanings of terms in the Combining Forms and Terminology sections of the text. Personally, I like *Miller-Keene Dictionary of Allied Health* (7th edition) for excellent explanations of terms and *Mosby's Medical Nursing & Allied Health Dictionary* (7th edition) for good images to illustrate terminology.

- Encourage good study skills. The more times students *write* out words, over and over again, the faster and better they will learn them. Listing difficult words in a separate notebook, making a file system of flash cards (medical term or word part on one side with its meaning on the other), testing and retesting themselves by covering one and then the other side of review sheets, and writing meanings and terms are *all* necessary to retention of the language. Some teachers encourage the use of a study buddy. Working together and testing each other is a good idea.

- Use visual aids. For classroom use you may want to convert the diagrams provided at the back of the manual into transparencies. This can be done by using a Xerox machine to copy a diagram onto a transparency acetate. The acetate can then be projected on a screen or wall and used during class in teaching, labeling of diagrams, and illustrating terms. I have a collection of models (skeleton, female pelvis, heart, kidney) that I bring into class to illustrate anatomy. I also share my brother's gallstones, my chest x-ray (when I had pneumonia), a bone marrow biopsy needle (my daughter was a medical student), and assorted other visual aids that are enormously helpful for students to *see* terminology in action. Over the years I have collected old anatomical prints that are interesting to students as well.

- Give quizzes often. The tests motivate students to study and give the student, as well as the teacher, an indication as to how learning is proceeding. Often I will allow a student to retake his or her test in order to encourage mastery of the material. In addition to quizzes, I give frequent spelling tests. Students write words that I pronounce aloud. On other occasions I ask students to spell terms that are dictated and then we go over the terms and their meanings as a review of the vocabulary or combining forms and terminology lists. In the chapter sections of this manual, I have provided several different types of quizzes for use in classes. These quizzes are:

  1. **Multiple Choice Quiz**. These are easy to grade, but may not be as comprehensive as other types of tests with more and different types of questions.

  2. **Exercise Quiz**. These are taken from exercises at the end of each chapter; my students find this helpful in knowing exactly what to study.

3. **Dictation and Comprehension Quiz**. I use this type of quiz often to quickly test spelling and understanding of terms after each chapter. I may also add short answer questions depending on what I have covered in each chapter.

4. **Spelling Quiz**. These contain misspellings as well as the correct spelling. Some teachers like this, others do not. I am including them for those instructors who find them useful.

5. **Pronunciation Quiz**. These are based on the terms in the Pronunciation of Terms list in each chapter. Students indicate the accented syllable in a term, match terms with their meanings, and complete the spelling of a term from its definition.

6. **Diagram Quiz**. Each of these quizzes contains a diagram from one of the systems chapters, with a list of terms. Students are asked to complete the labeling of the diagram with the given terms. I often use flow diagrams (with labels removed) and ask students to complete them as a quiz.

7. **NEW! Vocabulary Quiz**. These are based on the terms in the vocabulary section in each chapter.

8. **NEW! Review Sheet Quiz**. These quizzes are based on the terms presented in the Review Sheets throughout the text.

9. **Abbreviations Quiz**. These ask students to spell out each abbreviation and match it with an associated sentence that helps the student understand the meaning of the abbreviation.

10. **Crossword Puzzle Quiz**. These were created by Susan Webb of Vancouver Island, who designed them for her medical terminology classes. Her students complete them in class as a review before their regular quiz.

11. **Practical Applications Quiz**. These are short paragraphs with multiple choice questions. You may use them for extra credit or for discussion in class after completing each chapter.

- Evaluate your teaching experience and your methods after each course is completed. Ask students to give a written critique of the course. You might ask students questions such as "What helped most?" "What helped least?" "Was the pace too fast or too slow?" "Was the course relevant to your needs?"

Ancillary Products: Back-of-Book CD, Instant Translator, Instructor's Resource Manual

Student CD

In the back of each copy of the eighth edition of *The Language of Medicine* is a CD that contains activities and information that will reinforce the medical terminology taught in each chapter of the book. The purpose of the CD is to allow students to use their newly acquired knowledge of terminology in a way that is both fun and informative. A wide array of features— full-color images and photographs, video clips, animations, games, an assortment of interactive activities including case reports, vignettes, spelling bees, explanations of answers and hints to help students find correct responses—are made available in an attractive, easy-to-use format. In addition, pronunciation of all terms on the Pronunciation of Terms lists in every chapter is provided so that students have easy access to how each term sounds. Furthermore, the CD contains a glossary with definitions of all word parts, a glossary of additional images, and the answers to the Pronunciation of Terms lists.

When using the CD students should see (by testing themselves) how much they have already learned and at the same time acquire new knowledge from the interactive program. Thus, the CD is specifically tailored to work chapter by chapter with *The Language of Medicine* as an invaluable study aid.

Instant Translator

The *Medical Language Instant Translator*, 3rd edition, will help students while learning medical terminology and provide quick access to useful medically related information as a professional resource. It is a convenient, pocket-sized book containing the following features:

- Instructions on **how to analyze medical terms**
- **Word parts glossary** (medical terms to English and English to medical terms)
- Commonly used **abbreviations** and **symbols**
- Frequently encountered **acronyms** and their meanings
- **Professional designations** and their meanings
- How to form **plurals** of medical terms
- Common **hematological reference values** and their implications
- Explanations of familiar **diagnostic tests and procedures**
- The top 100 principal **diagnoses** and associated **procedures**
- The top 100 **prescription drugs** (and what they treat)
- **Classes of drugs** with examples in each class
- **Surgical terminology** easy-reference lists that provide quick access to surgical terms
    - Easy-reference lists that provide quick access to surgical terms
    - Photos of **surgical instruments** with their names and uses
- **NEW!** Listing of **complementary and alternative medicine terms**
- **Common medical terminology mistakes** that alert students to potential errors
- **Diagrams** of body systems figures and an index to reference each body part
- **NEW!** Medical records reference terms.

I hope that this handy reference book will help medical terminology students decipher new terms and medical information with ease.

Testbank and Image Collection

An Instructor's Electronic Resource is available to complement this eighth edition. It is a CD program with questions to use in creating exams for your students. This electronic test bank will allow you to create your own quizzes, tests, and exams very easily. The questions are grouped together by subject matter in accordance with the chapters in *The Language of Medicine*. To create a test, you can either select each question one-by-one or have the CD select them randomly. If desired, you can also edit questions or add your own. An instructor's "answer key" will print out with each test you generate to make grading that much easier.

Furthermore, the CD contains an electronic image collection of over 400 figures from *The Language of Medicine*, as well as a Power Point presentation.

Please note:

You will notice in *The Language of Medicine*, 8th edition, that the possessive form with eponyms is dropped throughout. While the possessive form with eponyms still remains acceptable, this text responds to a growing trend in medicine (i.e., Down syndrome, Tourette syndrome, Apgar score) as well as to a need for clarity and consistency.* Since medical dictionaries, wordbooks, and style manuals vary, the situation is often confusing for students and professionals. If you are uncomfortable with this change in tradition, you may advise your students to continue to be guided by sources such as *Dorland's Dictionary* or an appropriate medical or hospital reference.

*According to AAMT, when the noun is dropped (and implied), the possessive should be retained, i.e., "The patient was seen for Alzheimer's."

chapter 1

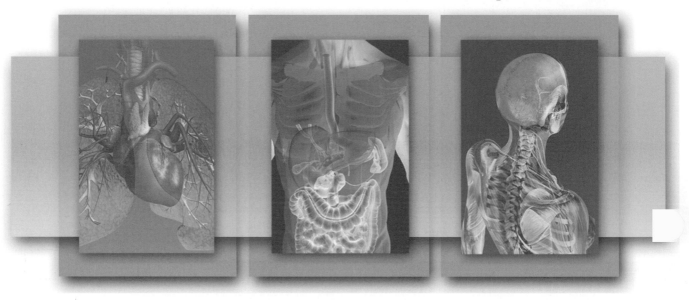

Chapter One

MULTIPLE CHOICE QUIZ

Name: _____

In the box write the letter of the choice that is the definition of the term or best answers the question. There is only one correct answer for each question.

1. **Gastrectomy:** .... ☐
   A. Gastric resection
   B. Intestinal incision
   C. Tumor of the stomach
   D. Incision of the stomach
   E. Resection of the intestine

2. **Osteitis:** .... ☐
   A. Incision of a bone
   B. Removal of a bone
   C. Incision of a joint
   D. Inflammation of a joint
   E. Inflammation of a bone

3. **Cystoscopy:** .... ☐
   A. Study of cells
   B. Visual examination of cells
   C. Removal of a sac of fluid
   D. Removal of the urinary bladder
   E. Visual examination of the
      urinary bladder

4. **Hepatoma:** .... ☐
   A. Incision of the kidney
   B. Tumor of the liver
   C. Blood mass
   D. Inflammation of the liver
   E. Red blood cell

5. **Which of the following is not
   an endocrine gland?** .... ☐
   A. Thyroid gland
   B. Adrenal gland
   C. Ovary
   D. Mammary gland
   E. Pituitary gland

6. **Iatrogenic:** .... ☐
   A. Pertaining to produced by treatment
   B. Produced by the mind
   C. Cancer producing
   D. Pertaining to producing a tumor
   E. Cutting into a tumor

7. **Electroencephalogram:** .... ☐
   A. Record of electricity in the brain
   B. Record of electricity in the heart
   C. X-ray of the brain
   D. Record of sound waves in the brain
   E. X-ray of the heart and brain

8. **Diagnosis:** .... ☐
   A. Is made after the prognosis
   B. Is a guess as to the patient's condition
   C. Is a prediction of the course of treatment
   D. Is made on the basis of complete
      knowledge about the patient's condition
   E. Is a treatment of the patient

9. **Cancerous tumor:** .... ☐
   A. Hematoma
   B. Adenoma
   C. Carcinoma
   D. Carcinogenic
   E. Neurotomy

10. **Microscopic examination of
    living tissue:** .... ☐
    A. Incision
    B. Pathology
    C. Biopsy
    D. Autopsy
    E. Resection

11. **Pertaining to the largest part
    of the brain:** .... ☐
    A. Cerebral
    B. Cephalic
    C. Renal
    D. Cardiac
    E. Neural

12. **Removal of a gland:** .... ☐
    A. Gastrotomy
    B. Gastric
    C. Hepatic resection
    D. Nephric section
    E. Adenectomy

13. **Decrease in numbers of red blood cells or hemoglobin within red blood cells:** .... ☐
   A. Anemia
   B. Erythrocytosis
   C. Thrombocytosis
   D. Leukemia
   E. Leukocytosis

14. **Pathologist:** .... ☐
   A. One who examines x-rays
   B. One who operates on the urinary tract
   C. One who performs autopsies and reads biopsies
   D. One who operates on the kidney
   E. One who treats diseases with chemicals

15. **Pain in a joint:** .... ☐
   A. Ostealgia
   B. Arthritis
   C. Osteoarthritis
   D. Arthroalgia
   E. Arthralgia

16. **Increase in numbers of malignant white blood cells:** .... ☐
   A. Leukocytosis
   B. Leukemia
   C. Erythremia
   D. Thrombocytosis
   E. Erythrocytosis

17. **Instrument to view the eye:** .... ☐
   A. Ophthalmoscopy
   B. Opthalmoscope
   C. Opthalmology
   D. Ophthalmoscope
   E. Opthalmoscopy

18. **A platelet:** .... ☐
   A. Hematoma
   B. Thrombosis
   C. Leukocyte
   D. Thrombocyte
   E. Erythrocyte

19. **Abnormal condition of the mind:** .... ☐
   A. Physchosis
   B. Psychosis
   C. Psychogenic
   D. Encephalopathy
   E. Adenoma

20. **Inflammation of the nose:** .... ☐
   A. Arthrosis
   B. Hepatitis
   C. Nephritis
   D. Dermatosis
   E. Rhinitis

21. **Study of cells:** .... ☐
   A. Pathology
   B. Cytology
   C. Cystology
   D. Dermatology
   E. Urology

22. **Pertaining to through the liver:** .... ☐
   A. Subrenal
   B. Transdermal
   C. Transhepatic
   D. Subhepatic
   E. Hepatoma

23. **Abnormal condition of the kidney:** .... ☐
   A. Neurologic
   B. Neuralgia
   C. Nephrotomy
   D. Neural
   E. Nephrosis

24. **Incision of a bone:** .... ☐
   A. Sarcoma
   B. Pathogenic
   C. Osteotomy
   D. Ostectomy
   E. Endoscopy

25. **High level of sugar in the blood:** .... ☐
   A. Hematoma
   B. Hypodermic
   C. Hypoglycemia
   D. Hyperglycemia
   E. Hypogastric

Chapter One
EXERCISE QUIZ

Name: _____

A. *Give meanings for the following combining forms:*

   1. arthr/o _____   4. aden/o _____

   2. cyst/o _____   5. cyt/o _____

   3. encephal/o _____   6. carcin/o _____

B. *Give meanings for the following suffixes:*

   7. -gram _____   10. -oma _____

   8. -itis _____   11. -scopy _____

   9. -opsy _____   12. -logy _____

C. *Using slashes, divide the following terms into parts and give the meaning of the entire term:*

   13. cerebral _____

   14. electrocardiogram _____

   15. dermatitis _____

   16. cephalic _____

D. *Complete the medical term from its meaning given below:*

   17. red blood cell: _____ cyte   19. white blood cell: _____ cyte

   18. mass of blood: _____ oma   20. pain of nerves: neur _____

E. *Underline the suffix in each term and give the meaning of the entire term:*

   21. nephrectomy _____   24. renal _____

   22. osteotomy _____   25. psychosis _____

   23. oncology _____   26. carcinogenic _____

F. *Give the meanings for the following prefixes:*

   27. hyper- _____   30. trans- _____

   28. peri- _____   31. hypo- _____

   29. epi- _____   32. dia- _____

G. Underline the prefix and give the meaning of the entire term:

33. subhepatic _____

34. hyperglycemia _____

35. pericardium _____

36. resection _____

37. prognosis _____

38. hypodermic _____

H. Match the English term in column I with its combining form in column II:

Column I English Term	Column II Combining Form
39. kidney _____	psych/o
40. disease _____	ophthalm/o
41. eye _____	path/o
42. nose _____	ren/o
43. flesh _____	rhin/o
44. bone _____	radi/o
45. mind _____	onc/o
46. tumor _____	sarc/o
47. clotting _____	thromb/o
48. urinary tract _____	ur/o
49. x-rays _____	oste/o
50. to cut _____	sect/o

Chapter One
DICTATION AND COMPREHENSION QUIZ

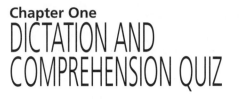

Name: _____

A. Dictation of Terms

1. _____   11. _____

2. _____   12. _____

3. _____   13. _____

4. _____   14. _____

5. _____   15. _____

6. _____   16. _____

7. _____   17. _____

8. _____   18. _____

9. _____   19. _____

10. _____   20. _____

B. Comprehension of Terms: Match the number of the above term with its meaning below.

_____ Pain of nerves

_____ Inflammation of bone

_____ Prediction about the outcome of treatment

_____ Microscopic examination of living tissue

_____ Blood cell that carries oxygen

_____ Physician who specializes in drug treatment of cancerous tumors

_____ Disease of a gland

_____ Resection of a kidney

_____ A platelet

_____ Process of visual examination of the urinary bladder

_____ Pertaining to an abnormal condition produced by a treatment

_____ Incision of the stomach

_____ Pertaining to producing cancer

_____ An instrument to visually examine the eye

_____ High blood sugar: diabetes mellitus

_____ Λ physician who examines dead bodies to determine the cause of death

_____ Pain of a joint

_____ Mass or collection of blood

_____ Slight increase in numbers of white blood cells as a response to infection

_____ Increase in abnormal, immature white blood cells; a malignant condition

Chapter One
SPELLING QUIZ

Name: _____

A. *Circle the term that is spelled correctly and write its meaning in the space provided:*

1. luekocyte   leukocyte _____

2. neuralgia   nueralgia _____

3. biospy   biopsy _____

4. gynocology   gynecology _____

5. erythrocyte   erthyrocyte _____

6. opthalmoscopy   ophthalmoscopy _____

7. pathogenic   pathojenic _____

8. thrombocyte   thrombocyt _____

9. sacroma   sarcoma _____

10. psychology   physcology _____

B. *Circle the term that is spelled correctly. The meaning of each term is given.*

11.	resection of a nerve .... neruotomy	neurectomy	neurotomy
12.	pertaining to produced by treatment........ iatrogenic	iatragenic	itarogenic
13.	pertaining to the brain .... cerebrol	serebral	cerebral
14.	cancerous tumor .... carcinoma	carsinoma	karsinoma
15.	collection of blood .... hepatoma	hematoma	hepitoma
16.	high blood sugar...................................... hypoglycemia	hyperglicemia	hyperglycemia
17.	membrane surrounding the heart .... perycardium	pericardium	pericardum
18.	instrument to examine within .... endoscope	endoskope	endoscopy
19.	disease of the intestines........................... entrapathy	interopathy	enteropathy
20.	inflammation of the urinary bladder .... cytitis	cystitis	sistitis

Chapter One
PRONUNCIATION QUIZ

Name: _____

A. *Underline the accented syllable in the following terms (for example: an<u>e</u>mia, diag<u>no</u>sis, <u>e</u>ndocrine):*

1. arthrotomy
2. cystoscopy
3. gastrectomy
4. endocrinology
5. neuralgia
6. pericarditis
7. ophthalmoscope
8. hepatoma
9. retrogastric
10. cytology

B. *Match the term in Column I with its meaning in Column II:*

Column I

1. encephalopathy _____
2. carcinogenic _____
3. oncology _____
4. dermatosis _____
5. psychiatry _____
6. leukemia _____
7. hypoglycemia _____
8. iatrogenic _____
9. gastric resection _____
10. leukocytosis _____

Column II

A. Low levels of blood sugar.
B. Treatment of the mind.
C. Study of tumors.
D. Excision of the stomach.
E. Pertaining to producing cancer.
F. Abnormal condition (slight increase) of white blood cells.
G. Brain disease.
H. Abnormal condition of the skin.
I. Cancerous condition of white blood cells.
J. Pertaining to produced by treatment.

C. *Complete the following terms from their definitions:*

1. pro _____   Prediction about the outcome of a disease; "before knowledge."

2. _____ itis   Inflammation of the kidney.

3. patho _____   Pertaining to producing disease.

4. _____ ology   Study of women and female diseases.

5. electro _____   Record of electricity in the brain.

6. thrombocyt _____   Abnormal condition of clotting cells.

7. bi _____   Examination of living tissue under a microscope.

8. _____ al   Pertaining to the largest part of the brain.

9. _____ oma   Tumor of a gland (benign).

10. _____ arthritis   Inflammation of bone and joint.

Chapter One
REVIEW SHEET QUIZ

Name: _____

A. *Give meanings for the following combining forms:*

1. cephal/o _____

2. cerebr/o _____

3. cyt/o _____

4. encephal/o _____

5. enter/o _____

6. hepat/o _____

7. ped/o _____

8. ren/o _____

9. ur/o _____

10. cis/o _____

B. *Give combining forms for the following meanings:*

1. heart _____

2. skin _____

3. sugar _____

4. woman, female _____

5. x-rays _____

6. mind _____

7. nose _____

8. flesh _____

C. *Give meanings for the following suffixes and prefixes:*

1. hypo- _____

2. dia- _____

3. -scopy _____

4. -gram _____

5. -globin _____

6. trans- _____

7. sub- _____

8. retro- _____

9. epi- _____

10. end-, endo- _____

Chapter One
CROSSWORD PUZZLE

Name: _____

Fill in the crossword puzzle below using the clues listed underneath it.

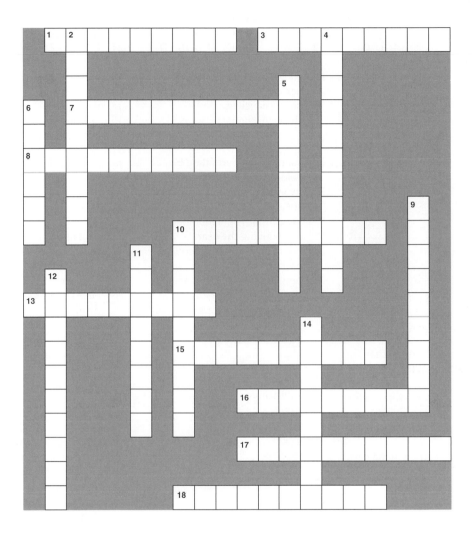

Across Clues

1. Process of cutting back (removal).
3. Complete knowledge.
7. Red blood cell.
8. Pertaining to above the stomach.
10. Study of women's diseases.
13. White blood cell.
15. Pertaining to produced by treatment.
16. Inflammation of the liver.
17. Pertaining to under the skin.
18. Pertaining to below the liver.

Down Clues

2. Inflammation of the small intestine.
4. Removal of the stomach.
5. Study of nerves.
6. Blood condition of low numbers of erythrocytes or deficient hemoglobin in the red blood cell.
9. Before knowledge (prediction about the outcome of treatment).
10. Inflammation of the stomach.
11. Process to cut into a part of the body.
12. Study of the kidney.
14. Mass of blood under the skin.

Chapter One
ANSWERS TO THE QUIZZES

Multiple Choice Quiz

1. A	4. B	7. A	10. C	13. A	16. B	19. B	22. C	25. D
2. E	5. D	8. D	11. A	14. C	17. D	20. E	23. E	
3. E	6. A	9. C	12. E	15. E	18. D	21. B	24. C	

Exercise Quiz

A
1. joint
2. urinary bladder
3. brain
4. gland
5. cell
6. cancer

B
7. record
8. inflammation
9. to view
10. tumor
11. process of visual examination
12. study of

C
13. cerebral—pertaining to the cerebrum (largest part of the brain)
14. electrocardiogram—record of the electricity in the heart
15. dermatitis—inflammation of the skin
16. cephalic—pertaining to the head

D
17. erythrocyte
18. hematoma
19. leukocyte
20. neuralgia

E
21. nephrectomy—removal of the kidney
22. osteotomy—incision of a bone
23. oncology—study of tumors (cancerous)
24. renal—pertaining to the kidney
25. psychosis—abnormal condition of the mind
26. carcinogenic—pertaining to producing cancer

F
27. excessive; above
28. surrounding
29. above
30. across; through
31. below; deficient
32. through; complete

G
33. subhepatic—pertaining to below the liver
34. hyperglycemia—excessive blood sugar
35. pericardium—membrane surrounding the heart
36. resection—process of cutting back (removal)
37. prognosis—prediction about the outcome of treatment
38. hypodermic—pertaining to under the skin

H
39. ren/o
40. path/o
41. ophthalm/o
42. rhin/o
43. sarc/o
44. oste/o
45. psych/o
46. onc/o
47. thromb/o
48. ur/o
49. radi/o
50. sect/o

Dictation and Comprehension Quiz

A
1. adenopathy
2. arthralgia
3. biopsy
4. carcinogenic
5. cystoscopy
6. erythrocyte
7. gastrotomy
8. hematoma
9. hyperglycemia
10. iatrogenic
11. leukemia
12. leukocytosis
13. nephrectomy
14. neuralgia
15. oncologist
16. ophthalmoscope
17. osteitis
18. pathologist
19. prognosis
20. thrombocyte

B
14 Pain of nerves
17 Inflammation of bone
19 Prediction about the outcome of treatment
3   Microscopic examination of living tissue
6   Blood cell that carries oxygen
15 Physician who specializes in drug treatment of cancerous tumors
1   Disease of a gland
13 Resection of a kidney
20 A platelet
5   Process of visual examination of the urinary bladder
10 Pertaining to an abnormal condition produced by a treatment
7   Incision of the stomach
4   Pertaining to producing cancer
16 An instrument to visually examine the eye
9   High blood sugar: diabetes mellitus
18 A physician who examines dead bodies to determine the cause of death
2   Pain of a joint
8   Mass or collection of blood
12 Slight increase in numbers of white blood cells as a response to infection
11 Increase in abnormal, immature white blood cells; a malignant condition

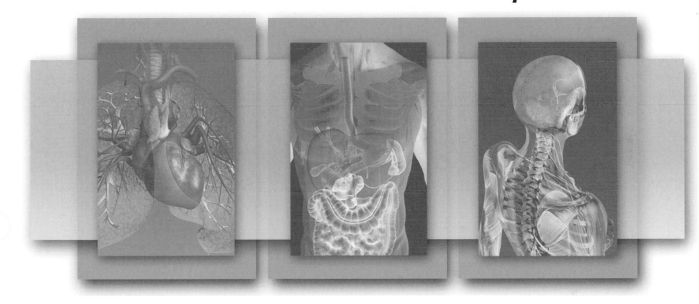

chapter 2

Chapter Two
MULTIPLE CHOICE QUIZ

Name: _____

In the box write the letter of the choice that is the definition of the term or best answers the question. There is only one correct answer for each question.

1. **The process by which food is burned to release energy:** ☐
   A. Nuclear energy
   B. Anabolism
   C. Phagocytosis
   D. Catabolism
   E. Protein synthesis

2. **Part of the cell where formation of proteins occurs:** ☐
   A. Genes
   B. Chromosomes
   C. Endoplasmic reticulum
   D. Cartilage
   E. Cell membrane

3. **Sum of the chemical processes in a cell:** ☐
   A. Anabolism
   B. Metabolism
   C. Protein synthesis
   D. Catabolism
   E. A and C

4. **Picture of nuclear structures arranged in numerical order:** ☐
   A. Biopsy
   B. X-ray
   C. Electroencephalogram
   D. Sonogram
   E. Karyotype

5. **Part of a cell where catabolism primarily occurs:** ☐
   A. Cell membrane
   B. Nucleus
   C. Mitochondria
   D. Genes
   E. Endoplasmic reticulum

6. **Allows materials to pass into and out of the cell:** ☐
   A. Cytoplasm
   B. Cell membrane
   C. Chromosomes
   D. Mitochondria
   E. Nucleus

7. **Genes are composed of:** ☐
   A. Chromosomes
   B. Ribosomes
   C. Hemoglobin
   D. Deoxyribonucleic acid (DNA)
   E. Mitochondria

8. **Muscular wall separating the abdominal and thoracic cavities:** ☐
   A. Mediastinum
   B. Diaphragm
   C. Pleura
   D. Pericardium
   E. Peritoneum

9. **The space in the chest between the lungs is the:** ☐
   A. Peritoneum
   B. Esophagus
   C. Pleural cavity
   D. Mediastinum
   E. Retroperitoneal space

10. **Adipose means pertaining to:** ☐
    A. Cartilage
    B. Bone
    C. Fat
    D. Skin
    E. Nervous tissue

11. **Throat:** ☐
    A. Trachea
    B. Coccyx
    C. Larynx
    D. Esophagus
    E. Pharynx

12. **Sarcoma:** ☐
    A. Part of the backbone
    B. Flesh tumor; benign
    C. Malignant tumor of flesh tissue
    D. Mass of blood
    E. Skin tumor of epithelial cells

13. **Craniotomy:** .... ☐
    A. Incision of the skull
    B. Pertaining to the skull
    C. Pertaining to the brain
    D. Incision of the chest
    E. Pertaining to the head

14. **A histologist studies:** .... ☐
    A. Drugs
    B. X-rays
    C. Tissues
    D. The backbone
    E. The spinal cord

15. **An epithelial cell is a(an):** .... ☐
    A. Skin cell
    B. Nerve cell
    C. Fat cell
    D. Organ
    E. Muscle cell

16. **The pleural cavity is the:** .... ☐
    A. Space within the abdomen
    B. Space within the backbones
    C. Space surrounding the hip
    D. Space between the membranes around
       the lungs
    E. Space within the skull

17. **Viscera:** .... ☐
    A. Cells in the blood
    B. Internal organs
    C. Parts of cells
    D. Cavities of the body
    E. Tissues composed of cartilage

18. **The pituitary gland is in which
    body cavity?** .... ☐
    A. Cranial
    B. Spinal
    C. Pelvic
    D. Abdominal
    E. Thoracic

19. **Voice box:** .... ☐
    A. Bronchial tube
    B. Pharynx
    C. Esophagus
    D. Larynx
    E. Tongue

20. **The tailbone is the:** .... ☐
    A. Sacrum
    B. Cervix
    C. Ilium
    D. Coccyx
    E. Cranium

21. **Supine means:** .... ☐
    A. Lying on the back
    B. Conducting toward a structure
    C. In front of the body
    D. Lying on the belly
    E. Pertaining to the side

22. **The upper lateral regions of the
    abdomen, beneath the ribs, are the:** ..... ☐
    A. Hypogastric regions
    B. Inguinal regions
    C. Lumbar regions
    D. Umbilical regions
    E. Hypochondriac regions

23. **The RUQ contains the:** .... ☐
    A. Liver
    B. Appendix
    C. Lung
    D. Spleen
    E. Heart

24. **Pertaining to a plane that divides the
    body into right and left portions:** .... ☐
    A. Coronal
    B. Transverse
    C. Frontal
    D. Sagittal
    E. Distal

25. **A disk is:** .... ☐
    A. Part of the hip bone
    B. A piece of cartilage between backbones
    C. A piece of bony tissue connecting the
       joints in the back
    D. An abnormal structure in the back
    E. A pad of fatty tissue between backbones

Chapter Two
EXERCISE QUIZ

Name: _____

A. *Use medical terms to complete the following sentences:*

1. Control center of the cell, containing chromosomes _____

2. The process of building up proteins in a cell is called _____

3. The total of the chemical processes in a cell is known as _____

4. A scientist who studies tissues is called a(an) _____

5. Regions of DNA within a chromosome _____

B. *Match the part of the body listed with its description below:*

adipose tissue   pharynx   ureter
cartilage   pleura   urethra
larynx   trachea

6. throat _____

7. collection of fat cells _____

8. windpipe _____

9. tube from the kidney to the urinary bladder _____

10. voice box _____

11. membrane surrounding the lungs _____

12. flexible connective tissue at joints _____

13. tube from the urinary bladder to outside of body _____

C. *Name the five cavities of the body:*

14. cavity surrounded by the skull _____

15. cavity in the chest surrounded by ribs _____

16. cavity surrounded by the hip bone _____

17. cavity surrounded by the backbones _____

18. cavity below the chest containing digestive organs _____

D. *Name the five divisions of the back:*

19. region of the neck _____   22. region of the sacrum _____

20. region of the chest _____   23. region of the tailbone _____

21. region of the waist _____

E. Give opposites of the following terms:

24. deep _____   26. supine _____

25. proximal _____   27. dorsal _____

F. Select from the following to complete the sentences below:

distal   lateral   sagittal   transverse
inferior (caudal)   proximal   superior   vertebra

28. The left lung lies _____ to the heart.

29. The _____ end of the humerus is at the shoulder.

30. The liver lies _____ to the intestines.

31. A backbone is called a (an) _____ .

32. The _____ end of the thigh bone (femur) joins with the knee cap.

33. The _____ plane divides the body into upper and lower portions.

34. The _____ plane divides the body into right and left portions.

35. The diaphragm lies _____ to the organs in the thoracic cavity.

G. Give meanings for the following terms:

36. craniotomy _____   39. umbilical _____

37. epigastric _____   40. posterior _____

38. chondroma _____   41. intervertebral _____

H. Complete each term from its meaning:

42. Space between the lungs: media _____

43. Endocrine gland at the base of the brain: _____ ary gland

44. Sausage-shaped cellular structures in which catabolism takes place: mito _____

45. Pertaining to skin (surface) cells: epi _____

46. Tumor of flesh tissue (malignant): _____ oma

47. Pertaining to internal organs: _____ al

48. Picture of the chromosomes in the cell nucleus: _____ type

I. Give meanings for the following abbreviations:

49. RUQ _____   50. L5-S1 _____

Chapter Two
DICTATION AND COMPREHENSION QUIZ

Name: _____

A. Dictation of Terms

1. _____   11. _____

2. _____   12. _____

3. _____   13. _____

4. _____   14. _____

5. _____   15. _____

6. _____   16. _____

7. _____   17. _____

8. _____   18. _____

9. _____   19. _____

10. _____   20. _____

B. Comprehension of Terms: Match the number of the above term with its meaning below.

_____ Incision of the skull

_____ Pertaining to the groin

_____ Malignant tumor of connective (flesh) tissue

_____ Picture of nuclear structures

_____ Pertaining to internal organs

_____ Study of tissues

_____ Secretory organ in the neck

_____ Flexible connective tissue at joints

_____ Divides the body horizontally

_____ Tube from the urinary bladder to the outside of the body

_____ Cytoplasmic structures where catabolism takes place

_____ Throat

_____ Divides the body laterally into right and left parts

_____ Secretory organ at the base of the brain

_____ Voice box

_____ Pertaining to the navel

_____ Pertaining to the windpipe

_____ Pertaining to fat tissue

_____ Line external body surface and internal surface of organs

_____ Rod-shaped nuclear structures

Chapter Two
SPELLING QUIZ

Name: _____

A. Circle the term that is spelled correctly and write its meaning in the space provided (optional).

1. abdomin   abdomen _____

2. cartiledge   cartilage _____

3. chromosome   chromosone _____

4. diaphram   diaphragm _____

5. saggital   sagittal _____

6. larynx   larnyx _____

7. cervecal   cervical _____

8. chrondroma   chondroma _____

9. nucleus   neucleus _____

10. traychea   trachea _____

B. Circle the term that is spelled correctly. The meaning of each term is given.

11. internal organs .... viscera   vicsera   vissera

12. malignant tumor of flesh
    (connective tissue) .... sacroma   sarcoma   sarkoma

13. pertaining to the chest .... thoracic   thorasic   thoroacic

14. lying on the back .... surpine   supin   supine

15. pertaining to the abdomen .... abdominel   abdominal   abdomineal

16. picture of the chromosomes
    in the nucleus .... karyotype   karryotype   kariotype

17. membrane surrounding the lungs .... pleura   ploora   plura

18. space between the lungs .... mediastinim   mediastinam   mediastinum

19. pertaining to skin (surface) cells .... epitheleal   epithelial   epithelal

20. endocrine gland at the base
    of the brain .... pituitary   pituitary   pituitery

Chapter Two
PRONUNCIATION QUIZ

Name: _____

A. *Underline the accented syllable in the following terms (for example: anemia, diagnosis, endocrine):*

1. cephalic
2. posterior
3. proximal

4. thoracotomy
5. hypochondriac
6. cranial

7. catabolism
8. chondrosarcoma
9. pharynx

10. viscera

B. *Match the term in Column I with its meaning in Column II:*

Column I

1. karyotype   _____
2. epithelium   _____
3. cartilage   _____
4. anabolism   _____
5. diaphragm   _____
6. vertebra   _____
7. sagittal   _____
8. supine   _____
9. mitochondria   _____
10. larynx   _____

Column II

A. A backbone.

B. The voice box.

C. Skin cells.

D. Vertical plane dividing the body into a right and left portion.

E. The throat.

F. Classification of chromosomes.

G. Lying on one's back.

H. Muscle dividing the thoracic and abdominal cavities.

I. Connective tissue at the joints.

J. Lying on one's belly.

K. Structures in a cell where food is burned to produce energy.

L. Building-up process in a cell; proteins are synthesized for use in the body.

C. *Complete the following terms from their definitions:*

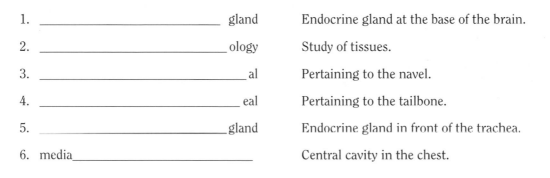

1. _____ gland   Endocrine gland at the base of the brain.

2. _____ ology   Study of tissues.

3. _____ al   Pertaining to the navel.

4. _____ eal   Pertaining to the tailbone.

5. _____ gland   Endocrine gland in front of the trachea.

6. media _____   Central cavity in the chest.

7. _____ vertebral   Pertaining to between the backbones.

8. _____ tomy   Incision of the skull.

9. _____ somes   Bodies in the nucleus of a cell; contain DNA.

10. peri _____   Membrane surrounding the abdominal cavity.

Chapter Two
DIAGRAM QUIZ

Name: _____

Label the diagram below using the terms listed below:

BODY CAVITIES

Abdominal
Cranial
Pelvic
Spinal
Thoracic

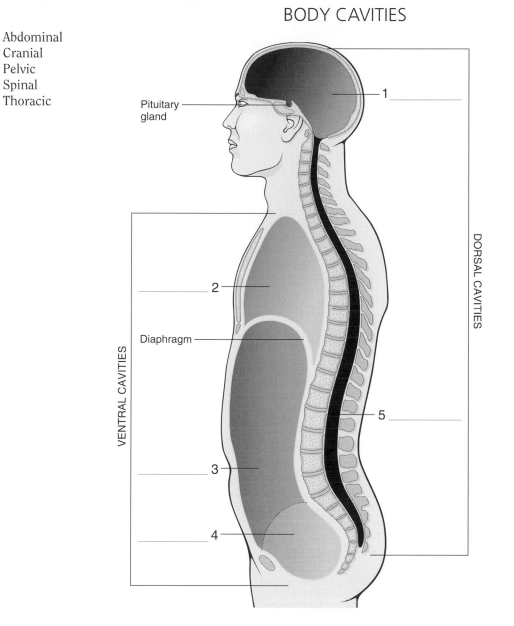

Chapter Two

REVIEW SHEET QUIZ

Name: _____

A. *Give meanings for the following combining forms:*

   1. crani/o _____

   2. cervic/o _____

   3. sacr/o _____

   4. trache/o _____

   5. inguin/o _____

   6. viscer/o _____

   7. sarc/o _____

   8. chondr/o _____

   9. thorac/o _____

  10. hist/o _____

B. *Give meanings for the following word parts:*

   1. inter- _____

   2. hypo- _____

   3. ana- _____

   4. -ose _____

   5. -eal _____

   6. epi- _____

   7. -ectomy _____

   8. kary/o _____

   9. -tomy _____

C. *Name the 5 divisions of the spinal column:*

   1. C1-C7 _____

   2. T1-T12 _____

   3. L1-L5 _____

   4. S1-S5 _____

   5. tailbone region _____

D. *Name the plane of the body described below:*

   1. horizontal plane dividing the body into superior and inferior parts:_____

   2. vertical plane dividing the body into right and left parts: _____

   3. vertical plane dividing the body into anterior and posterior parts: _____

E. *Give the positional or directional term:*

   1. on the surface of the body _____

   2. lying on the back _____

   3. below another structure _____

4. pertaining to the side _____

5. pertaining to the middle _____

6. lying on the belly _____

7. above another structure _____

8. near the point of attachment to the trunk or near the beginning of a structure _____

9. away from the surface of the body _____

10. far from the point of attachment to the trunk or far from the beginning of a structure _____

F. *Give the name of the structure described below:*

1. membrane surrounding abdominal viscera _____

2. a backbone _____

3. membrane surrounding the lungs _____

4. pad of cartilage between each backbone _____

5. space between the lungs containing the heart, trachea, aorta _____

Chapter Two

CROSSWORD PUZZLE

Name: _____

Fill in the crossword puzzle below using the clues listed underneath it.

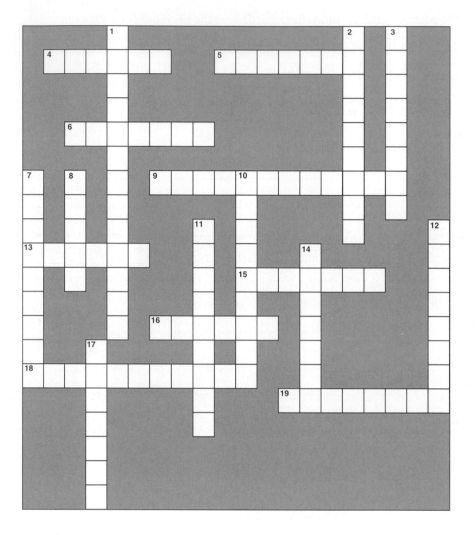

Across Clues

4. Voice box.
5. Collection of fat cells.
6. Control center of a cell.
9. Structures in cytoplasm where food is burned to release energy.
13. A double-layered membrane surrounding each lung.
15. Throat.
16. Loin (waist) region.
18. Area between the lungs.
19. Vertical plane dividing body into right and left sides.

Down Clues

1. Upper right and left regions beneath the ribs.
2. Backbones.
3. Lower right and left regions near the groin.
7. Muscle separating the abdominal and thoracic cavities.
8. Regions of DNA within each chromosome.
10. All the material that is outside the nucleus yet within the cell membrane.
11. Stomach, small and large intestines, spleen, liver, gallbladder, and pancreas.
12. Bones and joints; musculo_____ system.
14. Tube from the urinary bladder to the outside of the body.
17. Internal organs.

Chapter Two
ANSWERS TO THE QUIZZES

Multiple Choice Quiz

1. D	4. E	7. D	10. C	13. A	16. D	19. D	22. E	25. B
2. C	5. C	8. B	11. E	14. C	17. B	20. D	23. A	
3. B	6. B	9. D	12. C	15. A	18. A	21. A	24. D	

Exercise Quiz

A
1. nucleus
2. anabolism
3. metabolism
4. histologist
5. genes

B
6. pharynx
7. adipose tissue
8. trachea
9. ureter
10. larynx
11. pleura
12. cartilage
13. urethra

C
14. cranial
15. thoracic
16. pelvic
17. spinal
18. abdominal

D
19. cervical
20. thoracic
21. lumbar
22. sacral
23. coccygeal

E
24. superficial
25. distal
26. prone
27. ventral (anterior)

F
28. lateral
29. proximal
30. superior
31. vertebra
32. distal
33. transverse
34. sagittal
35. inferior (caudal)

G
36. incision of the skull
37. pertaining to above the stomach
38. tumor of cartilage (benign)
39. pertaining to the navel
40. pertaining to the back
41. pertaining to between vertebrae

H
42. mediastinum
43. pituitary gland
44. mitochondria
45. epithelial
46. sarcoma
47. visceral
48. karyotype

I
49. right upper quadrant (of the abdomen)
50. between the 5th lumbar and the 1st sacral vertebrae

Dictation and Comprehension Quiz

A
1. adipose
2. cartilage
3. chondrosarcoma
4. chromosomes
5. craniotomy
6. epithelial cells
7. histology
8. inguinal
9. karyotype
10. larynx
11. mitochondria
12. pharynx
13. pituitary gland
14. sagittal plane
15. thyroid gland
16. tracheal
17. transverse plane
18. umbilical
19. urethra
20. visceral

B
5 Incision of the skull
8 Pertaining to the groin
3 Malignant tumor of connective (flesh) tissue
9 Picture of nuclear structures
20 Pertaining to internal organs
7 Study of tissues
15 Secretory organ in the neck
2 Flexible connective tissue at joints
17 Divides the body horizontally
19 Tube from the urinary bladder to the outside of the body
11 Cytoplasmic structures where catabolism takes place
12 Throat
14 Divides the body laterally into right and left parts
13 Secretory organ at the base of the brain
10 Voice box
18 Pertaining to the navel
16 Pertaining to the windpipe
1 Pertaining to fat tissue
6 Line external body surface and internal surface of organs
4 Rod-shaped nuclear structures

Spelling Quiz

A
1. abdomen—area under the chest containing the stomach, intestines, liver, gallbladder
2. cartilage—flexible connective tissue between joints
3. chromosome—contains genetic material in nucleus of a cell
4. diaphragm—muscular wall separating the chest and abdomen
5. sagittal—vertical plane dividing the body into right and left portions
6. larynx—voice box
7. cervical—pertaining to the neck
8. chondroma—tumor of cartilage (benign)

9. nucleus—control center of the cell
10. trachea—windpipe

B

11. viscera
12. sarcoma
13. thoracic
14. supine
15. abdominal
16. karyotype
17. pleura
18. mediastinum
19. epithelial
20. pituitary

Pronunciation Quiz

A

1. cephalic
2. posterior
3. proximal
4. thoracotomy
5. hypochondriac
6. cranial
7. catabolism
8. chondrosarcoma
9. pharynx
10. viscera

B

1. F
2. C
3. I
4. L
5. H
6. A
7. D
8. G
9. K
10. B

C

1. pituitary
2. histology
3. umbilical
4. coccygeal
5. thyroid
6. mediastinum
7. intervertebral
8. craniotomy
9. chromosomes
10. peritoneum

Diagram Quiz

1. Cranial
2. Thoracic
3. Abdominal
4. Pelvic
5. Spinal

Review Sheet Quiz

A

1. skull
2. neck
3. sacrum
4. trachea, windpipe
5. groin
6. internal organs
7. flesh
8. cartilage
9. chest
10. tissue

B

1. between
2. below
3. up
4. pertaining to, full of
5. pertaining to
6. above
7. removal, excision, resection
8. picture, classification
9. cut into, incision, section

C

1. cervical
2. thoracic
3. lumbar

4. sacral
5. coccygeal

D

1. transverse, axial
2. sagittal, lateral
3. frontal, coronal

E

1. superficial
2. supine
3. inferior, caudal
4. lateral
5. medial
6. prone
7. superior, cephalic
8. proximal
9. deep
10. distal

F

1. peritoneum
2. vertebra
3. pleura
4. disk
5. mediastinum

Crossword Puzzle

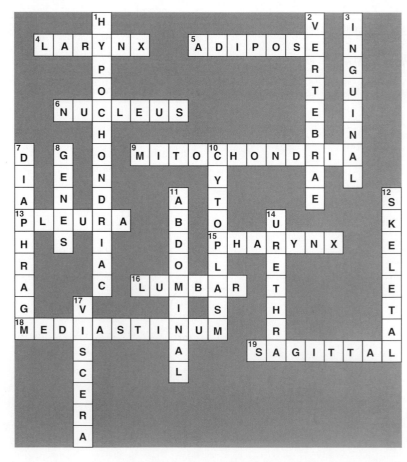

Chapter Three
MULTIPLE CHOICE QUIZ

Name: _____

In the box write the letter of the choice that is the definition of the term or best answers the question. There is only one correct answer for each question.

1. **Amniocentesis:** .... ☐
   A. Incision of the abdomen
   B. Paracentesis
   C. Surgical puncture to remove fluid from the abdomen
   D. Puncture of the chest region
   E. Surgical puncture to remove fluid from the sac around the embryo

2. **Inflammation of lymph tissue in the throat:** .... ☐
   A. Bronchitis
   B. Laryngitis
   C. Pharyngeal
   D. Tonsilitis
   E. Tonsillitis

3. **Prolapse:** .... ☐
   A. -pathy
   B. -ptosis
   C. -trophy
   D. -plasty
   E. -plasm

4. **Blood is held back from an area:** .... ☐
   A. Thrombocyte
   B. Anemia
   C. Ischemia
   D. Hematoma
   E. Hemolysis

5. **Death:** .... ☐
   A. neur/o
   B. nephr/o
   C. neutr/o
   D. nucle/o
   E. necr/o

6. **Acromegaly:** .... ☐
   A. Exocrine disorder of bone enlargement
   B. Enlargement of extremities after puberty due to pituitary gland problem
   C. Abnormal growth of bones before puberty
   D. Endocrine gland problem in young children
   E. Fear of extremities (heights)

7. **Pain in the ear:** .... ☐
   A. Pleurodynia
   B. Otitis
   C. Otalgia
   D. Osteitis
   E. Neuralgia

8. **Continuing over a long period of time:** .... ☐
   A. Chronic
   B. Acute
   C. Chromic
   D. Relapse
   E. Remission

9. **Small artery:** .... ☐
   A. Capillary
   B. Arteriole
   C. Venule
   D. Lymph vessel
   E. Blood vessel leading from the heart

10. **Instrument to visually examine:** .... ☐
    A. -scope
    B. -scopy
    C. -opsy
    D. -stasis
    E. -tomy

11. **Hernia of the urinary bladder:** .... ☐
    A. Rectocele
    B. Inguinal hernia
    C. Hiatal hernia
    D. Rectalgia
    E. Cystocele

12. **Tumor of bone marrow (cancerous):** .... ☐
    A. Myosarcoma
    B. Multiple myeloma
    C. Osteogenic sarcoma
    D. Adenocarcinoma
    E. Metastasis

13. **X-ray record of the spinal cord:** .... ☐
    A. Electroencephalogram
    B. Bone scan
    C. Myogram
    D. Myelogram
    E. Electromyogram

14. **Berry-shaped (spheroidal)**
    bacteria: .... ☐
    A. staphyl/o
    B. pneum/o
    C. -cele
    D. strept/o
    E. -cocci

15. **Neutrophil:** .... ☐
    A. Lymphocyte
    B. Polymorphonuclear leukocyte
    C. Monocyte
    D. Mononuclear agranulocyte
    E. Platelet

16. **Instrument to record:** .... ☐
    A. -gram
    B. -scopy
    C. -scope
    D. -graph
    E. -graphy

17. **Resembling:** .... ☐
    A. -osis
    B. -eal
    C. lith/o
    D. -oid
    E. -ic

18. **An eosinophil is a/an:** .... ☐
    A. Erythrocyte
    B. Leukocyte
    C. Mononuclear cell
    D. Platelet
    E. Lymphocyte

19. **Removal of the voice box:** .... ☐
    A. Larnygectomy
    B. Pharyngotomy
    C. Pharynostomy
    D. Laryngectomy
    E. Trachectomy

20. **Angioplasty means:** .... ☐
    A. Pertaining to fat
    B. Fear of extremities
    C. Therapy with chemicals
    D. Surgical puncture of a blood vessel
    E. Surgical repair of a blood vessel

21. **A blood cell that produces**
    antibodies: .... ☐
    A. Erythrocyte
    B. Platelet
    C. Lymphocyte
    D. Monocyte
    E. Basophil

22. **The opposite of -malacia is:** .... ☐
    A. -megaly
    B. -sclerosis
    C. -emia
    D. -plasia
    E. -lysis

23. **Excessive development:** .... ☐
    A. Hypoplasia
    B. Dystrophy
    C. Achondroplasia
    D. Morphology
    E. Hypertrophy

24. **Treatment:** .... ☐
    A. -therapy
    B. -genic
    C. -plasty
    D. -osis
    E. -stasis

25. **Surgical creation of a permanent**
    opening to the outside
    of the body: .... ☐
    A. -stomy
    B. -tomy
    C. -ectomy
    D. Section
    E. Resection

Chapter Three

EXERCISE QUIZ

Name: _____

A. *Give meanings for the following suffixes:*

1. -cele _____
4. -genesis _____

2. -coccus _____
5. -graphy _____

3. -centesis _____
6. -emia _____

B. *Using the following combining forms and your knowledge of suffixes, build medical terms for the definitions below:*

amni/o	cyst/o	laryng/o	myel/o	thorac/o
angi/o	isch/o	my/o	staphyl/o	

7. record of the spinal cord _____

8. process of recording blood vessels _____

9. pain of a muscle _____

10. surgical puncture to remove fluid from the chest _____

11. berry-shaped (spheroidal) bacteria in clusters _____

12. resection of the voice box _____

13. holding back of blood (from cells) _____

14. hernia of the urinary bladder _____

C. *Match the following terms that describe blood cells with their meanings below:*

erythrocyte	thrombocyte	monocyte
eosinophil	neutrophil	lymphocyte

15. a clotting cell; platelet _____

16. a red blood cell _____

17. a granulocytic white blood cell that destroys cells by engulfing and digesting them; polymorphonuclear leukocyte _____

18. a mononuclear leukocyte that is a phagocyte _____

19. a mononuclear leukocyte that destroys foreign cells by making antibodies _____

20. a leukocyte whose granules turn red with stain and whose numbers are elevated in allergic reactions _____

D. *Give meanings for the following suffixes:*

21. -lysis _____   26. -phobia_____

22. -pathy _____   27. -plasty _____

23. -penia _____   28. -stasis_____

24. -malacia_____   29. -plasia_____

25. -megaly _____   30. -sclerosis _____

E. *Using the following combining forms and your knowledge of suffixes, build medical terms for the definitions below:*

acr/o	cardi/o	morph/o	myel/o
blephar/o	chondr/o	my/o	sarc/o

31. fear of heights (extremities) _____

32. flesh (malignant) tumor of muscle _____

33. study of the shape (of cells) _____

34. inflammation of an eyelid _____

35. softening of cartilage _____

36. tumor of bone marrow_____

37. disease of heart muscle _____

F. *Give meanings for the following suffixes:*

38. -ptosis _____   43. -trophy _____

39. -stomy_____   44. -oid _____

40. -tomy_____   45. -ole _____

41. -ule _____   46. -opsy _____

42. -genic _____   47. -ectomy _____

G. *Underline the suffix in the following terms and give the meaning of each term:*

48. pulmonary _____

49. necrotic _____

50. inguinal _____

Chapter Three
DICTATION AND COMPREHENSION QUIZ

Name: _____

A. Dictation of Terms

1. _____   11. _____

2. _____   12. _____

3. _____   13. _____

4. _____   14. _____

5. _____   15. _____

6. _____   16. _____

7. _____   17. _____

8. _____   18. _____

9. _____   19. _____

10. _____   20. _____

B. Comprehension of Terms: Match the number of the above term with its meaning below.

_____ Pertaining to the groin

_____ Prolapse of an eyelid

_____ Disease of heart muscle

_____ Resection of a breast

_____ Ear pain

_____ Pertaining to the voice box

_____ Formation of blood vessels

_____ Pertaining to the membrane surrounding the abdomen

_____ Destruction of blood (RBCs)

_____ Incision of the abdomen

_____ Spread of a malignant tumor

_____ Holding back blood from tissues

_____ Fear of heights

_____ New opening of the windpipe to the outside of the body

_____ Abnormal condition of death of cells

_____ Hernia of the urinary bladder

_____ Record of the electricity in the brain

_____ Deficiency of clotting cells (platelets)

_____ Removal of living tissue and examination under a microscope

_____ Abnormal condition of fluid (water) in the kidney

Chapter Three
SPELLING QUIZ

Name: _____

A. *Circle the term that is spelled correctly and write its meaning in the space provided:*

1. pericardeum   pericardium _____

2. arteriosclerosis   arteriosklerosis _____

3. myleogram   myelogram _____

4. hepatomeagaly   hepatomegaly _____

5. trachostomy   tracheostomy _____

6. tonsillitis   tonsilitis _____

7. abdominocentesis   adbominocentesis _____

8. ploorodinia   pleurodynia _____

9. ophthalmology   opthalmology _____

10. staphylococci   staphlococci _____

B. *Circle the term that is spelled correctly. The meaning of each term is given.*

11. beyond control (spread of a cancerous tumor)	metastesis	metastasis	metastatis
12. pertaining to the voice box	larnygeal	laryngeal	laryngel
13. condition (disease) of the lung	pneumonia	pneumoneia	pnuemonia
14. hernia of the urinary bladder	cytocele	cystocele	cystosele
15. deficiency in white blood cells	leukopenia	luekopenia	lucopinea
16. excessive development	hypertropy	hypertrophy	hypertrofe
17. pertaining to the groin	inguinal	ingiuinal	ingwanal
18. clotting cell	platelete	platlet	platelet
19. incision of a vein	pilbotomy	phlebotomy	plebotomy
20. small vein	venule	vanule	venuel

Chapter Three
PRONUNCIATION QUIZ

Name: _____

A. *Underline the accented syllable in the following terms (for example: anemia, diagnosis, endocrine):*

1. arteriole
2. hypertrophy
3. osteomalacia
4. necrosis
5. carcinogenesis
6. laparoscopy
7. arteriosclerosis
8. thrombocytopenia
9. abdominocentesis
10. hydrotherapy

B. *Match the suffix in Column I with its meaning in Column II:*

Column I

1. -malacia _____
2. -phobia _____
3. -plasia _____
4. -ptosis _____
5. -pathy _____
6. -plasty _____
7. -emia _____
8. -penia _____
9. -trophy _____
10. -megaly _____

Column II

A. Prolapse.
B. Surgical repair.
C. Nourishment or development.
D. Fear.
E. Blood condition.
F. Formation.
G. Enlargement.
H. Softening.
I. Disease condition.
J. Deficiency.

C. *Complete the following terms from their definitions:*

1. _____ oma   Tumor of bone marrow.
2. _____ cocci   Berry-shaped (spheroidal) bacteria in twisted chains.
3. _____ cele   Hernia of the urinary bladder.
4. colo_____   New opening from the colon to the outside of the body.
5. staphylo_____   Berry-shaped (spheroidal) bacteria in clusters.
6. _____phobia   Fear of heights.
7. _____ology   Study of the eye.
8. _____ule   Small vein.
9. arterio_____   Hardening of arteries.
10. hemo_____   Destruction of blood.

Chapter Three
REVIEW SHEET QUIZ

Name: _____

A. *Give meanings for the following noun suffixes:*

1. -centesis _____

2. -dynia _____

3. -stasis _____

4. -plasty _____

5. -genesis _____

6. -cyte _____

7. -penia _____

8. -trophy _____

9. -emia _____

10. -graphy _____

B. *Give the suffixes for the following meanings:*

1. instrument to visually examine _____

2. fear _____

3. enlargement _____

4. prolapse _____

5. separation, destruction _____

6. softening _____

7. incision _____

8. treatment _____

9. excision _____

10. new opening _____

C. *Give meanings for the following combining forms:*

1. chondr/o _____

2. lapar/o _____

3. inguin/o _____

4. axill/o _____

5. blephar/o _____

6. mamm/o _____

7. angi/o _____

8. cyst/o _____

9. isch/o _____

10. adip/o _____

D. *Give the combining forms for the following meanings:*

1. liver _____

2. muscle _____

3. ear _____

4. tonsil _____

5. shape _____

6. lung _____

Chapter Three
CROSSWORD PUZZLE

Name: _____

Fill in the crossword puzzle below using the clues listed underneath it.

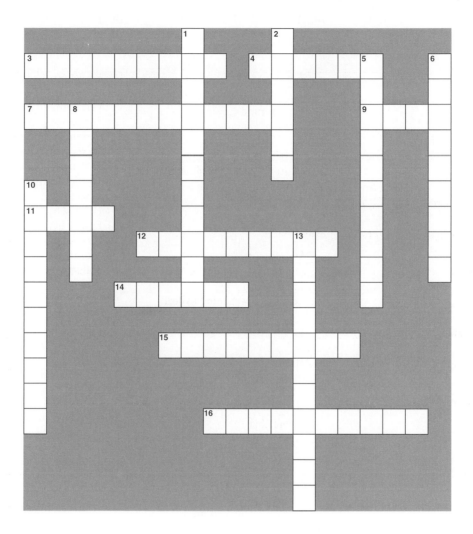

Across Clues

3. -malacia
4. -gram
7. -itis
9. -phobia
11. -algia
12. -therapy
14. -ule
15. -osis (abnormal _____)
16. -oid

Down Clues

1. -megaly
2. -cele
5. -penia
6. -sclerosis
8. -genesis
10. -ist
13. -trophy

Chapter Three
ANSWERS TO THE QUIZZES

Multiple Choice Quiz

1. E	4. C	7. C	10. A	13. D	16. D	19. D	22. B	25. A
2. E	5. E	8. A	11. E	14. E	17. D	20. E	23. E	
3. B	6. B	9. B	12. B	15. B	18. B	21. C	24. A	

Exercise Quiz

A

1. hernia
2. berry-shaped bacterium
3. surgical puncture to remove fluid
4. formation
5. process of recording
6. blood condition

B

7. myelogram
8. angiography
9. myalgia
10. thoracocentesis
11. staphylococci
12. laryngectomy
13. ischemia
14. cystocele

C

15. thrombocyte
16. erythrocyte
17. neutrophil
18. monocyte
19. lymphocyte
20. eosinophil

D

21. separation, destruction
22. disease condition
23. deficiency
24. softening
25. enlargement
26. fear
27. surgical repair
28. stop; control
29. formation
30. hardening

E

31. acrophobia
32. myosarcoma
33. morphology
34. blepharitis
35. chondromalacia
36. myeloma
37. cardiomyopathy

F

38. prolapse
39. new opening
40. incision
41. small; little
42. pertaining to producing
43. nourishment; development
44. resembling
45. small; little
46. to view
47. removal

G

48. pulmon<u>ary</u>—pertaining to the lungs
49. necrot<u>ic</u>—pertaining to death
50. inguin<u>al</u>—pertaining to the groin

Dictation and Comprehension Quiz

A

1. acrophobia
2. angiogenesis
3. biopsy
4. blepharoptosis
5. cardiomyopathy
6. cystocele
7. electroencephalogram
8. hemolysis
9. hydronephrosis
10. inguinal
11. ischemia
12. laparotomy
13. laryngeal
14. mastectomy
15. metastasis
16. necrosis
17. otalgia
18. peritoneal
19. thrombocytopenia
20. tracheostomy

B

10 Pertaining to the groin
4   Prolapse of an eyelid
5   Disease of heart muscle
14 Resection of a breast
17 Ear pain
13 Pertaining to the voice box
2   Formation of blood vessels
18 Pertaining to the membrane surrounding the abdomen
8   Destruction of blood (RBCs)
12 Incision of the abdomen
15 Spread of a malignant tumor
11 Holding back blood from tissues
1   Fear of heights
20 New opening of the windpipe to the outside of the body
16 Abnormal condition of death of cells
6   Hernia of the urinary bladder
7   Record of the electricity in the brain
19 Deficiency of clotting cells (platelets)
3   Removal of living tissue and examination under a microscope
9   Abnormal condition of fluid (water) in the kidney

Spelling Quiz

A

1. pericardium—lining (membrane) surrounding the heart
2. arteriosclerosis—hardening of arteries
3. myelogram—record (x-ray image) of spinal cord
4. hepatomegaly—enlargement of the liver
5. tracheostomy—new opening of the trachea to the outside of the body
6. tonsillitis—inflammation of the tonsils
7. abdominocentesis—surgical puncture to remove fluid from the abdomen (paracentesis)
8. pleurodynia—pain of the pleura (chest wall muscles)

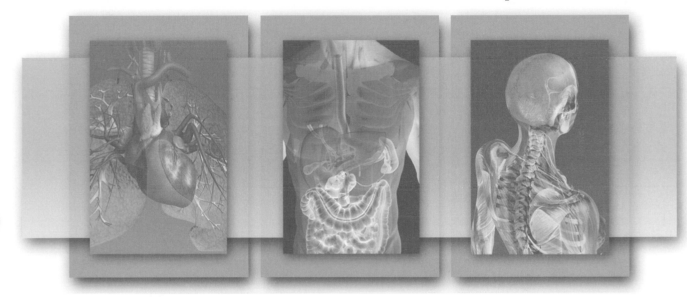

chapter 4

Chapter Four

MULTIPLE CHOICE QUIZ

Name: _____

In the box write the letter of the choice that is the definition of the term or best answers the question. There is only one correct answer for each question.

1. **Pertaining to between the ribs:** .... ☐
   A. Intracostal
   B. Infracostal
   C. Costochondral
   D. Mediastinal
   E. Intercostal

2. **Pertaining to the opposite side:** .... ☐
   A. Bilateral
   B. Contralateral
   C. Unilateral
   D. Contraindication
   E. Ipsilateral

3. **Protrusion of an eyeball:** .... ☐
   A. Cystocele
   B. Inguinal hernia
   C. Exopthalmos
   D. Ectopic
   E. Exophthalmos

4. **A congenital anomaly:** .... ☐
   A. Cerebral ischemia
   B. Pseudocyesis
   C. Hemiglossectomy
   D. Syndactyly
   E. Acromegaly

5. **Symbiosis:** .... ☐
   A. Parasitism is an example
   B. Symmetrical organs
   C. Biopsy
   D. Group of symptoms
   E. Prolapse of the uterus

6. **Symptoms precede an illness:** .... ☐
   A. Apnea
   B. Syndrome
   C. Euphoria
   D. Prodrome
   E. Prognosis

7. **Before meals:** .... ☐
   A. Prenatal
   B. Anti cibum
   C. Postpartum
   D. Antenatal
   E. Ante cibum

8. **Antibodies:** .... ☐
   A. Bacteria
   B. Protein substances made by leukocytes
   C. Phagocytes
   D. Produced by erythrocytes to fight disease
   E. Antibiotics

9. **Symphysis:** .... ☐
   A. Bifurcation
   B. Symptoms occur together
   C. Living organisms grow together for mutual benefit
   D. Bones grow together, as in the pelvis
   E. Synthesis of substances

10. **Ultrasonography:** .... ☐
    A. X-ray recording of sound waves
    B. Amniocentesis
    C. Sound waves and echoes are used to create an image
    D. Radioactive material is injected and sound waves are recorded
    E. Abdominal x-ray recording

11. **Metamorphosis:** .... ☐
    A. Paralysis of limbs
    B. Spread of a cancerous growth
    C. Precancerous
    D. Change in shape or form
    E. After death

12. **Hypertrophy:** .... ☐
    A. Underdeveloped
    B. Poor development
    C. Increase in cell size; increased development
    D. Increase in cell numbers
    E. Newborn

13. **Excessive sugar in the blood:** .... ☐
    A. Hypodermic
    B. Hypoglycemia
    C. Glycosuria
    D. Hematuria
    E. Hyperglycemia

14. **Retroperitoneal:**....................................☐
    A. Region of the stomach
    B. Within the chest
    C. Behind the abdomen
    D. Within the abdomen
    E. Below the pelvis

15. **Antigens:**............................☐
    A. Streptococci
    B. Antibiotics
    C. Antitoxins
    D. Produced by antibodies
    E. Penicillins

16. **Return of disease symptoms:**..............☐
    A. Prolapse
    B. Relapse
    C. Syndrome
    D. Prodrome
    E. Remission

17. **Dia-:**....................................☐
    A. Flow
    B. Down, lack of
    C. Complete, through
    D. Against
    E. Near

18. **Abductor muscle:**..........................☐
    A. Bending forward
    B. Located proximally
    C. Pertains to both sides
    D. Carries a limb toward the body
    E. Carries a limb away from the body

19. **Dyspnea:**..................................☐
    A. Abnormal formation
    B. Difficult breathing
    C. Not able to sleep
    D. Condition of lack of water
    E. Not able to breathe

20. **Brady-:**....................................☐
    A. Fast
    B. Bad
    C. Short
    D. Slow
    E. Large

21. **Located on the dorsal side of an endocrine gland in the neck:**..........☐
    A. Pituitary gland
    B. Parathyroid glands
    C. Adrenal glands
    D. Mammary glands
    E. Salivary glands

22. **Recombinant DNA:**............................☐
    A. Pregnancy that is out of place
    B. Artificial kidney machine
    C. Backward development
    D. Antibodies are made against normal tissue
    E. Gene from one organism is inserted into another organism

23. **Tachycardia:**..☐
    A. Bad, painful swallowing
    B. Inability to swallow
    C. Near the windpipe
    D. Rapid breathing
    E. Rapid heartbeat

24. **Epithelium:**......................................☐
    A. Surface cells that line internal organs and are found in the skin
    B. Membrane surrounding bone
    C. Connective tissue that binds muscles to bones
    D. Adipose tissue
    E. Above the stomach

25. **Percutaneous:**..................................☐
    A. Within a vein
    B. Through a vein
    C. Through the skin
    D. Surrounding cartilage
    E. Surrounding a bone

Chapter Four

EXERCISE QUIZ

Name: _____

A. *Give meanings for the following prefixes:*

1. ante- _____
2. anti- _____
3. ana- _____
4. brady- _____
5. con- _____

6. contra- _____
7. bi- _____
8. ad- _____
9. dys- _____
10. dia- _____

B. *Match the following terms with their meanings below:*

anoxia   antisepsis   congenital anomaly
anteflexion   apnea   contralateral
antepartum   bilateral   bilateral

11. against infection _____
12. not breathing _____
13. before birth _____

14. condition of no oxygen _____
15. irregularity at birth _____
16. pertaining to opposite side _____

C. *Give meanings of the following prefixes:*

17. epi- _____
18. eu- _____
19. intra- _____
20. de- _____

21. inter- _____
22. hypo- _____
23. hyper- _____
24. mal- _____

D. *Complete the following terms by supplying the word part that is called for:*

25. pregnancy that is out of place: _____ topic

26. good feeling (well-being): _____ phoria

27. condition of abnormal formation (of cells): dys _____

28. pertaining to within the windpipe: endo _____

29. pertaining to below the ribs: infra _____

30. blood condition of less than normal sugar: _____ glycemia

E. Match the following terms with their meanings below:

dialysis   exophthalmos   malignant   metastasis   ptosis
diarrhea   malaise   metamorphosis   pancytopenia

31. condition of change of shape or form _____

32. vague feeling of bodily discomfort _____

33. deficiency of all blood cells _____

34. separation of wastes from the blood _____

35. spread of a cancerous tumor to a secondary organ or tissue _____

36. eyeballs that bulge outward _____

F. Give meanings for the following prefixes:

37. peri- _____   41. neo- _____

38. poly- _____   42. meta- _____

39. per- _____   43. para- _____

40. syn- _____   44. post- _____

G. Underline the prefix and give the meaning of the entire term:

45. retroperitoneal _____

46. transurethral _____

47. subcutaneous _____

48. tachypnea _____

49. unilateral _____

50. pseudocyesis _____

H. Match the terms with their meanings below:

neoplasm   parathyroid   relapse   syndactyly
paralysis   prodrome   remission   syndrome

51. loss of movement in muscles _____

52. symptoms that appear before an illness _____

53. symptoms lessen _____

54. disease or symptoms return _____

55. webbed fingers or toes _____

56. new growth (tumor) _____

Chapter Four
DICTATION AND COMPREHENSION QUIZ

Name: _____

A. *Dictation of Terms*

1. _____   11. _____
2. _____   12. _____
3. _____   13. _____
4. _____   14. _____
5. _____   15. _____
6. _____   16. _____
7. _____   17. _____
8. _____   18. _____
9. _____   19. _____
10. _____   20. _____

B. *Comprehension of Terms: Match the number of the above term with its meaning below.*

_____ Pertaining to below a rib

_____ New growth (tumor)

_____ Membrane surrounding a bone

_____ Condition of slow heartbeat

_____ Pertaining to under the skin

_____ Condition of deficiency of all (blood cells)

_____ Carrying away from (the body)

_____ Two endocrine glands, each above a kidney

_____ Condition of "no" oxygen (deficiency)

_____ Pertaining to through the tube leading from the bladder to the outside of the body

_____ A substance that acts against a poison

_____ Pertaining to within the windpipe

_____ Rapid breathing

_____ Pertaining to the opposite side

_____ Four endocrine glands in the neck region

_____ Feeling of well-being

_____ Removal of half of the tongue

_____ Pertaining to between the ribs

_____ Harmless, non-cancerous

_____ Pertaining to behind the membrane surrounding the abdominal organs

Chapter Four
SPELLING QUIZ

Name: _____

A. *Circle the term that is spelled correctly and write its meaning in the space provided:*

1. neonatal   neonatel _____

2. postmortum   postmortem _____

3. metastasis   metastesis _____

4. symdrone   syndrome _____

5. biforcation   bifurcation _____

6. antebody   antibody _____

7. antibiotic   antebiotic _____

8. diarrhea   diarhhea _____

9. symbiosis   symbyosis _____

10. benign   beningn _____

B. *Circle the term that is spelled correctly. The meaning of each term is given.*

11. slow heart beat.............................	bradicardia	bradycardia	bradicardea
12. both sides	bilateral	bilaterel	bilataral
13. lack of water	dehydrashun	dehidration	dehydration
14. without oxygen	anoxia	aoxyia	anocksia
15. against infection	antesepsis	antisepsis	antisespsis
16. before birth	antipartum	antipartem	antepartum
17. not breathing	apnea	aphnea	afpnea
18. foreign substance	antigene	antigen	antegen
19. feeling of well-being	euforia	uforea	euphoria
20. through the skin	pericutaneus	percutaneous	percutanous

Chapter Four
PRONUNCIATION QUIZ

Name: _____

A. *Underline the accented syllable in the following terms (for example: anemia, diagnosis, endocrine):*

1. symbiosis

4. congenital anomaly

7. polyneuritis

10. bifurcation

2. endotracheal

5. hyperplasia

8. antitoxin

3. metamorphosis

6. symphysis

9. malaise

B. *Match the prefix in Column I with its meaning in Column II:*

Column I

Column II

1. inter- _____

A. Together; with

2. intra- _____

B. Toward

3. infra- _____

C. Away from

4. contra- _____

D. Within

5. ad- _____

E. Surrounding

6. para- _____

F. Below

7. peri- _____

G. Above

8. per- _____

H. Against

9. syn- _____

I. Before

10. pro- _____

J. Between

K. Abnormal; near, beside

L. Through

C. *Complete the following terms from their definitions:*

1. _____ natal   Pertaining to after birth.

2. _____ cardia   Slow heart rate.

3. ec _____   Out of place.

4. inter _____   Pertaining to between the ribs.

5. _____ cytopenia   Deficiency in all (blood) cells.

6. _____ glycemia   Condition of increased blood sugar.

7. supra _____   Pertaining to above the kidney.

8. _____ plasia   Bad (abnormal) formation.

9. _____ partum   Before birth.

10. re _____   Return of disease symptoms.

Chapter Four
REVIEW SHEET QUIZ

Name: _____

A. *Give meanings for the following prefixes:*

1. ab- _____
2. ante- _____
3. cata- _____
4. contra- _____
5. epi- _____
6. eu- _____
7. hyper- _____
8. hypo- _____

9. poly- _____
10. post- _____
11. syn-, sym- _____
12. retro- _____
13. supra- _____
14. intra- _____
15. endo- _____

B. *Give prefixes for the following meanings:*

1. two _____
2. no, not, without _____
3. all _____
4. new _____
5. surrounding _____

6. half _____
7. between _____
8. small _____
9. fast _____
10. false _____

C. *Give meanings for the following prefixes:*

1. dys- _____
2. dia- _____
3. brady- _____
4. pro- _____
5. ultra- _____

6. con- _____
7. mal- _____
8. meta- _____
9. para- _____
10. anti- _____

D. *Give meanings for the following combining forms and suffixes:*

1. necr/o _____
2. carp/o _____
3. gloss/o _____
4. seps/o _____
5. cost/o _____

6. -rrhea _____
7. -plasia _____
8. -pnea _____
9. -partum _____
10. -trophy _____

Chapter Four
CROSSWORD PUZZLE

Name: _____

Fill in the crossword puzzle below using the clues listed underneath it.

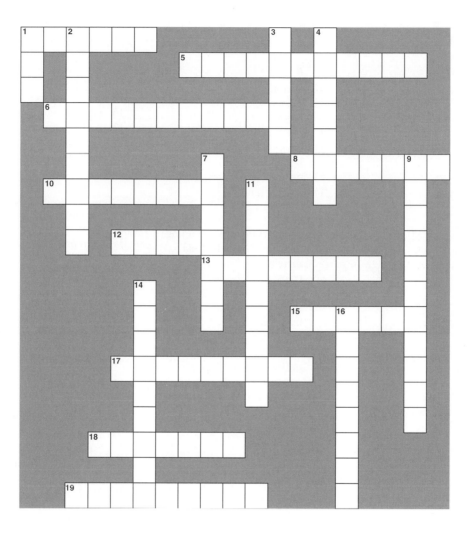

Across Clues

1. thyr/o (Greek, *thyreus*) means _____.
5. -trophy means development and _____.
6. -plasia means formation and _____.
8. contra- means opposite and _____.
10. trache/o means _____.
12. morph/o means form or _____.
13. para- means near, beside, or _____.
15. intra- means in or _____.
17. -cyesis means _____.
18. dactyl/o means toes or _____.
19. -rrhea means flow or _____.

Down Clues

1. -ptosis means prolapse or to _____.
2. seps/o means _____.
3. -partum means _____.
4. trans- means across or _____.
7. infra- means below or _____.
9. peri- means _____.
11. furc/o means forking or _____.
14. -blast means immature or _____.
16. con- means with or _____.

Chapter Four
ANSWERS TO THE QUIZZES

Multiple Choice Quiz

1. E	4. D	7. E	10. C	13. E	16. B	19. B	22. E	25. C
2. B	5. A	8. B	11. D	14. C	17. C	20. D	23. E	
3. E	6. D	9. D	12. C	15. A	18. E	21. B	24. A	

Exercise Quiz

A

1. before
2. against
3. up
4. slow
5. together; with
6. against; opposite
7. two
8. toward
9. bad, painful, difficult
10. complete; through

B

11. antisepsis
12. apnea
13. antepartum
14. anoxia
15. congenital anomaly
16. contralateral

C

17. above
18. good, normal
19. within
20. lack of, down
21. between
22. under, deficient
23. above, excessive
24. bad

D

25. ectopic
26. euphoria
27. dysplasia
28. endotracheal
29. infracostal
30. hypoglycemia

E

31. metamorphosis
32. malaise
33. pancytopenia
34. dialysis
35. metastasis
36. exophthalmos

F

37. surrounding
38. many, much
39. through
40. together, with
41. new
42. beyond; change
43. near, beside, abnormal
44. after, behind

G

45. retroperitoneal—pertaining to behind the abdominal membrane
46. transurethral—pertaining to across or through the urethra
47. subcutaneous—pertaining to under the skin
48. tachypnea—fast or rapid breathing
49. unilateral—pertaining to one side
50. pseudocyesis—false pregnancy

H

51. paralysis
52. prodrome
53. remission
54. relapse
55. syndactyly
56. neoplasm

Dictation and Comprehension Quiz

A

1. abduction
2. adrenal
3. anoxia
4. antitoxin
5. benign
6. bradycardia
7. contralateral
8. endotracheal
9. euphoria
10. hemiglossectomy
11. hypodermic
12. infracostal
13. intercostal
14. neoplasm
15. pancytopenia
16. parathyroid
17. periosteum
18. retroperitoneal
19. tachypnea
20. transurethral

B

12 Pertaining to below a rib
14 New growth (tumor)
17 Membrane surrounding a bone
6 Condition of slow heartbeat
11 Pertaining to under the skin
15 Condition of deficiency of all (blood cells)
1 Carrying away from (the body)
2 Two endocrine glands, each above a kidney
3 Condition of "no" oxygen (deficiency)
20 Pertaining to through the tube leading from the bladder to the outside of the body
4 A substance that works against a poison
8 Pertaining to within the windpipe
19 Rapid breathing
7 Pertaining to the opposite side
16 Four endocrine glands in the neck region
9 Feeling of well-being
10 Removal of half of the tongue
13 Pertaining to between the ribs
5 Harmless, non-cancerous
18 Pertaining to behind the membrane surrounding the abdominal organs

Spelling Quiz

A

1. neonatal—newborn
2. postmortem—after death
3. metastasis—beyond control (spread of tumor)

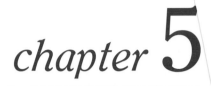

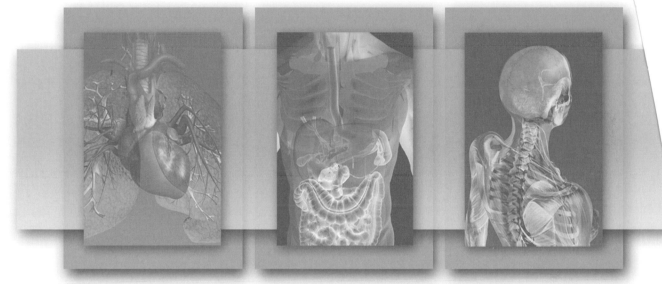

Chapter Five

MULTIPLE CHOICE QUIZ

Name: _____

In the box write the letter of the choice that is the definition of the term or best answers the question. There is only one correct answer for each question.

1. **The combining form of the first part of the large intestine is:** ....
   A. Ile/o
   B. Jejun/o
   C. Ili/o
   D. Duoden/o
   E. Cec/o

2. **Pertaining to the abdomen:** ....
   A. Gastric
   B. Celiac
   C. Colonic
   D. Pelvic
   E. Esophageal

3. **Muscular wave-like movement to transport food through the digestive system:** ....
   A. Mastication
   B. Regurgitation
   C. Emulsification
   D. Peristalsis
   E. Anastomosis

4. **Part of the tooth that contains a rich supply of nerves and blood vessels:** .....
   A. Enamel
   B. Dentin
   C. Pulp
   D. Cementum
   E. Periodontal membrane

5. **Gingiv/o means:** ....
   A. Tooth
   B. Stomach
   C. Intestine
   D. Chest
   E. Gums

6. **Buccal means:** ....
   A. Pertaining to the cheek
   B. Pertaining to the soft palate
   C. Pertaining to the tongue
   D. Pertaining to the teeth
   E. Pertaining to the throat

7. **High blood levels of a pigment released by the liver with bile:** ....
   A. Cholecystitis
   B. Hypoglycemia
   C. Hyperbilirubinemia
   D. Hematoma
   E. Steatorrhea

8. **Carries bile into the duodenum:** ....
   A. Cystic duct
   B. Portal vein
   C. Lymph duct
   D. Hepatic duct
   E. Common bile duct

9. **Enzyme to digest starch:** ....
   A. Lipase
   B. Amylase
   C. Glucose
   D. Bile
   E. Amino acid

10. **Chronic inflammation of the intestinal tract:** ....
   A. Crohn disease
   B. Colonic polyposis
   C. Irritable bowel syndrome
   D. Dysentery
   E. Achalasia

11. **Ring of muscles:** ....
   A. Uvula
   B. Rugae
   C. Papillae
   D. Myoma
   E. Sphincter

12. **Specialist in gums:** ....
   A. Endodontist
   B. Periodontist
   C. Orthodontist
   D. Pedodontist
   E. Proctologist

13. **Stomat/o means:** ....
   A. Roof of the mouth
   B. Mouth
   C. Cheek
   D. Stomach
   E. Tongue

14. **Cheil/o means the same as:** .... ☐
    A. Lingu/o
    B. Gingiv/o
    C. Gloss/o
    D. Palat/o
    E. Labi/o

15. **Stone in a salivary gland:** .... ☐
    A. Lithiasis
    B. Cholecystolithiasis
    C. Adenolithiasis
    D. Sialadenolithiasis
    E. Renal calculus

16. **Membrane that connects parts of
    small intestine:** .... ☐
    A. Anastomosis
    B. Ileum
    C. Mesentery
    D. Appendix
    E. Pylorus

17. **New opening from the large bowel
    to the surface of the body:** .... ☐
    A. Jejunostomy
    B. Jejunotomy
    C. Enterostomy
    D. Colostomy
    E. Duodenotomy

18. **Fats are improperly digested and
    appear in the feces:** .... ☐
    A. Adipose
    B. Steatorrhea
    C. Lipase
    D. Lipolysis
    E. Glycogenolysis

19. **Lack of appetite:** .... ☐
    A. Anorexia
    B. Aphthous stomatitis
    C. Leukoplakia
    D. Postprandial
    E. Achlorhydria

20. **Another term for jaundice:** .... ☐
    A. Achalasia
    B. Icterus
    C. Hypobilirubinemia
    D. Gallstones
    E. Melena

21. **Esophageal varices are:** .... ☐
    A. Hernias around the opening of the
       stomach
    B. Hemorrhoids
    C. Perianal fistulae
    D. Polyps
    E. Swollen, twisted veins

22. **Abnormal side pockets in a hollow
    organ, such as the intestine:** .... ☐
    A. Caries
    B. Ulcers
    C. Dysentery
    D. Diverticula
    E. Ascites

23. **Telescoping of the intestine:** .... ☐
    A. Volvulus
    B. Anal fistula
    C. Intussusception
    D. Ileus
    E. Hiatal hernia

24. **Difficulty in swallowing:** .... ☐
    A. Regurgitation
    B. Flatus
    C. Nausea
    D. Eructation
    E. Dysphagia

25. **White plaques on the mucosa of
    the mouth:** .... ☐
    A. Herpetic stomatitis
    B. Aphthous stomatitis
    C. Oral leukoplakia
    D. Rectocele
    E. Melena

Chapter Five
EXERCISE QUIZ

Name: _____

A. *Match the following digestive system structures with their meanings.*

cecum	duodenum	gallbladder	pancreas
colon	esophagus	ileum	pharynx

1. Third part of the small intestine _____

2. Organ under the stomach; produces insulin and enzymes _____

3. First part of the large intestine _____

4. Small sac under the liver; stores bile _____

5. Tube connecting the throat to the stomach _____

6. Large intestine _____

7. First part of the small intestine _____

8. Throat _____

B. *Complete the following:*

9. lapar/o and celi/o both mean _____

10. gloss/o and lingu/o both mean _____

11. or/o and stomat/o both mean _____

12. labi/o and cheil/o both mean _____

C. *Build medical terms:*

13. Enlargement of the liver _____

14. Study of the cause (of disease) _____

15. Incision of the common bile duct _____

16. Surgical repair of the roof of the mouth _____

17. After meals _____

18. New opening between the common bile duct and the jejunum _____

D. *Build medical terms to describe the following inflammations:*

19. Inflammation of the appendix _____

20. Inflammation of the membrane around the abdomen _____

21. Inflammation of the large intestine _____

22. Inflammation of the gallbladder _____

23. Inflammation of a salivary gland _____

24. Inflammation of the small and large intestines _____

25. Inflammation of the liver _____

26. Inflammation of the pancreas _____

27. Inflammation of the mouth _____

28. Inflammation of the gums _____

29. Inflammation of the third part of the small intestine _____

E. *Match the following pathological diagnoses with their definitions below:*

cholecystolithiasis	dysentery	ileus	ulcerative colitis
cirrhosis	hemorrhoids	irritable bowel syndrome	
diverticula	hepatitis	peptic ulcer	

30. Swollen, twisted veins in the rectal region _____

31. Chronic liver disease resulting from alcoholism and malnutrition _____

32. Failure of peristalsis _____

33. Calculi in the sac that stores bile _____

34. Sore or lesion of the mucous membrane in the stomach or duodenum _____

35. Painful, inflamed intestines often caused by bacterial infection _____

36. Inflammation of the liver caused by type A, type B, or type C virus _____

37. Chronic inflammation of the large bowel with ulcers _____

38. Abnormal side-pockets in the intestinal wall _____

39. Group of gastrointestinal symptoms associated with stress, but without inflammation of the intestines _____

F. *Give the names of the following gastrointestinal symptoms from their descriptions:*

40. Lack of appetite _____

41. Bright, fresh red blood in stools _____

42. Abnormal accumulation of fluid in the abdomen _____

43. Loose, watery stools _____

44. Gas expelled through the anus _____

45. Discharge of fat in the feces _____

G. Complete the spelling of the medical terms below:

46. Black, dark-brown, tarry stools: mel _____

47. Membrane that holds the intestines together: mes _____

48. Pertaining to under the tongue: sub _____

49. High levels of pigment in the blood (jaundice): hyper _____

50. New connection between two previously unconnected tubes: ana _____

Chapter Five

DICTATION AND COMPREHENSION QUIZ: VOCABULARY

Name: _____

A. Dictation of Terms

1. _____   11. _____

2. _____   12. _____

3. _____   13. _____

4. _____   14. _____

5. _____   15. _____

6. _____   16. _____

7. _____   17. _____

8. _____   18. _____

9. _____   19. _____

10. _____   20. _____

B. Comprehension of Terms: Match the number of the above term with its meaning below.

_____ Physical process of breaking down large fat globules into smaller parts

_____ Salivary gland near the ear

_____ Swallowing

_____ Small substances that are produced when proteins are digested

_____ Pigment released by the liver in bile

_____ Soft inner tissue within a tooth containing nerves and blood vessels

_____ Tiny microscopic projections in the walls of the small intestine

_____ Rhythm-like contractions of the tubes of the alimentary tract

_____ Hormone produced by the endocrine cells of the pancreas

_____ This tube carries bile from the liver and gallbladder into the duodenum

_____ Small nipple-like elevations on the tongue

_____ Soft tissue hanging from the roof of the mouth

_____ An enzyme that digests starch

_____ Chewing

_____ Simple sugar

_____ Substance produced by the stomach and necessary for digestion of foods

_____ Solid wastes; stools

_____ Pancreatic enzyme necessary to digest fats

_____ Ring of muscle at the distal region of the stomach

_____ Large fat molecules

Chapter Five

DICTATION AND COMPREHENSION QUIZ: PATHOLOGICAL SYMPTOMS

Name: _____

A. Dictation of Terms

1. _____   7. _____

2. _____   8. _____

3. _____   9. _____

4. _____   10. _____

5. _____   11. _____

6. _____   12. _____

B. Comprehension of Terms: Match the number of the above term with its meaning below.

_____ Feces containing fat

_____ Unpleasant sensation from the stomach with tendency to vomit

_____ Gas expelled through the anus

_____ Lack of appetite

_____ Bright, fresh, red blood from the rectum

_____ Difficult, delayed elimination of feces

_____ Black, tarry stools; feces containing blood

_____ Yellow-orange coloration of the skin; icterus

_____ Rumbling or gurgling noises produced by the movement of gas or fluid

_____ Difficulty in swallowing

_____ Loose, liquid stools

_____ Abnormal accumulation of fluid in the peritoneal cavity

Chapter Five

DICTATION AND COMPREHENSION QUIZ: PATHOLOGICAL CONDITIONS

Name: _____

A. Dictation of Terms

1. _____   11. _____

2. _____   12. _____

3. _____   13. _____

4. _____   14. _____

5. _____   15. _____

6. _____   16. _____

7. _____   17. _____

8. _____   18. _____

9. _____   19. _____

10. _____   20. _____

B. Comprehension of Terms: Match the number of the above term with its meaning below.

_____ Inflammation and degeneration of gums

_____ Twisting of the intestine upon itself

_____ Small benign growths protrude from the mucous membrane of the large bowel

_____ Telescoping of the intestines

_____ Solids and fluids return to the mouth from the stomach

_____ Gallbladder calculi

_____ Inflammation of the liver; viral etiology

_____ Chronic liver disease; etiology is often alcoholism and malnutrition

_____ Sore or lesion of the mucous membranes of the first part of the small intestine

_____ Abnormal tubelike passageway in the distal end of the alimentary tract

_____ Painful inflamed intestines; etiology is often bacterial

_____ Swollen, tortuous veins in the distal portion of the tube connecting the throat and stomach

_____ Inflammation of a gland behind the stomach; cysts may form

_____ Inflammation of small side-pockets in the intestinal wall

_____ Chronic inflammation of the large bowel with open sores of mucous membrane

_____ Chronic inflammation of the intestinal tract (terminal ileum)

_____ Failure of peristalsis

_____ Failure of the LES muscle to relax

_____ Inflammation of the mouth with open sores

_____ Tooth decay

Chapter Five
SPELLING QUIZ

Name: _____

A. *Circle the term that is spelled correctly and write its meaning in the space provided:*

1. pancreatitis   pancreasitis _____

2. anal fistula   anal fistulla _____

3. dental karies   dental caries _____

4. cholitis   colitis _____

5. ileus   ilius _____

6. assites   ascites _____

7. melana   melena _____

8. polyposis   poliposis _____

9. dysentery   dysentary _____

10. anarexia   anorexia _____

B. *Circle the term that is spelled correctly. The meaning of each term is given.*

11. membrane connecting the intestines	mesentary	mezentary	mesentery
12. gallbladder resection	cholocystectomy	cholecystectomy	colecystectomy
13. twisting of the intestine	vulvulus	volvulus	vulvulos
14. chronic intestinal inflammation	Chron disease	Chrohn disease	Crohn disease
15. pertaining to bile	billiary	biliary	billiery
16. yellow coloration of the skin	jaundice	jaundise	jawndice
17. salivary gland near the ear	perotid gland	parrotid gland	parotid gland
18. failure of muscles in the lower esophagus to relax	achalsia	achalasia	acalasia
19. nutrition is given other than through the intestine	parenteral	perinteral	perenteral
20. new opening between two previously unconnected tubes	anastomosis	anastomosus	anastamosis

Chapter Five
PRONUNCIATION QUIZ

Name: _____

A. *Underline the accented syllable in the following words:*

1. aphthous stomatitis
2. dysentery
3. choledocholithiasis
4. leukoplakia
5. esophageal varices
6. pyloric sphincter
7. biliary
8. cheilitis
9. diverticula
10. volvulus

B. *Match the term in Column I with its meaning in Column II:*

Column I

1. jejunum _____
2. pharynx _____
3. sigmoid colon _____
4. duodenum _____
5. uvula _____
6. amylase _____
7. cecum _____
8. ascites _____
9. intussusception _____
10. postprandial _____

Column II

A. Collection of fluid in the abdominal cavity.
B. First part of the small intestine.
C. First part of the colon.
D. The throat.
E. After meals.
F. Enzyme to digest starch.
G. Second part of the small intestine.
H. Soft tissue hanging from the roof of the mouth.
I. Telescoping of the intestines.
J. S-shaped portion of the large bowel.

C. *Complete the following terms from their definitions:*

1. _____ itis — Inflammation of the pancreas.
2. _____ ectomy — Removal of the gallbladder.
3. an_____ — Loss of appetite.
4. _____ itis — Inflammation of the third part of the small intestine.
5. _____ lithiasis — Abnormal condition of salivary stones.
6. enteric ana _____ — New opening between two previously unconnected parts of the intestine.
7. _____ plasty — Surgical repair of roof of the mouth.
8. _____ logist — One who studies the anus and rectum.
9. gluco _____ — Formation of new sugar from fats and protein.
10. peri _____ — Muscular, wave-like movement of digestive tract walls.

Chapter Five
DIAGRAM QUIZ

Name: _____

Label the diagram below using the terms listed below:

Anus	Descending colon	Ileum	Rectum
Appendix	Duodenum	Jejunum	Sigmoid colon
Ascending colon	Esophagus	Liver	Stomach
Cecum	Gallbladder	Pancreas	Transverse colon

Pharynx

Epiglottis

Larynx

1

Trachea

Lung

Diaphragm

4

Spleen

2

5

Splenic flexure

Hepatic flexure

6

3

7

12

13

11

8

Ileocecal valve

9

14

10

15

16

Chapter Five

VOCABULARY QUIZ

Name: _____

A. *Match the following terms with their meanings below:*

absorption	bilirubin	emulsification
amino acids	defecation	enamel
amylase	deglutition	fatty acids
bile	dentin	glucose

1. Swallowing _____

2. Pigment released by the liver in bile _____

3. Substances produced when proteins are digested _____

4. Major tissue composing teeth _____

5. Removal of waste material from the body _____

6. Passage of materials through villi into the blood _____

7. Enzyme secreted by the pancreas to digest starch _____

8. Hard, outermost layer of a tooth _____

9. Process of breaking up large fat globules _____

10. Simple sugar _____

11. Digestive juice made by the liver and stored in the gallbladder _____

12. Substances produced when fats are digested _____

B. *Match the following terms with their meanings below:*

feces	insulin	parotid gland
glycogen	LES	peristalsis
hydrochloric acid	lipase	portal vein
incisor	palate	protease

1. Contractions of the gastrointestinal tubes _____

2. Pancreatic enzyme necessary to digest fats _____

3. Starch; stored sugar _____

4. Solid wastes; stools _____

5. Roof of the mouth _____

6. Blood vessel bringing blood to the liver _____

7. Chemical produced by the stomach to aid digestion _____

8. Hormone produced by the pancreas _____

9. One of four front teeth _____

10. Enzyme that digests proteins _____

11. Ring of muscles between the esophagus and stomach _____

12. Secretes enzymes into the mouth _____

C. *Match the following terms with their meanings below:*

mastication   pyloric sphincter   uvula
papillae   rugae   villi
pulp   triglycerides

1. Soft tissue hanging from the soft palate _____

2. Microscopic projections in the walls of the small intestine _____

3. Ring of muscles at the distal region of the stomach _____

4. Small elevations on the tongue _____

5. Chewing _____

6. Ridges on the hard palate and wall of the stomach _____

7. Soft tissue within a tooth _____

8. Large fat molecules _____

Chapter Five
CROSSWORD PUZZLE

Name: _____

Fill in the crossword puzzle below using the clues listed underneath it.

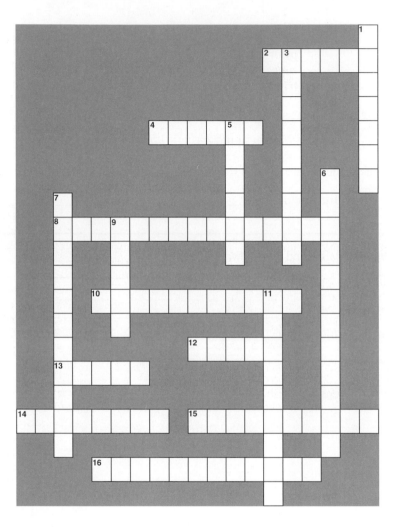

Across Clues

2. Decay.
4. Feces containing dark, tarry blood.
8. Telescoping of the intestines.
10. Swollen, twisted, varicose veins in the rectal region.
12. Failure of peristalsis.
13. Chronic inflammation of the terminal ileum is called _____ disease.
14. Twisting of the intestine upon itself.
15. Belching or raising gas from the stomach.
16. Lack of hydrochloric acid in the stomach.

Down Clues

1. Abnormal accumulation of fluid in the abdomen.
3. Failure of the muscles of the lower esophagus to relax during swallowing.
5. Unpleasant sensation from the stomach with a tendency to vomit.
6. Inflammation of the pancreas.
7. Abnormal side pockets in the intestinal wall.
9. Open sore or lesion of skin tissue.
11. Painful, inflamed intestines.

Chapter Five
ANSWERS TO THE QUIZZES

Multiple Choice Quiz

1. E	4. C	7. C	10. A	13. B	16. C	19. A	22. D	25. C
2. B	5. E	8. E	11. E	14. E	17. D	20. B	23. C	
3. D	6. A	9. B	12. B	15. D	18. B	21. E	24. E	

Exercise Quiz

A
1. ileum
2. pancreas
3. cecum
4. gallbladder
5. esophagus
6. colon
7. duodenum
8. pharynx

B
9. abdomen
10. tongue
11. mouth
12. lip

C
13. hepatomegaly
14. etiology
15. choledochotomy
16. palatoplasty
17. postprandial
18. choledochojejunostomy

D
19. appendicitis
20. peritonitis
21. colitis
22. cholecystitis
23. sialadenitis
24. enterocolitis
25. hepatitis
26. pancreatitis
27. stomatitis
28. gingivitis
29. ileitis

E
30. hemorrhoids
31. cirrhosis
32. ileus
33. cholecystolithiasis
34. ulcer
35. dysentery
36. hepatitis
37. ulcerative colitis

38. diverticula
39. irritable bowel syndrome

F
40. anorexia
41. hematochezia
42. ascites
43. diarrhea
44. flatus
45. steatorrhea

G
46. melena
47. mesentery
48. sublingual
49. hyperbilirubinemia
50. anastomosis

Dictation and Comprehension Quiz: Vocabulary

A
1. amino acids
2. amylase
3. bilirubin
4. common bile duct
5. deglutition
6. emulsification
7. feces
8. glucose
9. hydrochloric acid
10. insulin
11. lipase
12. mastication
13. papillae
14. parotid
15. peristalsis
16. pulp
17. pyloric sphincter
18. triglycerides
19. uvula
20. villi

B
6 Physical process of breaking down large fat globules into smaller parts

14 Salivary gland near the ear
5 Swallowing
1 Small substances that are produced when proteins are digested
3 Pigment released by the liver in bile
16 Soft inner tissue within a tooth containing nerves and blood vessels
20 Tiny microscopic projections in the walls of the small intestine
15 Rhythm-like contractions of the tubes of the alimentary tract
10 Hormone produced by the endocrine cells of the pancreas
4 This tube carries bile from the liver and gallbladder into the duodenum
13 Small nipple-like elevations on the tongue
19 Soft tissue hanging from the roof of the mouth
2 An enzyme that digests starch
12 Chewing
8 Simple sugar
9 Substance produced by the stomach and necessary for digestion of foods
7 Solid wastes; stools
11 Pancreatic enzyme necessary to digest fats
17 Ring of muscle at the distal region of the stomach
18 Large fat molecules

Dictation and Comprehension Quiz: Symptoms

A
1. anorexia
2. ascites
3. borborygmus
4. constipation
5. diarrhea
6. dysphagia

7. flatus
8. hematochezia
9. jaundice
10. melena
11. nausea
12. steatorrhea

B

12 Feces containing fat
11 Unpleasant sensation from the stomach with tendency to vomit
7 Gas expelled through the anus
1 Lack of appetite
8 Bright, fresh, red blood from the rectum
4 Difficult, delayed elimination of feces
10 Black, tarry stools; feces containing blood
9 Yellow-orange coloration of the skin; icterus
3 Rumbling or gurgling noises produced by the movement of gas or fluid
6 Difficulty in swallowing
5 Loose, liquid stools
2 Abnormal accumulation of fluid in the peritoneal cavity

Dictation and Comprehension Quiz: Pathological Conditions

A

1. achalasia
2. anal fistula
3. aphthous stomatitis
4. cholecystolithiasis
5. cirrhosis
6. colonic polyposis
7. Crohn disease
8. dental caries
9. diverticulitis
10. peptic ulcer
11. dysentery
12. esophageal varices
13. gastroesophageal reflux disease
14. hepatitis
15. ileus
16. intussusception
17. pancreatitis
18. periodontal disease
19. ulcerative colitis
20. volvulus

B

18 Inflammation and degeneration of gums
20 Twisting of the intestine upon itself

6 Small benign growths protrude from the mucous membrane of the large bowel
16 Telescoping of the intestines
13 Solids and fluids return to the mouth from the stomach
4 Gallbladder calculi
14 Inflammation of the liver; viral etiology
5 Chronic liver disease; etiology is often alcoholism and malnutrition
10 Sore or lesion of the mucous membrane of the first part of the small intestine
2 Abnormal tubelike passageway in the distal end of the alimentary tract
11 Painful inflamed intestines; etiology is often bacterial
12 Swollen, tortuous veins in the distal portion of the tube connecting the throat and stomach
17 Inflammation of a gland behind the stomach; cysts may form
9 Inflammation of small side-pockets in the intestinal wall
19 Chronic inflammation of the large bowel with open sores of mucous membranes
7 Chronic inflammation of the intestinal tract (terminal ileum)
15 Failure of peristalsis
1 Failure of the LES muscle to relax
3 Inflammation of the mouth with open sores
8 Tooth decay

Spelling Quiz

A

1. pancreatitis—inflammation of the pancreas
2. anal fistula—abnormal tube-like opening in the anus
3. dental caries—tooth decay
4. colitis—inflammation of the colon
5. ileus—intestinal obstruction
6. ascites—abnormal collection of fluid in the abdomen
7. melena—dark, tarry blood in the feces
8. polyposis—abnormal condition of polyps (small growths)
9. dysentery—abnormal, painful intestines
10. anorexia—loss of appetite

B

11. mesentery
12. cholecystectomy
13. volvulus
14. Crohn disease
15. biliary
16. jaundice
17. parotid gland
18. achalasia
19. parenteral
20. anastomosis

Pronunciation Quiz

A

1. aphthous stomatitis
2. dysentery
3. choledocholithiasis
4. leukoplakia
5. esophageal varices
6. pyloric sphincter
7. biliary
8. cheilitis
9. diverticula
10. volvulus

B

1. G
2. D
3. J
4. B
5. H
6. F
7. C
8. A
9. I
10. E

C

1. pancreatitis
2. cholecystectomy
3. anorexia
4. ileitis
5. sialolithiasis
6. enteric anastomosis
7. palatoplasty
8. proctologist
9. gluconeogenesis
10. peristalsis

Diagram Quiz

1. Esophagus
2. Stomach
3. Duodenum
4. Liver
5. Gallbladder
6. Pancreas
7. Jejunum
8. Ileum

Chapter Six
MULTIPLE CHOICE QUIZ

Name: _____ _____

In the box write the letter of the choice that is the definition of the term or best answers the question. There is only one correct answer for each question.

1. **Spitting up blood from the respiratory tract and lungs:** .... ☐
   A. Hyperemesis
   B. Hematemesis
   C. Hemorrhage
   D. Hemoptysis
   E. Hemolysis

2. **Suture:** .... ☐
   A. -rrhapy
   B. -rrhagia
   C. -ectasis
   D. -stasis
   E. -rrhaphy

3. **New opening between two parts of the jejunum:** .... ☐
   A. Jejunojejunostomy
   B. Duodenostomy
   C. Duodenojejunostomy
   D. Jejunostomy
   E. Jejunocecal anastomosis

4. **Dilation of a lymph vessel:** .... ☐
   A. Cholecystolithiasis
   B. Lymphangiography
   C. Lymphocytosis
   D. Lymphangiectasis
   E. Choledocholithiasis

5. **Difficult digestion:** .... ☐
   A. Deglutition
   B. Dysphagia
   C. Aphagia
   D. Polyphagia
   E. Dyspepsia

6. **Pyloric stenosis:** .... ☐
   A. Gastric ulcer
   B. Narrowing of the opening between the stomach and intestine
   C. Hiatal hernia
   D. Cardiospasm
   E. Achalasia

7. **Which test would tell the presence of melena?** .... ☐
   A. Barium enema
   B. Upper GI series
   C. Stool culture
   D. Stool guaiac
   E. Abdominal ultrasonography

8. **An ulcer would most likely be detected by which of the following tests?** .... ☐
   A. Cholecystography
   B. Serum hepatitis B surface antigen
   C. Intravenous cholangiogram
   D. Gastroscopy
   E. Abdominal CT scan

9. **Esophageal atresia:** .... ☐
   A. New opening of the esophagus into the stomach
   B. Esophagus is dilated
   C. Esophageal sphincter will not relax
   D. Esophagus does not open to the stomach at birth
   E. Twisted veins around the esophagus

10. **Bursting forth of blood from the spleen:** .... ☐
    A. Spleenorrhagia
    B. Splenorrhagia
    C. Splenomegaly
    D. Spleenomegaly
    E. Spleenectasis

11. **Lipase is:** .... ☐
    A. An enzyme that digests starch
    B. An enzyme that digests protein
    C. An enzyme that digests fat
    D. A breakdown product of fat digestion
    E. A hormone secreted by the pancreas

12. **Palatoplasty:** .... ☐
    A. Surgical repair of the roof of the mouth
    B. Overgrowth of gum tissue
    C. Surgical repair of the tongue
    D. Cleft palate
    E. Prolapse of the palate

13. **Which test is NOT a liver function test?** .... □
   A. Serum bilirubin
   B. ALP (alkaline phosphatase)
   C. Endoscopic retrograde cholangiopancreatography (ERCP)
   D. AST (SGOT)
   E. ALT (SGPT)

14. **Which test would demonstrate choledocholithiasis?** .... □
   A. Transhepatic cholangiography
   B. Barium enema
   C. Gastric intubation
   D. Upper GI series
   E. Gastric endoscopy

15. **Opposite of -ectasis:** .... □
   A. -stenosis
   B. -ptysis
   C. -spasm
   D. -stasis
   E. -lysis

16. **Flow, discharge:** .... □
   A. -ptysis
   B. -emesis
   C. -rrhaphy
   D. -rrhea
   E. -phagia

17. **Anastomosis:** .... □
   A. Ileostomy
   B. Duodenorrhaphy
   C. Cholecystojejunostomy
   D. Colostomy
   E. Gingivectomy

18. **Common bile duct:** .... □
   A. Cholecyst/o
   B. Celi/o
   C. Cholelith/o
   D. Choledoch/o
   E. Cheil/o

19. **Forward protrusion of the eye:** .... □
   A. Oropharynx
   B. Proptosis
   C. Blepharoptosis
   D. Rectocele
   E. Herniorrhaphy

20. **Surgical puncture to remove fluid from the abdomen:** .... □
   A. Cholestasis
   B. Dyspepsia
   C. Hemostasis
   D. Ascites
   E. Paracentesis

21. **Twisting of part of the intestine upon itself:** .... □
   A. Proctosigmoidoscopy
   B. Cecal volvulus
   C. Pyloric stenosis
   D. Biliary atresia
   E. Rectal stenosis

22. **Periodontal procedure:** .... □
   A. Glossotomy
   B. Glycolysis
   C. Gingivectomy
   D. Biliary lithotripsy
   E. Cheilostomatoplasty

23. **Heavy menstrual discharge:** .... □
   A. Menorrhea
   B. Hemorrhage
   C. Dysmenorrhea
   D. Menorrhagia
   E. Hematemesis

24. **Visual examination of the abdomen:** ... □
   A. Laparoscopy
   B. Colonoscopy
   C. Liver scan
   D. Colectomy
   E. Enterorrhaphy

25. **Salivary stones:** .... □
   A. Lithotripsy
   B. Cholecystolithiasis
   C. Sialolithiasis
   D. Renal calculi
   E. Nephroptosis

Chapter Six
EXERCISE QUIZ

Name: _____

A. *Give the meanings for the following suffixes:*

1. -pepsia _____

2. -ptysis _____

3. -emesis _____

4. -ptosis _____

5. -rrhagia _____

6. -phagia _____

7. -plasty _____

8. -rrhaphy _____

9. -ectasis _____

10. -stenosis _____

11. -stasis _____

12. -lysis _____

13. -ptosis _____

14. -rrhea _____

B. *Give meanings for the following terms:*

15. polyphagia _____

16. odynophagia _____

17. proptosis _____

18. esophageal atresia _____

C. *Match the following surgical procedures with their meanings below:*

blepharoplasty   gastroduodenal anastomosis   paracentesis
cecostomy   gingivectomy   sphincterotomy
cholecystectomy   herniorrhaphy

19. surgical repair of the eyelid _____

20. incision of a ring of muscles _____

21. removal of the gallbladder _____

22. suture of a weakened muscular wall _____

23. new surgical connection between the
    stomach and the first part of the small intestine _____

24. new opening of the first part of the colon to the outside of the body _____

25. removal of gum tissue _____

26. surgical puncture of the abdomen for withdrawal of fluid _____

D. *Build medical terms:*

27. difficult swallowing _____   30. discharge of fat (in feces) _____

28. pertaining to the cheek _____   31. pertaining to under the tongue _____

29. enlargement of the liver _____   32. pertaining to the common bile duct _____

E. *Give meanings for the following terms:*

33. aphthous stomatitis _____

34. lipase _____

35. cheilosis _____

36. sialadenectomy _____

37. periodontal membrane _____

38. colectomy _____

F. *Match name of laboratory test or clinical procedure with its description:*

abdominal ultrasonography   liver biopsy   serum bilirubin
barium enema   liver scan   stool culture
CT of the abdomen   nasogastric intubation   stool guaiac (Hemoccult)
endoscopic retrograde   percutaneous transhepatic   upper gastrointestinal series
   cholangiopancreatography   cholangiography

39. tube is inserted through the nose into the stomach _____

40. measurement of bile pigment in the blood _____

41. x-ray examination of the lower gastrointestinal tract _____

42. test to reveal hidden blood in feces _____

43. sound waves are used to image abdominal organs _____

44. feces are placed in a growth medium for bacterial analysis _____

45. percutaneous removal of liver tissue followed by microscopic analysis _____

46. contrast material is injected through an endoscope and x-rays are taken of the
    pancreas and bile ducts _____

47. radioactive material is injected and image recorded of uptake in liver cells _____

48. transverse x-ray pictures of abdominal organs _____

49. x-ray images of the esophagus, stomach, and small intestine
    after administering barium by mouth _____

50. contrast material is injected through the liver and x-rays
    are taken of bile vessels _____

Chapter Six
DICTATION AND COMPREHENSION QUIZ

Name: _____

A. Dictation of Terms

1. _____
2. _____
3. _____
4. _____
5. _____
6. _____
7. _____
8. _____
9. _____
10. _____

11. _____
12. _____
13. _____
14. _____
15. _____
16. _____
17. _____
18. _____
19. _____
20. _____

B. Comprehension of Terms: Match the number of the above term with its meaning below.

_____ Difficult digestion

_____ Vomiting blood

_____ Forward protrusion of the eye

_____ Discharge of pus (gingivitis)

_____ Dilation of a tube leading into the lung

_____ Food tube is not connected to the stomach from birth

_____ Suture of an abdominal protrusion

_____ Surgical repair of the lip and mouth

_____ Removal of the large bowel

_____ Pertaining to the common bile duct

_____ Spitting up blood

_____ Pertaining to the cheek

_____ An anastomosis

_____ Difficult swallowing

_____ Removal of gum tissue

_____ Removal of the gallbladder

_____ Painful menstruation

_____ Narrowing of a ring of muscles

_____ Ulcers and inflammation of the mouth

_____ Pertaining to the tongue and throat

Chapter Six
SPELLING QUIZ

Name: _____

A. *Circle the term that is spelled correctly and write its meaning in the space provided:*

1. herniorrhapy   herniorrhaphy _____
2. hematemesis   hematemisis _____
3. hemmorhage   hemorrhage _____
4. colestasis   cholestasis _____
5. menorrhagia   mennorhagia _____
6. lymphangectasis   lymphangiectasis _____
7. blepharophlasty   blepharoplasty _____
8. choleductal   choledochal _____
9. glossotomy   glosotomy _____
10. stenosis   stanosis _____

B. *Circle the term that is spelled correctly. The meaning of each term is given.*

11. Abnormal condition of the lip...........	cheilosis	chielosis	cielosis
12. Pertaining to the cheek....................	buckel	buckal	buccal
13. Drooping, sagging, prolapse	tossis	tosis	ptosis
14. Record of bile vessels........................	colangiogram	cholangiogram	choleangiogram
15. Not open..	treesia	atresia	atrezia
16. Spitting up blood..............................	hemmoptsyis	hemotisis	hemoptysis
17. Enlargement of the liver	hepatomeagaly	hepatomegaly	hepatomegely
18. Difficult swallowing...........................	dysfagia	disphagia	dysphagia
19. Destruction of blood...........................	hemolysis	hemmolysis	hemolisis
20. Pertaining to the abdomen	cieliac	celiac	sealiac

Chapter Six
PRONUNCIATION QUIZ

Name: _____

A. *Underline the accented syllable in the following terms:*

1. hemoptysis	4. dysmenorrhea	7. glycolysis	10. lipase
2. gingivectomy	5. bronchiectasis	8. cholecystolithiasis	
3. cholestasis	6. herniorrhaphy	9. colonoscopy	

B. *Match the term in Column I with its meaning in Column II:*

Column I   Column II

1. -rrhagia   _____   A. New opening

2. -rrhea   _____   B. Suture

3. -tomy   _____   C. Flow; discharge

4. -phagia   _____   D. Narrowing

5. -ptosis   _____   E. Widening; dilation

6. -spasm   _____   F. Discharge of blood

7. -rrhaphy   _____   G. Prolapse

8. -stenosis   _____   H. Swallowing, eating

9. -stomy   _____   I. Involuntary muscular twitching

10. -ectasis   _____   J. Incision

                              K. Removal

C. *Complete the following terms from their definitions:*

1. dys _____   Difficult digestion.

2. dys _____   Difficult swallowing.

3. hemat _____   Vomiting blood.

4. gloss _____   Incision of the tongue.

5. _____ al   Pertaining to the cheek.

6. _____ orrhea   Discharge of fat.

7. hepato _____   Enlargement of the liver.

8. entero _____   Suture of the small intestine.

9. a _____   No opening.

10. a _____ stomatitis   Inflammation of the mouth with small ulcers.

Chapter Six
REVIEW SHEET QUIZ

Name: _____

A. *Give meanings for the following combining forms:*

1. amyl/o _____
2. an/o _____
3. appendic/o _____
4. bil/i _____
5. bronch/o _____
6. celi/o _____
7. cheil/o _____
8. cholangi/o _____
9. cib/o _____
10. col/o _____

11. dent/i _____
12. duoden/o _____
13. enter/o _____
14. esophag/o _____
15. eti/o _____
16. gloss/o _____
17. glyc/o _____
18. hem/o _____
19. herni/o _____
20. lapar/o _____

B. *Give combining forms for the following meanings:*

1. cheek _____
2. gallbladder _____
3. common bile duct _____
4. stomach _____
5. liver _____

6. ileum _____
7. jejunum _____
8. stone _____
9. pancreas _____
10. throat _____

C. *Give meanings for the following combining forms:*

1. labi/o _____
2. lingu/o _____
3. lip/o _____
4. lymphangi/o _____
5. mandibul/o _____
6. men/o _____

7. odont/o _____
8. odyn/o _____
9. or/o _____
10. peritone/o _____
11. proct/o _____
12. prote/o _____

13. pylor/o _____

14. rect/o _____

15. sialaden/o _____

16. sigmoid/o _____

17. splen/o _____

18. steat/o _____

19. stomat/o _____

20. tonsill/o _____

D. Give meanings for the following suffixes:

1. -ase _____

2. -centesis _____

3. -chezia _____

4. -ectasia _____

5. -ectomy _____

6. -spasm _____

7. -emia _____

8. -genesis _____

9. -graphy _____

10. -iasis _____

11. -lysis _____

12. -megaly _____

13. -orexia _____

14. -pathy _____

15. -pepsia _____

16. -phagia _____

17. -plasty _____

18. -prandial _____

19. -ptosis _____

20. -tresia _____

E. Give suffixes for the following meanings:

1. bursting forth of blood _____

2. suture _____

3. flow, discharge _____

4. process of visual examination _____

5. narrowing, tightening _____

6. new opening _____

7. to stop, control _____

8. incision _____

9. spitting _____

10. vomiting _____

Chapter Six
CROSSWORD PUZZLE

Name: _____

Fill in the crossword puzzle below using the clues listed underneath it.

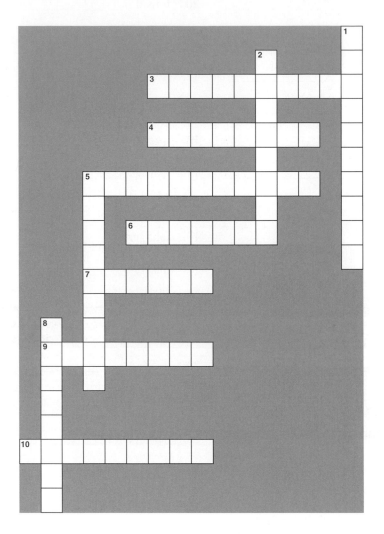

Across Clues

3. -phagia
4. -ectasis means stretching, widening, or _____
5. -lysis means separation or _____
6. -tresia
7. -rrhaphy
9. -ptosis means to sag or _____
10. -rrhea means flow or _____

Down Clues

1. -stenosis means narrowing or
2. -emesis
5. -pepsia
8. -ptysis

Chapter Six

PRACTICAL APPLICATIONS

Name: _____

History and Plan   cc: Leonard Smith, M.D.

Identifying Data:

This 72-year-old female presents with a biopsy-proven adenocarcinoma of the sigmoid colon at 20 cm.

History of Present Illness:

The patient has been noted to have some bright, red bleeding intermittently for approximately 8 months, initially presumable of a hemorrhoidal basis. She recently has had intensification of the rectal bleeding but no weight loss, anorexia, or obstructive pain. No significant diarrhea or constipation. Some low back pain, probably unrelated. Recent colonoscopy by Dr. Scoma revealed a large sessile (attached by a broad base) polyp, which was partially excised at the 20 cm level, showing infiltrating adenocarcinoma at the base. The patient is to enter the hospital at this time, after home antibiotic and mechanical bowel prep, to undergo sigmoid colectomy and possible further resection.

Questions

1. **The patient has had which of the following chronic symptoms:** ....
    A. Loss of appetite
    B. Melena
    C. Hematochezia
    D. Loose stools

2. **The cause of her chronic symptom was:** ....
    A. Glandular tumor of the stomach
    B. Swollen rectal veins
    C. Ulcerative colitis
    D. Malignant tumor of the colon

3. **What procedure did she have recently that diagnosed her condition?** ....
    A. Visual examination of her large intestine
    B. Removal of her sigmoid colon
    C. Low anterior resection of the large intestine
    D. Hemorrhoidectomy

4. **The patient is scheduled for which of the following procedures?** ....
    A. Biopsy of the sigmoid colon
    B. Excision of polyp in her colon
    C. Removal of the sigmoid colon and possible excision of additional colon tissue
    D. Removal of 20 cm of colon, including the sigmoid colon

Chapter Six
ANSWERS TO THE QUIZZES

Multiple Choice Quiz

1. D	4. D	7. D	10. B	13. C	16. D	19. B	22. C	25. C
2. E	5. E	8. D	11. C	14. A	17. C	20. E	23. D	
3. A	6. B	9. D	12. A	15. A	18. D	21. B	24. A	

Exercise Quiz

A

1. digestion
2. spitting
3. vomiting
4. prolapse, sagging
5. bursting forth of blood
6. eating, swallowing
7. surgical repair
8. suture
9. widening, dilation
10. narrowing
11. stop, control
12. separation; destruction
13. prolapse
14. flow, discharge

B

15. excessive eating
16. painful swallowing
17. abnormal protrusion (prolapse) of the eyeball (exophthalmos)
18. the esophagus is not open to the stomach at birth

C

19. blepharoplasty
20. sphincterotomy
21. cholecystectomy
22. herniorrhaphy
23. gastroduodenal anastomosis
24. cecostomy
25. gingivectomy
26. paracentesis

D

27. dysphagia
28. buccal
29. hepatomegaly
30. steatorrhea
31. sublingual or hypoglossal
32. choledochal

E

33. inflammation of the mouth with small ulcers
34. enzyme to digest fat
35. abnormal condition of the lip
36. removal of a salivary gland
37. tissue surrounding a tooth
38. removal of the colon

F

39. nasogastric intubation
40. serum bilirubin
41. barium enema
42. stool guaiac (Hemoccult)
43. abdominal ultrasonography
44. stool culture
45. liver biopsy
46. endoscopic retrograde cholangiopancreatography
47. liver scan
48. CT of the abdomen
49. upper gastrointestinal series
50. percutaneous transhepatic cholangiography

Dictation and Comprehension Quiz

A

1. aphthous stomatitis
2. bronchiectasis
3. buccal
4. cheilostomatoplasty
5. cholecystectomy
6. cholecystojejunostomy
7. choledochal
8. colectomy
9. congenital esophageal atresia
10. dysmenorrhea
11. dyspepsia
12. dysphagia
13. gingivectomy
14. glossopharyngeal
15. hematemesis
16. hemoptysis
17. herniorrhaphy
18. proptosis
19. pyloric stenosis
20. periodontal disease

B

11 Difficult digestion
15 Vomiting blood
18 Forward protrusion of the eye
20 Discharge of pus (gingivitis)
2   Dilation of a tube leading into the lung
9   Food tube is not connected to the stomach from birth
17 Suture of an abdominal protrusion
4   Surgical repair of the lip and mouth
8   Removal of the large bowel
7   Pertaining to the common bile duct
16 Spitting up blood
3   Pertaining to the cheek
6   An anastomosis
12 Difficult swallowing
13 Removal of gum tissue
5   Removal of the gallbladder
10 Painful menstruation
19 Narrowing of a ring of muscles
1   Ulcers and inflammation of the mouth
14 Pertaining to the tongue and throat

Spelling Quiz

A

1. herniorrhaphy—suture (repair) of a hernia
2. hematemesis—vomiting blood
3. hemorrhage—bursting forth of blood
4. cholestasis—stoppage of flow of bile
5. menorrhagia—heavy menstrual flow
6. lymphangiectasis—dilation of lymph vessels
7. blepharoplasty—surgical repair of the eyelids
8. choledochal—pertaining to the common bile duct
9. glossotomy—incision of the tongue
10. stenosis—narrowing, tightening

B

11. cheilosis
12. buccal
13. ptosis
14. cholangiogram
15. atresia
16. hemoptysis
17. hepatomegaly
18. dysphagia
19. hemolysis
20. celiac

Pronunciation Quiz

A

1. hemoptysis
2. gingivectomy
3. cholestasis
4. dysmenorrhea
5. bronchiectasis
6. herniorrhaphy
7. glycolysis
8. cholecystolithiasis
9. colonoscopy
10. lipase

B

1. F
2. C
3. J
4. H
5. G
6. I
7. B
8. D
9. A
10. E

C

1. dyspepsia
2. dysphagia
3. hematemesis
4. glossotomy
5. buccal
6. steatorrhea
7. hepatomegaly
8. enterorrhaphy
9. atresia
10. aphthous stomatitis

Review Sheet Quiz

A

1. starch
2. anus
3. appendix
4. bile
5. bronchial tube
6. belly, abdomen
7. lip
8. bile vessel
9. meal
10. colon
11. tooth
12. duodenum
13. intestine (usually small intestine)
14. esophagus
15. cause
16. tongue
17. sugar
18. blood
19. hernia
20. abdomen

B

1. bucc/o
2. cholecyst/o
3. cholangi/o
4. gastr/o
5. hepat/o
6. ile/o
7. jejun/o
8. lith/o
9. pancreat/o
10. pharyng/o

C

1. lip
2. tongue
3. fat
4. lymph vessel
5. mandible (lower jaw bone)
6. menses, menstruation
7. tooth
8. painful
9. mouth
10. peritoneum
11. anus and rectum
12. protein

13. pylorus
14. rectum
15. salivary gland
16. sigmoid colon
17. spleen
18. fat
19. mouth
20. tonsils

D

1. enzyme
2. surgical puncture to remove fluid
3. defecation
4. dilation, stretching, widening
5. removal, excision, resection
6. sudden, involuntary contraction of muscles
7. blood condition
8. formation
9. process of recording
10. abnormal condition
11. breakdown, destruction
12. enlargement
13. appetite
14. disease condition
15. digestion
16. eating, swallowing
17. surgical repair
18. meal
19. drooping, sagging, prolapse
20. opening

E

1. -rrhage, -rrhagia
2. -rrhaphy
3. -rrhea
4. -scopy
5. -stenosis
6. -stomy
7. -stasis
8. -tomy
9. -ptysis
10. -emesis

Crossword Puzzle

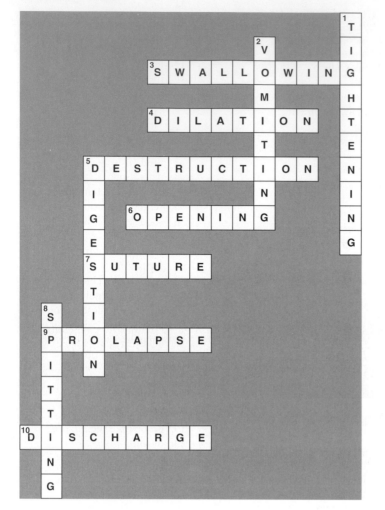

Practical Applications

1. C
2. D
3. A
4. C

chapter 7

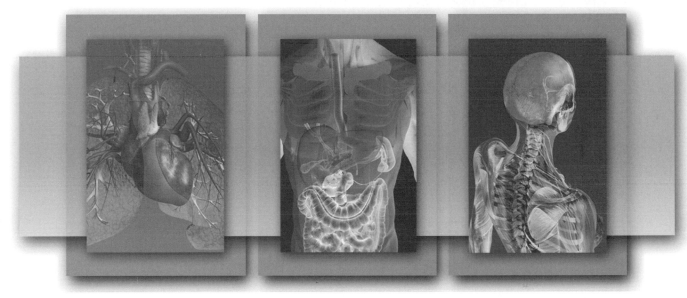

Chapter Seven
MULTIPLE CHOICE QUIZ

Name: _____

In the box write the letter of the choice that is the definition of the term or best answers the question. There is only one correct answer for each question.

1. **Portion of the urinary bladder:** ....
   A. Hilum
   B. Pylorus
   C. Fundus
   D. Medulla
   E. Trigone

2. **Glomerular:** ....
   A. Pertaining to a tube leading from the kidney to the bladder
   B. Pertaining to small balls of capillaries in the kidney
   C. Pertaining to a tube in the bladder
   D. Pertaining to a collecting chamber in the kidney
   E. Pertaining to the urinary bladder

3. **Meatal stenosis:** ....
   A. Enlargement of an opening
   B. Stoppage of blood flow to the kidney
   C. Incision of an opening
   D. Widening of the bladder orifice
   E. Narrowing of the urethral opening to the outside of the body

4. **Electrolyte:** ....
   A. Bilirubin
   B. Creatinine
   C. Albumin
   D. Sodium
   E. Glucose

5. **Nitrogenous waste:** ....
   A. Creatinine
   B. Fatty acid
   C. Lipid
   D. Carbon dioxide
   E. Sugar

6. **Renal pelvis:** ....
   A. nephr/o
   B. cyst/o
   C. ren/o
   D. py/o
   E. pyel/o

7. **A term that means no urine production is:** ....
   A. Diuresis
   B. Anuria
   C. Voiding
   D. Micturition
   E. Nocturia

8. **Surrounding the urinary bladder:** ....
   A. Suprarenal
   B. Infrarenal
   C. Perivisceral
   D. Perivesical
   E. Perinephric

9. **Uremia:** ....
   A. Azotemia
   B. Hematuria
   C. Dysuria
   D. Cystitis
   E. Hemorrhage

10. **X-ray of the urinary tract:** ....
    A. Renal ultrasonography
    B. KUB
    C. BUN
    D. Cystoscopy
    E. Renal dialysis

11. **Oliguria:** ....
    A. Nocturia
    B. Polyuria
    C. Scanty urination
    D. Bacteriuria
    E. Pus in the urine

12. **Diabetes insipidus is characterized by all of the following EXCEPT:** ....
    A. Polydipsia
    B. Glycosuria
    C. Polyuria
    D. Pituitary gland malfunction
    E. Insufficient ADH

13. **Hernia of the tube connecting the kidney and urinary bladder:**.................. ☐
    A. Herniorrhaphy
    B. Urethrocele
    C. Ureterocele
    D. Urethroileostomy
    E. Urethrostomy

14. **Artificial kidney machine:** .... ☐
    A. Renal biopsy
    B. CAPD
    C. Lithotripsy
    D. Hemodialysis
    E. Renal transplantation

15. **Nephrolithotomy:** .... ☐
    A. Hardening of a stone
    B. Removal of the urinary bladder and kidney stones
    C. Removal of the kidney and stones
    D. Bladder calculi
    E. Incision to remove a renal calculus

16. **Protein in the urine:** .... ☐
    A. Ketonuria
    B. Acetonuria
    C. Hyperbilirubinemia
    D. Bilirubinuria
    E. Albuminuria

17. **Renal abscess may lead to:** .... ☐
    A. Diabetes mellitus
    B. Pyuria
    C. Nephroptosis
    D. Ascites
    E. Diabetes insipidus

18. **Alkaline:** .... ☐
    A. Acidic
    B. pH
    C. Basic
    D. Acetone
    E. Water

19. **A group of symptoms marked by edema, proteinuria, and hypoalbuminemia:** .... ☐
    A. Renal ischemia
    B. Essential hypertension
    C. Polycystic kidney
    D. Nephrotic syndrome
    E. Diabetes mellitus

20. **High levels of ketones in the blood can lead to:** .... ☐
    A. High pH of urine
    B. Acidosis
    C. Excessive elimination of fats
    D. Diabetes insipidus
    E. Low specific gravity

21. **Childhood renal carcinoma:** .... ☐
    A. Hypernephroma
    B. Polycystic kidney
    C. Glomerulonephritis
    D. Wilms tumor
    E. Phenylketonuria

22. **Urine is held in the bladder:** .... ☐
    A. Urinary incontinence
    B. Pyuria
    C. Polyuria
    D. Nocturia
    E. Urinary retention

23. **Test that measures the amount of urea in the blood:** .... ☐
    A. CT scan
    B. RP
    C. BUN
    D. VCU
    E. Creatinine clearance test

24. **Nephrosclerosis:** .... ☐
    A. Hardening of blood vessels in the kidney
    B. Loss of protein in the urine
    C. A test of kidney function
    D. Prolapse of the kidney
    E. Excess fluid in the kidney

25. **Lithotripsy:** .... ☐
    A. Renal transplant
    B. Shock waves crush urinary tract stones
    C. Radioscopic study
    D. Panendoscopy
    E. Foley catheterization

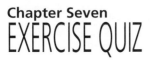

Chapter Seven
EXERCISE QUIZ

Name: _____

A. *Using the following terms, trace the path of urine formation from afferent renal arterioles to the point at which urine leaves the body:*

renal pelvis   renal tubule   urinary meatus   Bowman capsule
glomerulus   ureter   urinary bladder   urethra

1. _____   5. _____

2. _____   6. _____

3. _____   7. _____

4. _____   8. _____

B. *Give the meanings for the following medical terms:*

9. caliceal _____   12. medullary _____

10. urinary meatal stenosis _____   13. cystocele _____

11. creatinine _____   14. vesicoureteral reflux _____

C. *Match the following terms that pertain to urinalysis with their meanings below:*

bilirubinuria   hematuria   pH   pyuria
glycosuria   ketonuria   proteinuria   sediment

15. Sugar in the urine; a symptom of diabetes mellitus _____

16. Color of the urine is smoky red owing to presence of blood _____

17. Urine is turbid (cloudy) owing to presence of WBCs and pus_____

18. Abnormal particles are present in urine—cells, bacteria, casts _____

19. Urine test that reflects the acidity or alkalinity of urine_____

20. Dark pigment accumulates in urine as a result of liver disease _____

21. High levels of acids and acetones accumulate in urine _____

22. Leaky glomeruli can produce this accumulation of albumin in urine_____

D. *Give the meanings for the following terms that relate to urinary symptoms:*

23. azotemia _____   28. urinary retention_____

24. polydipsia _____   29. polyuria _____

25. nocturia_____   30. anuria_____

26. oliguria _____   31. bacteriuria _____

27. dysuria_____   32. enuresis _____

E. Match the following terms with their meanings below:

abscess   edema   secondary hypertension
catheter   essential hypertension   stricture
diabetes insipidus   hypernephroma

33. high blood pressure that is idiopathic _____

34. malignant tumor of the kidney _____

35. high blood pressure caused by kidney disease _____

36. a tube for withdrawing or giving fluid _____

37. collection of pus _____

38. swelling, fluid in tissues _____

39. inadequate secretion of ADH _____

40. a narrowed area in a tube _____

F. Identify the following tests, procedures, or abbreviations:

41. C&S _____

42. BUN _____

43. cysto _____

44. Na^+ _____

45. UTI _____

46. MRI _____

47. hemodialysis _____

48. CAPD _____

49. renal biopsy _____

50. renal angiography _____

Chapter Seven
DICTATION AND COMPREHENSION QUIZ

Name: _____

A. Dictation of Terms

1. _____   11. _____

2. _____   12. _____

3. _____   13. _____

4. _____   14. _____

5. _____   15. _____

6. _____   16. _____

7. _____   17. _____

8. _____   18. _____

9. _____   19. _____

10. _____   20. _____

B. Comprehension of Terms: Match the number of the above term with its meaning below.

_____ X-ray record of the renal pelvis and urinary tract

_____ Blood is held back from the kidney

_____ A tube for withdrawing and inserting fluid

_____ Act of urination

_____ Hormone secreted by the kidney to increase production of red blood cells

_____ Narrowing of the opening of the urinary tract to the outside of the body

_____ Sodium and potassium are examples

_____ High blood pressure due to kidney disease

_____ Swelling or fluid in tissue spaces

_____ Collection of pus

_____ Hardening of arterioles in the kidney

_____ Visual examination of the urinary bladder

_____ Protein in the urine

_____ High levels of nitrogenous waste in the blood

_____ Inability to hold urine in the bladder

_____ A nitrogenous waste excreted in the urine

_____ Renal calculi

_____ Inflammation of the small balls of capillaries in the kidney

_____ Blood in the urine

_____ An anastomosis

Chapter Seven
SPELLING QUIZ

Name: _____

A. *Circle the term that is spelled correctly and write its meaning in the space provided:*

1. nitrogenous   nitrogenius _____

2. urinalysis   urinanalysis _____

3. meatis   meatus _____

4. dysuria   dysurea _____

5. abcess   abscess _____

6. dyalysis   dialysis _____

7. medulla   medula _____

8. pyleogram   pyelogram _____

9. vesicorectal   visicorectal _____

10. creatinine   cretatinine _____

B. *Circle the term that is spelled correctly. The meaning of each term is given.*

11. Swelling; fluid in tissues	ademia	edema	edemia
12. Visual examination of the bladder	sistoscopy	cystascopy	cystoscopy
13. Hardening of vessels in the kidney	nephroscherosis	nephrosclerosis	neferosclerosis
14. Protein in the urine	albuminuria	albuminurea	albumenuria
15. Stone	calkulus	calculus	calculis
16. Excessive thirst	polydipsia	polydypsia	polidipsia
17. Collecting area in the kidney	calics	kalyx	calyx
18. Inability to hold urine in bladder..............	incontenence	incontinence	incontinance
19. Chemical that carries an electrical charge...	electrolite	electricolyte	electrolyte
20. Hormone secreted by the kidney to increase red blood cells	erithropoeitin	erythropoietin	erythropoeitin

Chapter Seven
PRONUNCIATION QUIZ

Name: _____

A. *Underline the accented syllables in the following terms:*

1. cystourethrogram	4. hilum	7. urethroplasty	10. creatinine
2. meatotomy	5. nephrolithotomy	8. ureterocele	
3. edema	6. trigone	9. glycosuria	

B. *Match the term in Column I with its meaning in Column II:*

Column I

1. hematuria	_____
2. diuresis	_____
3. abscess	_____
4. uremia	_____
5. perivesical	_____
6. dysuria	_____
7. cortical	_____
8. medullary	_____
9. renal cell carcinoma	_____
10. enuresis	_____

Column II

A. Painful urination.

B. Bedwetting.

C. Collection of pus.

D. Pertaining to the outer section of an organ.

E. Blood in the urine.

F. Excessive urination.

G. Pertaining to the inner section of an organ.

H. Excessive urea in the bloodstream.

I. Malignant tumor of the kidney.

J. Pertaining to surrounding the urinary bladder.

C. *Complete the following terms from their definitions:*

1.	cali_____	Dilation of a calyx.
2.	_____ uria	Scanty urination.
3.	nephro_____	Disease of the kidney.
4.	bacteri_____	Bacteria in the urine.
5.	poly _____	Excessive thirst.
6.	_____ lithotomy	Incision to remove a stone from the renal pelvis.
7.	_____ uria	Protein in the urine.
8.	_____ scopy	Visual examination of the urinary bladder.
9.	litho_____	Crushing of a stone.
10.	_____ uria	Sugar in the urine.

Chapter Seven

DIAGRAM QUIZ

Name: _____

Label the diagram below using the terms listed below:

Hilum
Kidney
Prostate gland
Trigone
Ureter
Urethra
Urinary bladder
Urinary meatus

Large vein to heart —————————— Aorta

Adrenal gland —————

Renal vein ————

Hilum ————

Renal artery ————

———— Cortex

———— Medulla

————1 _____

————1_____

————2_____

2_____

Trigone —————— 3 _____

Prostate gland —————

4 _____

Urinary
meatus

Chapter Seven
VOCABULARY QUIZ

Name: _____

A. *Match the following terms with their meanings below:*

arteriole	nephron	ureter
calyx	renal tubule	urethra
hilum	trigone	
meatus	renal vein	

1. Tube carrying urine from each kidney to the urinary bladder _____

2. Cuplike collecting region of the renal pelvis _____

3. Opening or canal _____

4. Microscopic tube in the kidney where urine is formed after filtration _____

5. Small artery _____

6. Functional unit of the kidney; about one million in each kidney _____

7. Tube leading from the urinary bladder to the outside of the body _____

8. Triangular area in the urinary bladder _____

9. Blood vessel that carries blood away from the kidney _____

10. Depression or hollow in that part of an organ (such as the kidney)
    where blood vessels and nerves enter and leave _____

B. Match the following terms with their meanings below:

catheter   erythropoietin   urinary bladder
cortex   glomerulus   voiding
creatinine   medulla
electrolyte   renal pelvis

1. Central collecting region in the kidney _____

2. Chemical element carrying an electrical charge when dissolved in
    water; sodium and potassium are examples _____

3. Tube for injecting or removing fluids _____

4. Hormone secreted by the kidney to stimulate production of
    red blood cells by bone marrow _____

5. Inner region of an organ _____

6. Outer region of an organ _____

7. Tiny ball of capillaries in outer area of kidney _____

8. Urination; micturition _____

9. Nitrogenous waste product of muscle metabolism excreted in urine _____

10. Hollow, muscular sac that holds and stores urine _____

Chapter Seven
REVIEW SHEET QUIZ

Name: _____

A. *Give meanings for the following combining forms:*

1. cyst/o _____
2. pyel/o _____
3. vesic/o _____
4. lith/o _____
5. ren/o _____

6. albumin/o _____
7. hydr/o _____
8. py/o _____
9. azot/o _____
10. olig/o _____

B. *Give meanings for the following suffixes:*

1. -ptosis _____
2. -tripsy _____
3. -stenosis _____
4. -lysis _____
5. -ectasis _____

6. -megaly _____
7. -poietin _____
8. -uria _____
9. -sclerosis _____
10. -ole _____

C. *Give meanings for the following prefixes:*

1. anti- _____
2. peri- _____
3. retro- _____
4. poly- _____

5. dys- _____
6. dia- _____
7. en- _____
8. a-, an- _____

D. *Give suffixes or combining forms for the following:*

1. new opening _____
2. incision _____
3. disease condition _____
4. removal _____
5. record _____

6. surgical repair _____
7. blood condition _____
8. thirst _____
9. night _____
10. blood vessel _____

Chapter Seven
CROSSWORD PUZZLE

Name: _____

Fill in the crossword puzzle below using the clues listed underneath it.

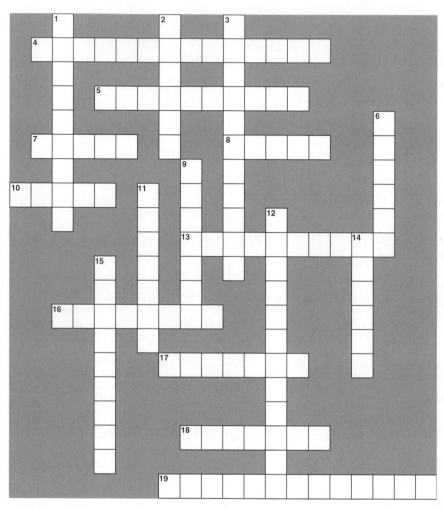

Across Clues

4. Secreted by the kidney to stimulate red blood cell production.
5. Process whereby some substances pass through the walls of a glomerulus.
7. Notch on the medial surface of the kidney where blood vessels and nerves enter and leave.
8. Substance made in the kidney that increases blood pressure.
10. Cuplike collecting region of the renal pelvis.
13. Tiny ball of capillaries in cortex of the kidney.
16. Tube for injecting fluids into or removing fluids from the urinary tract.
17. Tube leading from the bladder to the outside of the body.
18. Expelling urine.
19. Malignant tumor of the kidney: another term for renal cell carcinoma.

Down Clues

1. A small artery.
2. The outer region of the kidney is the renal _____.
3. Another term for urination.
6. Opening or canal.
9. Triangular area in the bladder where the ureters enter and urethra exits.
11. Sac that holds urine.
12. The process of accepting again or taking back; substances needed by the body pass from the renal tubules back into the blood stream.
14. One of two tubes leading from the kidney to the urinary bladder.
15. Urine cannot leave the bladder; urinary _____.

Chapter Seven

PRACTICAL APPLICATIONS

Name: _____

A. Patient History

The patient is a 75-year-old male with a history of hematuria, dysuria, chronic UTIs, and benign prostatic hyperplasia. At present, he has nocturia three times per night with slow urinary stream. A CT scan showed a distended urinary bladder with large postvoid residual. In the kidney there was evidence of cortical renal cysts. Cystoscopy was performed, revealing a diverticulum of the bladder with a neoplastic lesion within the diverticulum. A biopsy was performed, and it showed ulceration and chronic cystitis, but no malignancy.

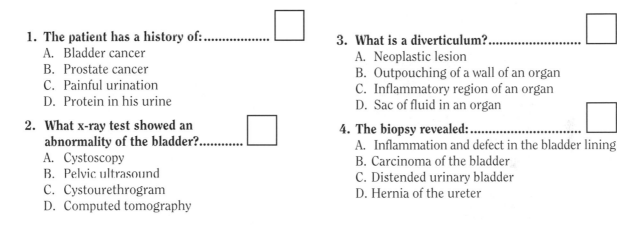

1. The patient has a history of: ....
  A. Bladder cancer
  B. Prostate cancer
  C. Painful urination
  D. Protein in his urine

2. What x-ray test showed an abnormality of the bladder? ....
  A. Cystoscopy
  B. Pelvic ultrasound
  C. Cystourethrogram
  D. Computed tomography

3. What is a diverticulum? ....
  A. Neoplastic lesion
  B. Outpouching of a wall of an organ
  C. Inflammatory region of an organ
  D. Sac of fluid in an organ

4. The biopsy revealed: ....
  A. Inflammation and defect in the bladder lining
  B. Carcinoma of the bladder
  C. Distended urinary bladder
  D. Hernia of the ureter

B. UTI in Children

The symptoms of urinary tract infections in older children are similar to those seen in adults. Cystitis is manifest by suprapubic discomfort, burning, urgency, and polyuria. An upper UTI such as pyelonephritis is manifest by chills, fever, and flank (the sides of the body, between the ribs and the ilium) pain. Any child previously toilet-trained who suddenly develops enuresis or day-time wetting should be evaluated. However, many UTIs in children are asymptomatic, and the younger the child, the more obscure the signs and symptoms. An infant with a UTI may present only with fever, lethargy, irritability, and/or failure to thrive.

1. A symptom of cystitis is: ....
  A. Inability to urinate
  B. Frequent urination
  C. Chest pain
  D. Jaundice and itching

2. An example of an upper UTI is: ....
  A. Nephrosclerosis
  B. Flank pain
  C. Lithotripsy
  D. Anuria
  E. Inflammation of the renal pelvis

3. Enuresis is: ....
  A. Bedwetting
  B. Nocturia
  C. Anuria
  D. Strong sensation of having to urinate throughout the day

4. What type of symptoms do young children with UTIs frequently manifest? ....
  A. Blood in the urine
  B. Protein in the urine
  C. Often no symptoms
  D. Elevated BUN

Chapter Seven
ANSWERS TO THE QUIZZES

Multiple Choice Quiz

1. E	4. D	7. B	10. B	13. C	16. E	19. D	22. E	25. B
2. B	5. A	8. D	11. C	14. D	17. B	20. B	23. C	
3. E	6. E	9. A	12. B	15. E	18. C	21. D	24. A	

Exercise Quiz

A

1. glomerulus
2. Bowman capsule
3. renal tubule
4. renal pelvis
5. ureter
6. urinary bladder
7. urethra
8. urinary meatus

B

9. pertaining to a calyx
10. narrowing of the opening of the urethra to the outside of the body
11. nitrogenous waste
12. pertaining to the inner section of an organ
13. hernia of the urinary bladder
14. backflow of urine from the urinary bladder to the ureter

C

15. glycosuria
16. hematuria
17. pyuria
18. sediment
19. pH
20. bilirubinuria
21. ketonuria
22. proteinuria

D

23. nitrogenous wastes in the blood
24. excessive thirst
25. frequent urination at night
26. scanty urination
27. painful urination
28. urine is held in the bladder
29. excessive urination
30. no urination
31. bacteria in the urine
32. bedwetting

E

33. essential hypertension
34. hypernephroma
35. secondary hypertension
36. catheter
37. abscess
38. edema
39. diabetes insipidus
40. stricture

F

41. culture and sensitivity
42. blood, urea, nitrogen
43. cystoscopy
44. sodium
45. urinary tract infection
46. magnetic resonance imaging
47. separation of wastes from the blood by removing the blood and filtering it through a machine
48. continuous ambulatory peritoneal dialysis
49. removal of tissue from the kidney and microscopic examination
50. x-ray record of the blood vessels in the kidney

Dictation and Comprehension Quiz

A

1. abscess
2. albuminuria
3. catheter
4. creatinine
5. cystoscopy
6. edema
7. electrolyte
8. erythropoietin
9. glomerulonephritis
10. hematuria
11. meatal stenosis
12. micturition
13. nephrolithiasis
14. nephrosclerosis
15. pyelography
16. renal ischemia
17. secondary hypertension
18. uremia
19. ureteroneocystostomy
20. urinary incontinence

B

15 X-ray record of the renal pelvis and urinary tract
16 Blood is held back from the kidney
3 A tube for withdrawing and inserting fluid
12 Act of urination
8 Hormone secreted by the kidney to increase production of red blood cells
11 Narrowing of the opening of the urinary tract to the outside of the body
7 Sodium and potassium are examples
17 High blood pressure due to kidney disease
6 Swelling or fluid in tissue spaces
1 Collection of pus
14 Hardening of arterioles in the kidney
5 Visual examination of the urinary bladder
2 Protein in the urine
18 High levels of nitrogenous waste in the blood
20 Inability to hold urine in the bladder
4 A nitrogenous waste excreted in the urine
13 Renal calculi
9 Inflammation of the small balls of capillaries in the kidney
10 Blood in the urine
19 An anastomosis

Spelling Quiz

A

1. nitrogenous—pertaining to nitrogen
2. urinalysis—examination of urine
3. meatus—opening or canal

4. dysuria—painful urination
5. abscess—collection of pus
6. dialysis—separation of wastes from blood
7. medulla—inner section of an organ
8. pyelogram—x-ray record of the renal pelvis
9. vesicorectal—pertaining to the bladder and rectum
10. creatinine—nitrogen-containing waste

B

11. edema
12. cystoscopy
13. nephrosclerosis
14. albuminuria
15. calculus
16. polydipsia
17. calyx
18. incontinence
19. electrolyte
20. erythropoietin

Pronunciation Quiz

A

1. cystou<u>re</u>throgram
2. mea<u>to</u>tomy
3. e<u>de</u>ma
4. <u>hi</u>lum
5. nephroli<u>tho</u>tomy
6. <u>tri</u>gone
7. urethro<u>plas</u>ty
8. u<u>re</u>terocele
9. glyco<u>su</u>ria
10. cre<u>at</u>inine

B

1. E
2. F
3. C
4. H
5. J
6. A
7. D
8. G
9. I
10. B

C

1. caliectasis
2. oliguria
3. nephropathy
4. bacteriuria
5. polydipsia
6. pyelolithotomy
7. albuminuria; proteinuria
8. cystoscopy
9. lithotripsy
10. glycosuria

Diagram Quiz

1. Kidney
2. Hilum
3. Ureter
4. Urinary bladder
5. Trigone
6. Prostate gland
7. Urethra
8. Urinary meatus

Vocabulary Quiz

A

1. ureter
2. calyx
3. meatus
4. renal tubule
5. arteriole
6. nephron
7. urethra
8. trigone
9. renal vein
10. hilum

B

1. renal pelvis
2. electrolyte
3. catheter
4. erythropoietin
5. medulla
6. cortex
7. glomerulus
8. voiding
9. creatinine
10. urinary bladder

Review Sheet Quiz

A

1. urinary bladder
2. renal pelvis
3. urinary bladder
4. stone
5. kidney
6. protein; albumin
7. water
8. pus
9. nitrogen
10. scanty

B

1. prolapse
2. crushing
3. narrowing
4. destruction; separation
5. widening; stretching; dilation
6. enlargement
7. formation
8. urine condition
9. hardening
10. small; little

C

1. against
2. surrounding
3. back; behind
4. much; many
5. bad; painful; difficult; abnormal
6. complete; through
7. in; within
8. no; not; without

D

1. -stomy
2. -tomy
3. -pathy
4. -ectomy
5. -gram
6. -plasty
7. -emia
8. dips/o or -dipsia
9. noct/o
10. angi/o

Crossword Puzzle

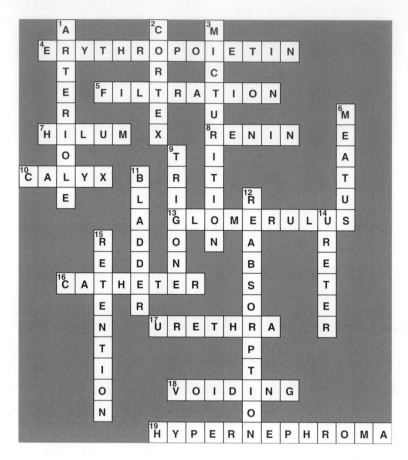

Practical Applications

A	B
1. C	1. B
2. D	2. D
3. B	3. A
4. A	4. C

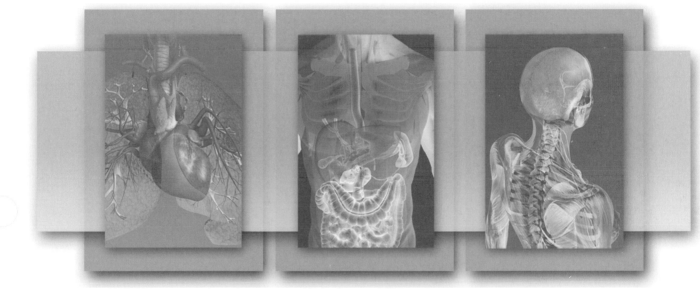

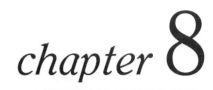
chapter 8

Chapter Eight
MULTIPLE CHOICE QUIZ

Name: _____

In the box write the letter of the choice that is the definition of the term or best answers the question. There is only one correct answer for each question.

1. **The ovum is the:** .... ☐
   A. Female gonad
   B. Female gamete
   C. Embryo
   D. Fertilized egg cell
   E. Fetus

2. **Pregnancy:** .... ☐
   A. Lactation
   B. Micturition
   C. Parturition
   D. Ovulation
   E. Gestation

3. **Area between the uterus and the rectum:** .... ☐
   A. Cul-de-sac
   B. Peritoneum
   C. Labia minora
   D. Clitoris
   E. Perineum

4. **Part of the vulva:** .... ☐
   A. Uterine cervix
   B. Fallopian tubes
   C. Labia majora
   D. Ovaries
   E. All of the above

5. **Adnexa uteri:** .... ☐
   A. Fetus
   B. Chorion
   C. Ovaries and fallopian tubes
   D. Bartholin glands
   E. Vagina

6. **Ovarian sac:** .... ☐
   A. Endometrium
   B. Corpus luteum
   C. Amnion
   D. Chorion
   E. Placenta

7. **Respiratory disorder in the neonate:** .... ☐
   A. Pyloric stenosis
   B. Hydrocephalus
   C. Hemolytic disease
   D. Melena
   E. Hyaline membrane disease

8. **Incision of the perineum during childbirth:** .... ☐
   A. Episiotomy
   B. Colpotomy
   C. Perineoplasty
   D. Laparotomy
   E. Perineorrhaphy

9. **Fingerlike ends of the fallopian tubes are called:** .... ☐
   A. Ligaments
   B. Papillae
   C. Cysts
   D. Fimbriae
   E. Labia

10. **The study and treatment of newborns is called:** .... ☐
    A. Obstetrics
    B. Neonatology
    C. Gynecology
    D. Pediatrics
    E. Endocrinology

11. **Sac containing the egg cell is the:** .... ☐
    A. Corpus luteum
    B. Ovarian cyst
    C. Amnion
    D. Ovarian follicle
    E. Placenta

12. **Hormone produced by an endocrine gland located below the brain:** .... ☐
    A. HCG
    B. Progesterone
    C. Estrogen
    D. Follicle-stimulating hormone
    E. Erythropoietin

13. **Removal of the fallopian tubes and ovaries:** .... ☐
    A. Total hysterectomy
    B. Conization
    C. Bilateral salpingo-oophorectomy
    D. Salpingectomy
    E. Partial hysterectomy

14. **Premature separation of placenta:** .... ☐
    A. Ectopic pregnancy
    B. Placenta previa
    C. Abruptio placentae
    D. Pseudocyesis
    E. Dyspareunia

15. **A woman who has had 3 miscarriages and 2 live births:** .... ☐
    A. Grav. 3, para 2
    B. Grav. 5, para 2
    C. Grav. 2, para 3
    D. Grav. 5, para 3
    E. Grav. 2, para 5

16. **Endometrial carcinoma may be detected by:** .... ☐
    A. Cryocauterization
    B. Ovarian biopsy
    C. D & C
    D. Cesarean section
    E. Cystoscopy

17. **Removal of internal and reproductive organs in the region of the hip:** .... ☐
    A. Tubal ligation
    B. Abortion and D & C
    C. Pelvic exenteration
    D. Gonadal resection
    E. Bilateral oophorectomy

18. **Physician's effort to turn the fetus during delivery:** .... ☐
    A. Involution
    B. Retroflexion
    C. Retroversion
    D. Cephalic version
    E. Presentation

19. **Gynecomastia:** .... ☐
    A. Occurs after lactation in females
    B. Abnormal development of breast tissue in males
    C. Abnormal discharge of milk from the breast
    D. Abnormal condition of pregnancy
    E. Lumpectomy and chemotherapy are treatments

20. **Excessive flow of blood from the uterus between menstrual periods:** ..... ☐
    A. Menorrhea
    B. Menorrhagia
    C. Metrorrhagia
    D. Oligomenorrhea
    E. Dysmenorrhea

21. **Painful labor and delivery:** .... ☐
    A. Dystocia
    B. Eutocia
    C. Dyspareunia
    D. Eclampsia
    E. Endometriosis

22. **Menarche:** .... ☐
    A. Last menstrual period
    B. First menstrual period
    C. Absence of menstruation
    D. Painful menstruation
    E. Frequent menstrual periods

23. **Ms. Sally Ping has vaginal discharge, pain in the LLQ and RLQ, dysmenorrhea, and a gonococcal infection. A likely diagnosis is:** .... ☐
    A. Ovarian carcinoma
    B. Choriocarcinoma
    C. Fibroids
    D. Pelvic inflammatory disease
    E. Vulvovaginitis

24. **Pieces of the inner lining of the uterus are ectopic:** .... ☐
    A. Endocervicitis
    B. Ectopic pregnancy
    C. Endometriosis
    D. Cystadenocarcinoma
    E. Fibrocystic disease of the breast

25. **Leukorrhea is associated with which of the following conditions?** .... ☐
    A. Ovarian cysts
    B. Menorrhagia
    C. Eclampsia
    D. Cervicitis
    E. Oophoritis

Chapter Eight
EXERCISE QUIZ

Name: _____

A. *Match the following terms for structures or tissues with their meanings below:*

amnion   endometrium   ovaries
areola   fallopian tubes   perineum
cervix   fimbriae   placenta
clitoris   mammary papilla   vulva

1. inner lining of the uterus _____

2. nipple of the breast _____

3. innermost membrane around the developing embryo _____

4. dark-pigmented area around the breast nipple _____

5. external genitalia of female (perineum, labia, hymen, clitoris) _____

6. area between the anus and vagina in females _____

7. female gonads; producing ova and hormones _____

8. blood-vessel-filled organ that develops during pregnancy _____

9. uterine tubes _____

10. organ of sensitive erectile tissue in females _____

11. finger-like ends of the fallopian tube _____

12. lower, neck-like portion of the uterus _____

B. *Give short answers for the following:*

13. galact/o and lact/o mean _____

14. colp/o and vagin/o mean _____

15. oophor/o and ovari/o mean _____

16. mamm/o and mast/o mean _____

17. metr/o and hyster/o mean _____

18. -cyesis and gravid/o mean _____

19. episi/o and vulv/o mean _____

20. ovul/o and o/o mean _____

C. *Give meanings for the following gynecologic symptoms:*

21. leukorrhea _____

22. metrorrhagia _____

23. amenorrhea _____

24. dyspareunia _____

25. pyosalpinx _____

D. *Give the medical term for the following:*

26. pertaining to newborn _____

27. surgical puncture to remove fluid from the cul-de-sac _____

28. inflammation of the cervix _____

29. first menstrual period _____

30. rapid labor _____

E. *Match the following terms with their meanings below:*

abruptio placentae   cystadenocarcinoma   placenta previa
carcinoma in situ   endometrial carcinoma   preeclampsia
choriocarcinoma   endometriosis

31. malignant tumor of the pregnant uterus _____

32. condition during pregnancy; hypertension, proteinuria, edema, and uremia _____

33. malignant condition of the inner lining of the uterus _____

34. malignant tumor; often of the ovary _____

35. displaced placenta; implantation in lower region of uterus _____

36. uterine tissue is located outside the uterus _____

37. cancerous tumor cells are localized in a small area _____

38. premature separation of a normally implanted placenta _____

F. *Give the name of the test or procedure described below:*

39. visual examination of the vagina _____

40. withdrawal of fluid by suction with a needle _____

41. cold temperatures are used to destroy tissue _____

42. cone-shaped section of the cervix is removed _____

43. HCG is measured in urine or blood _____

44. widening the cervical opening and scraping the uterine lining _____

G. *Give medical terms for the following.*

45. benign muscle tumors in the uterus _____

46. accessory organs of the uterus _____

47. ovarian hormone that sustains pregnancy _____

48. removal of an ovary _____

49. inflammation of the vulva and vagina _____

50. reproductive organs _____

Chapter Eight
DICTATION AND COMPREHENSION QUIZ: VOCABULARY AND TERMINOLOGY

Name: _____

A. Dictation of Terms

1. _____   11. _____

2. _____   12. _____

3. _____   13. _____

4. _____   14. _____

5. _____   15. _____

6. _____   16. _____

7. _____   17. _____

8. _____   18. _____

9. _____   19. _____

10. _____   20. _____

B. Comprehension of Terms: Match the number of the above term with its meaning below.

_____ Woman who has had more than one live birth

_____ Painful sexual intercourse

_____ Outermost membrane surrounding the developing embryo

_____ Tissue lying between the anus and vagina

_____ First menstrual period

_____ Hormone secreted by the ovary during pregnancy

_____ Ovary and fallopian tubes; accessory uterine structures

_____ An opening

_____ Pigmented area around the nipple of the breast

_____ Inner lining of the uterus

_____ Visual examination of the vagina

_____ Practice of caring for women during pregnancy and delivering neonates

_____ Pertaining to no egg production

_____ Surgical puncture to remove fluid from the membrane surrounding the embryo

_____ Excessive discharge of blood from the uterus (not during menstruation)

_____ Pus in the fallopian tubes

_____ Difficult labor and delivery

_____ Removal of a breast

_____ Reproductive organs

_____ Female organ of sexual stimulation; located anterior to the urethra

Chapter Eight
DICTATION AND COMPREHENSION QUIZ: PATHOLOGICAL CONDITIONS, CLINICAL TESTS, AND PROCEDURES

Name: _____

A. Dictation of Terms

1. _____   11. _____

2. _____   12. _____

3. _____   13. _____

4. _____   14. _____

5. _____   15. _____

6. _____   16. _____

7. _____   17. _____

8. _____   18. _____

9. _____   19. _____

10. _____   20. _____

B. Comprehension of Terms: Match the number of the above term with its meaning below.

_____ Tissue from the inner lining of the uterus is found in abnormal locations

_____ Benign tumor in the uterus; fibroid

_____ Visual examination of the abdomen; minimally invasive surgery

_____ Examination by touch

_____ Fluid is removed by a needle

_____ Type of bacteria found as a common cause of pelvic inflammatory disease

_____ Malignant tumor that is localized and not invasive

_____ X-ray examination of the breast

_____ Narrowing of the opening of the stomach to the intestine in a newborn

_____ Condition during pregnancy marked by hypertension, proteinuria, and edema

_____ Tying off the fallopian tubes; sterilization procedure

_____ Accumulation of fluid in the spaces of the brain; can occur in a neonate

_____ Widening the cervix and scraping the lining of the uterus

_____ Burning tissue with chemicals or an electrically heated instrument

_____ Abnormal growth of tissue in the neck of the uterus

_____ Removal of an infant through an incision of the abdominal wall

_____ Abnormal location of the organ connecting the infant and the mother

_____ X-ray examination of the uterus and the fallopian tubes

_____ Embryo is not implanted in the uterus

_____ Removal of a cone-shaped section of the cervix for biopsy

Chapter Eight

SPELLING QUIZ

Name: _____

A. *Circle the term that is spelled correctly and write its meaning in the space provided:*

1. amenorhea   amenorrhea _____

2. oophoritis   oopheritis _____

3. menarchy   menarche _____

4. cervisitis   cervicitis _____

5. areola   aereola _____

6. pappila   papilla _____

7. progesterone   progestrone _____

8. esterogen   estrogen _____

9. dialation   dilation _____

10. carsinoma en situ   carcinoma in situ _____

B. *Circle the term that is spelled correctly. The meaning of each term is given.*

11. Secreted by the anterior pituitary   leutinizing   luteinizing   lutienizing
     gland to promote ovulation............................. hormone   hormone   hormone

12. Muscular tube leading from the uterus .... vagina   vajina   vigina

13. Reproductive organs .... genatalia   genitalia   genitailia

14. Scraping of tissue .... currettage   curettage   cruettage

15. Development of female breasts
     in a male .... gynecomastia   gynomastia   gynacomastia

16. Instrument to visually examine the
     tube leading from the uterus .... culposcope   colposcope   coldoscope

17. Act of giving birth .... parrition   parturition   partrition

18. Organ in the pregnant female's
     uterus that provides nourishment
     for the fetus... placenta   plasenta   plecenta

19. Monthly discharge of blood from
     the lining of the uterus .... menstration   menstruation   menstrashun

20. Innermost membrane around
     the developing embryo .... amnion   amneoin   amneon

Chapter Eight
PRONUNCIATION QUIZ

Name: _____

A. *Underline the accented syllables in the following terms:*

1. fimbriae   4. menarche   7. perineum   10. endometriosis
2. genitalia   5. gravida   8. areola
3. primipara   6. pelvimetry   9. gamete

B. *Match the term in Column I with its meaning in Column II:*

Column I   Column II

1. gestation   _____   A. Fluid accumulation in the head

2. cauterization _____   B. Period of pregnancy

3. dilation   _____   C. Scraping to remove tissue

4. coitus   _____   D. Sexual intercourse

5. parturition   _____   E. Burning to remove tissue

6. hydrocephalus _____   F. Hormone necessary during pregnancy

7. progesterone   _____   G. Widening

8. curettage   _____   H. To examine by touch

9. palpation   _____   I. Act of giving birth

10. menstruation   _____   J. Monthly discharge of blood and cells from the uterus

C. *Complete the following terms from their definitions:*

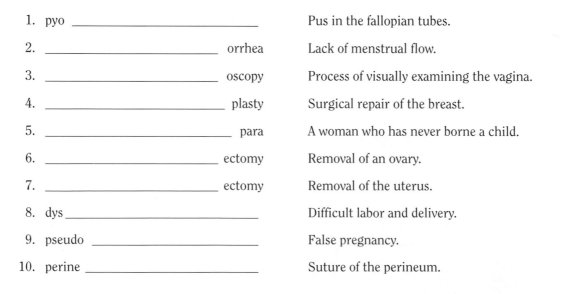

1. pyo _____   Pus in the fallopian tubes.

2. _____ orrhea   Lack of menstrual flow.

3. _____ oscopy   Process of visually examining the vagina.

4. _____ plasty   Surgical repair of the breast.

5. _____ para   A woman who has never borne a child.

6. _____ ectomy   Removal of an ovary.

7. _____ ectomy   Removal of the uterus.

8. dys_____   Difficult labor and delivery.

9. pseudo _____   False pregnancy.

10. perine _____   Suture of the perineum.

Chapter Eight
DIAGRAM QUIZ

Name: _____

Label the diagram below using the terms listed below:

Bartholin glands
Clitoris
Cul-de-sac
Fallopian tube
Ovary
Perineum
Uterus
Vagina

Abdominal cavity

Pelvic cavity

1

2

3

4

Urinary bladder

Cervix

Pubic bone

Urethra

5

6

7

8

Rectum

Anus

ANTERIOR

POSTERIOR

Chapter Eight
VOCABULARY QUIZ

Name: _____

A. *Match the following terms with their meanings below:*

adnexa uteri   cervix   corpus luteum
amnion   chorion   cul-de-sac
areola   clitoris
Bartholin glands   coitus

1. Lower, neck-like portion of the uterus _____

2. Sexual intercourse _____

3. Innermost membranous sac surrounding the developing fetus _____

4. Fallopian tubes, ovaries, and supporting ligaments _____

5. Region in the lower abdomen midway between the rectum and uterus _____

6. Empty ovarian follicle that secretes progesterone _____

7. Dark-pigmented area surrounding the breast nipple _____

8. Sensitive erectile tissue anterior to the opening of the female urethra _____

9. Outermost layer of two membranes surrounding the embryo _____

10. Small mucus-secreting glands at the vaginal orifice _____

B. *Match the following terms with their meanings below:*

embryo   fertilization   gamete
endometrium   fetus   genitalia
estrogen   fimbriae
fallopian tube   follicle-stimulating hormone

1. Finger or fringe like projections at the end of the fallopian tubes_____

2. Hormone produced by the ovaries; promotes female secondary sex characteristics _____

3. Union of the sperm cell and ovum _____

4. Stage in prenatal development from 2 to 6 weeks _____

5. Reproductive organs _____

6. Stage in prenatal development from 6 to 39–40 weeks _____

7. Hormone secreted by the pituitary gland to stimulate maturation of the ovum _____

8. Inner, mucous membrane lining of the uterus _____

9. Male or female sexual reproductive cell; ovum and sperm _____

10. One of a pair of ducts through which the ovum travels to the uterus _____

C. Match the following terms with their meanings below:

gestation   labia   menarche
gonad   lactiferous ducts   menopause
gynecology   luteinizing hormone
hCG   mammary papilla

1. Tubes carrying milk within the breast _____

2. Hormone produced by the placenta to sustain pregnancy _____

3. Breast nipple _____

4. Study of female reproductive organs and breast _____

5. Lips of the vagina _____

6. Female or male reproductive organ _____

7. Gradual ending of menstruation _____

8. Pituitary gland secretion; promotes ovulation _____

9. Beginning of the first menstrual period _____

10. Pregnancy _____

D. Match the following terms with their meanings below:

menstruation   orifice   parturition
myometrium   ovarian follicle   perineum
neonatology   ovulation
obstetrics   ovum

1. Study of the care of newborns _____

2. Egg cell _____

3. Area between the anus and the vagina _____

4. Branch of medicine concerned with pregnancy and childbirth _____

5. Release of an egg cell from the ovary _____

6. Muscle layer of the uterus _____

7. An opening _____

8. Monthly shedding of the uterine lining _____

9. Act of giving birth _____

10. Sac enclosing each egg cell within the ovary _____

E. Match the following terms with their meanings below:

ovary	progesterone	vulva
pituitary gland	puberty	zygote
placenta	uterine serosa	
pregnancy	vagina	

1. Stage in prenatal development from fertilization and weeks implantation to 2 _____

2. Outermost layer of the uterus _____

3. Hormone produced by the corpus luteum and placenta of pregnant women _____

4. Period of life when the ability to reproduce begins _____

5. Vascular organ that develops in the uterine wall as communication between maternal and fetal bloodstreams _____

6. One of a pair of female gonads; produces egg cells and hormones _____

7. Muscular, mucosal tube extending from the uterus to the exterior of the body _____

8. Endocrine gland at the base of the brain; secretes FSH and LH _____

9. Condition in a female of sustaining a developing embryo/fetus in her uterus. _____

10. External female genitalia that includes labia, hymen, clitoris, and vaginal orifice _____

Chapter Eight
REVIEW SHEET QUIZ

Name: _____

A. *Give meanings for the following combining forms:*

1. metr/o _____
2. olig/o _____
3. myom/o _____
4. galact/o _____
5. mast/o _____

6. colp/o _____
7. episi/o _____
8. oophor/o _____
9. hyster/o _____
10. perine/o _____

B. *Give meanings for the following suffixes:*

1. -stenosis _____
2. -pareunia _____
3. -plasty _____
4. -ectasis _____
5. -cele _____

6. -rrhaphy _____
7. -stomy _____
8. -gravida _____
9. -rrhagia _____
10. -parous _____

C. *Give meanings for the following prefixes:*

1. intra- _____
2. retro- _____
3. peri- _____
4. uni- _____
5. multi- _____

6. dys- _____
7. nulli- _____
8. pre- _____
9. pseudo- _____
10. endo- _____

Chapter Eight
CROSSWORD PUZZLE

Name: _____

Fill in the crossword puzzle below using the clues listed underneath it.

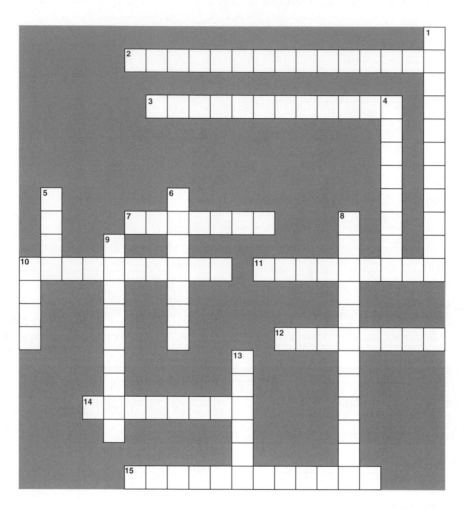

Across Clues

2. Malignant tumor of the pregnant uterus.
3. A condition during pregnancy marked by high blood pressure, proteinuria, and edema.
7. Female gonads.
10. The muscle layer lining the uterus.
11. Pseudocyesis means false _____.
12. Benign tumors in the uterus.
14. Finger-like ends of the fallopian tubes.
15. Hormone secreted by the ovaries to sustain pregnancy.

Down Clues

1. Process of taking x-rays of the breast.
4. Premature termination of pregnancy before embryo or fetus is able to exist on its own.
5. Multi- means _____.
6. A small, nipple-shaped projection or elevation; the mammary _____.
8. The monthly shedding of the uterine lining.
9. Reproductive organs.
10. Galact/o means _____.
13. Womb.

Chapter Eight
PRACTICAL APPLICATIONS

Name: _____

Operative Report

Preoperative Diagnosis:	Menorrhagia, Leiomyomata.
Anesthetic:	General
Material Forwarded to Laboratory for Examination:	A. Endocervical curettings B. Endometrial curettings

Operation Performed: Dilation and Curettage of the Uterus

With the patient in the dorsal lithotomy position (legs are flexed on the thighs, thighs flexed on the abdomen and abducted) and sterilely prepped and draped, manual examination of the uterus revealed it to be 6–8 week size, retroflexed; no adnexal masses noted. The anterior lip of the cervix was then grasped with a tenaculum (hooklike surgical instrument for grasping and holding parts). The cervix was dilated up to a #20 Hank dilator. The uterus was sounded (widened) up to 4 inches. A sharp curettage of the endocervix showed only a scant amount of tissue. With a sharp curettage, the uterus was curetted in a clockwise fashion with an irregularity noted in the posterior floor. A large amount of hyperplastic endometrial tissue was removed. The patient tolerated the procedure well.

Operative diagnosis:

1. The preoperative diagnosis indicated: .... ☐
   A. Excessive bleeding between menstrual periods
   B. Possibility of malignancy in the uterine lining
   C. Fibroids and excessive bleeding during menstruation
   D. Pelvic inflammatory disease

2. The operation described is: .... ☐
   A. Scraping and burning the lining of the uterus
   B. Surgical removal of a malignant tumor
   C. Freezing and aspirating tissue from the cervix and uterus
   D. Widening the cervix and scraping the lining of the uterus

3. What materials were sent to the laboratory for analysis? .... ☐
   A. Tissue samples from vaginal and perineal region
   B. Cervical and uterine tissue samples
   C. Ovarian and abdominal tissue
   D. Uterine and ovarian tissue

Leiomyomata uteri:

4. What were characteristics of the uterus upon examination by hand? ..... ☐
   A. Bent forward and prepregnancy size
   B. Bent backward and early pregnancy size
   C. Narrowed and bent forward
   D. Filled with hyperplastic tissue

5. An adnexal mass would be located in the: .... ☐
   A. Uterus
   B. Vagina
   C. Cervix
   D. Ovaries and/or fallopian tubes

6. The diagnosis following the operative procedure indicated: .... ☐
   A. Endometriosis
   B. Endocervicitis and endometritis
   C. Benign growths in the uterus
   D. Malignant fibroid tumors

FYI: When your Pap smear is positive

The Pap smear is a test for cervical cancer, but the causes of an abnormal Pap smear are more likely to be a yeast infection or STD with human papillomavirus (HPV). The following are five categories of Pap smear abnormalities:

1. **ASCUS** (atypical squamous cells of unknown significance) means that the Pap smear wasn't completely normal, but did not meet diagnostic criteria for a lesion. A gynecologist may recommend repeating the Pap smear in 3 to 6 months, test for HPV, or perform colposcopy in high-risk women.
2. **LSIL** (low-grade squamous intraepithelial lesion) is a precancerous lesion caused by HPV. Physicians perform colposcopy for exact diagnosis (often mild dysplasia or cervical intraepithelial neoplasia [CIN-1]) and most of these lesions disappear on their own within 2 years.
3. **HSIL** (high-grade squamous intraepithelial lesion) is a serious precancerous lesion caused by HPV. Colposcopy is recommended, and abnormal tissue (moderate dysplasia or CIN-11) is destroyed. Conization for biopsy will rule out cervical cancer.
4. **AGCUS** (atypical glandular cells of undetermined significance) indicates precancerous or cancerous condition of the cervix or uterus. Colposcopy and conization are performed for biopsy and treatment to remove abnormal tissue.
5. **Adenocarcinoma** is cancerous glandular tissue of the cervix or uterus. Treatment is removal of the cervix and uterus and additional therapy with radiation.

Chapter Eight
ANSWERS TO THE QUIZZES

Multiple Choice Quiz

1. B	4. C	7. E	10. B	13. C	16. C	19. B	22. B	25. D
2. E	5. C	8. A	11. D	14. C	17. C	20. C	23. D	
3. A	6. B	9. D	12. D	15. B	18. D	21. A	24. C	

Exercise Quiz

A

1. endometrium
2. mammary papilla
3. amnion
4. areola
5. vulva
6. perineum
7. ovaries
8. placenta
9. fallopian tubes
10. clitoris
11. fimbriae
12. cervix

B

13. milk
14. vagina
15. ovary
16. breast
17. uterus
18. pregnancy
19. vulva
20. egg cell

C

21. yellowish-white discharge from the vagina
22. excessive discharge of blood from the uterus between menstrual periods
23. no menstrual period
24. painful sexual intercourse
25. pus in a fallopian tube

D

26. neonatal
27. culdocentesis
28. cervicitis
29. menarche
30. oxytocia

E

31. choriocarcinoma
32. preeclampsia
33. endometrial carcinoma
34. cystadenocarcinoma

35. placenta previa
36. endometriosis
37. carcinoma in situ
38. abruptio placentae

F

39. colposcopy
40. aspiration
41. cryocauterization
42. conization
43. pregnancy test
44. dilation and curettage

G

45. fibroids
46. adnexa uteri
47. progesterone
48. oophorectomy
49. vulvovaginitis
50. genitalia

Dictation and Comprehension Quiz: Vocabulary and Terminology

A

1. adnexa
2. anovulatory
3. areola
4. chorion
5. clitoris
6. colposcopy
7. culdocentesis
8. dyspareunia
9. dystocia
10. endometrium
11. genitalia
12. mastectomy
13. menarche
14. metrorrhagia
15. multipara
16. obstetrics
17. orifice
18. perineum
19. progesterone
20. pyosalpinx

B

15 Woman who has had more than one live birth
8 Painful sexual intercourse
4 Outermost membrane surrounding the developing embryo
18 Tissue lying between the anus and vagina
13 First menstrual period
19 Hormone secreted by the ovary during pregnancy
1 Ovary and fallopian tubes; accessory uterine structures
17 An opening
3 Pigmented area around the nipple of the breast
10 Inner lining of the uterus
6 Visual examination of the vagina
16 Practice of caring for women during pregnancy and delivering neonates
2 Pertaining to no egg production
7 Surgical puncture to remove fluid from the membrane surrounding the embryo
14 Excessive discharge of blood from the uterus (not during menstruation)
20 Pus in the fallopian tubes
9 Difficult labor and delivery
12 Removal of a breast
11 Reproductive organs
5 Female organ of sexual stimulation; located anterior to the urethra

Dictation and Comprehension Quiz: Pathological Conditions, Clinical Tests, and Procedures

A

1. aspiration
2. carcinoma in situ
3. cauterization

4. cervical dysplasia
5. cesarean section
6. Chlamydia
7. conization
8. dilation and curettage
9. ectopic pregnancy
10. endometriosis
11. hydrocephalus
12. hysterosalpingography
13. laparoscopy
14. leiomyoma
15. mammography
16. palpation
17. placenta previa
18. preeclampsia
19. pyloric stenosis
20. tubal ligation

B

10 Tissue from the inner lining of the uterus is found in abnormal locations
14 Benign tumor in the uterus; fibroid
13 Visual examination of the abdomen; minimally invasive surgery
16 Examination by touch
1   Fluid is removed by a needle
6   Type of bacteria found as a common cause of pelvic inflammatory disease
2   Malignant tumor that is localized and not invasive
15 X-ray examination of the breast
19 Narrowing of the opening of the stomach to the intestine in a newborn
18 Condition during pregnancy marked by hypertension, proteinuria, and edema
20 Tying off the fallopian tubes; sterilization procedure
11 Accumulation of fluid in the spaces of the brain; can occur in a neonate
8   Widening the cervix and scraping the lining of the uterus
3   Burning tissue with chemicals or an electrically heated instrument
4   Abnormal growth of tissue in the neck of the uterus
5   Removal of an infant through an incision of the abdominal wall
17 Abnormal location of the organ connecting the infant and the mother
12 X-ray examination of the uterus and the fallopian tubes

9 Embryo is not implanted in the uterus
7 Removal of a cone-shaped section of the cervix for biopsy

Spelling Quiz

A

1. amenorrhea—no menstrual flow
2. oophoritis—inflammation of an ovary
3. menarche—first menstrual period
4. cervicitis—inflammation of the cervix
5. areola—pigmented area around breast nipple
6. papilla—nipple
7. progesterone—ovarian hormone; for pregnancy
8. estrogen—ovarian hormone; for secondary sex characteristics
9. dilation—widening
10. carcinoma in situ—localized malignancy

B

11. luteinizing hormone
12. vagina
13. genitalia
14. curettage
15. gynecomastia
16. colposcope
17. parturition
18. placenta
19. menstruation
20. amnion

Pronunciation Quiz

A

1. fimbriae
2. genitalia
3. primipara
4. menarche
5. gravida
6. pelvimetry
7. perineum
8. areola
9. gamete
10. endometriosis

B

1. B
2. E
3. G
4. D
5. I
6. A

7. F
8. C
9. H
10. J

C

1. pyosalpinx
2. amenorrhea
3. colposcopy
4. mammoplasty
5. nullipara
6. oophorectomy
7. hysterectomy
8. dystocia
9. pseudocyesis
10. perineorrhaphy

Diagram Quiz

1. Ovary
2. Fallopian tube
3. Uterus
4. Cul-de-sac
5. Vagina
6. Bartholin glands
7. Clitoris
8. Perineum

Vocabulary Quiz

A

1. cervix
2. coitus
3. amnion
4. adnexa uteri
5. cul-de-sac
6. corpus luteum
7. areola
8. clitoris
9. chorion
10. Bartholin glands

B

1. fimbriae
2. estrogen
3. fertilization
4. embryo
5. genitalia
6. fetus
7. follicle-stimulating hormone
8. endometrium
9. gamete
10. fallopian tube

C

1. lactiferous ducts
2. hCG (human chorionic gonadotropin)
3. mammary papilla
4. gynecology
5. labia

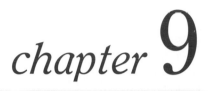

chapter 9

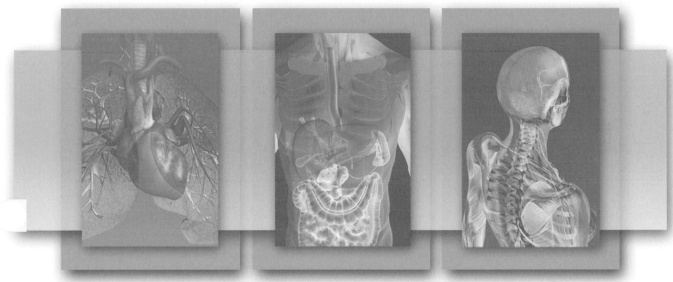

Chapter Nine

MULTIPLE CHOICE QUIZ

Name: _____

In the box write the letter of the choice that is the definition of the term or best answers the question. There is only one correct answer for each question.

1. **The male gonad:** .... ☐
   A. Sperm cell
   B. Scrotum
   C. Testis
   D. Penis
   E. Epididymis

2. **A gland below the bladder and surrounding the urethra:** .... ☐
   A. Vas deferens
   B. Bulbourethral
   C. Bartholin
   D. Seminal vesicle
   E. Prostate

3. **Tissue that produces sperm cells:** .... ☐
   A. Seminiferous tubules
   B. Endometrium
   C. Urethra
   D. Ureters
   E. Interstitial

4. **Hair-like tail region of the sperm is called:** .... ☐
   A. Cilia
   B. Sperm head
   C. Flagellum
   D. Fimbriae
   E. Calyx

5. **Tube that leads from the epididymis to the urethra:** .... ☐
   A. Ureter
   B. Seminiferous tubule
   C. Cowper duct
   D. Vas deferens
   E. Bulbourethral duct

6. **Foreskin:** .... ☐
   A. Perineum
   B. Phimosis
   C. Prepuce
   D. Glans penis
   E. Scrotum

7. **Male castration would result from which of the following operations?** ...... ☐
   A. Bilateral orchiectomy
   B. TURP
   C. Vasectomy
   D. Bilateral oophorectomy
   E. Unilateral orchidectomy

8. **Inflammation of the glans penis:** .... ☐
   A. Orchitis
   B. Hydrocele
   C. Varicocele
   D. Balanitis
   E. Epididymitis

9. **A chancre is the primary lesion in which of the following conditions?** ...... ☐
   A. Pelvic inflammatory disease
   B. Genital herpes
   C. Non-gonococcal urethritis
   D. Gonorrhea
   E. Syphilis

10. **An androgen:** .... ☐
    A. Luteinizing hormone
    B. hCG
    C. Testosterone
    D. Estrogen
    E. Progesterone

11. **Testosterone is produced by:** .... ☐
    A. Interstitial cells of the testes
    B. Prostate gland
    C. Cowper glands
    D. Seminiferous tubules
    E. Seminal vesicles

12. **Undescended testicles:** .... ☐
    A. Anorchism
    B. Phimosis
    C. Epispadias
    D. Cryptorchism
    E. Orchiotomy

13. **Benign prostatic hyperplasia is characterized by:**.................... ☐
    A. Adenocarcinoma of the prostate
    B. Overgrowth of glandular tissue
    C. Hydrocele
    D. Urinary incontinence
    E. Varicocele

14. **Testicular carcinoma:** .... ☐
    A. BPH
    B. Seminoma
    C. Hypernephroma
    D. PID
    E. Chlamydia

15. **Sterilization procedure:** .... ☐
    A. Vasectomy
    B. Circumcision
    C. Orchiotomy
    D. TURP
    E. Left orchiectomy

16. **The sac containing the male gonad:** .... ☐
    A. Perineum
    B. Peritoneum
    C. Epididymis
    D. Scrotum
    E. Seminal vesicle

17. **Congenital condition of the male urethra:**.................... ☐
    A. Varicocele
    B. Phimosis
    C. Circumcision
    D. Hypospadias
    E. Hydrocele

18. **Parenchymal tissue in the testes:** .... ☐
    A. Seminiferous tubules
    B. Bulbourethral fluid
    C. Vas deferens
    D. Connective tissue
    E. Interstitial tissue

19. **Congenital absence of a testicle:**.......... ☐
    A. Azoospermia
    B. Cryptorchism
    C. Aspermia
    D. Oligospermia
    E. Anorchism

20. **A spermolytic substance:** .... ☐
    A. Produces sperm cells
    B. Destroys sperm cells
    C. Is used for benign prostatic hyperplasia
    D. Increases potency
    E. Is produced by the testes

21. **Orchiopexy:**.................... ☐
    A. Removal of a testicle
    B. Incision and removal of a piece of the vas deferens
    C. Fixation of an undescended testicle
    D. Removal of the prepuce
    E. Prolapse of a testicle

22. **Swollen, twisted veins near the testes:** .... ☐
    A. Varicocele
    B. Hydrocele
    C. Hypospadias
    D. Herpes genitalis
    E. Testicular torsion

23. **Non-gonococcal urethritis is most often caused by:**.................... ☐
    A. Prostatitis
    B. Syphilis
    C. Herpes genitalis
    D. Chlamydial infection
    E. Castration

24. **Treating tissue with cold temperatures is called:**.......................... ☐
    A. Aspiration
    B. Purulent
    C. Ejaculation
    D. Curettage
    E. Cryogenic surgery

25. **Which of the following is not an STD:** .... ☐
    A. HSV
    B. Gonorrhea
    C. BPH
    D. Syphilis
    E. Chlamydia

Chapter Nine
EXERCISE QUIZ

Name: _____

A   *Build medical terms:*

1. inflammation of the testes _____

2. resection of the prostate gland _____

3. condition of scanty sperm _____

4. process of forming (producing) sperm cells _____

5. fixation of an undescended testicle _____

B. *Give meanings for the following medical terms:*

6. parenchyma _____

7. androgen _____

8. testicular teratoma _____

9. stroma _____

10. azoospermia _____

C. *Give medical terms for the descriptions below:*

11. pair of sacs; secrete fluid into ejaculatory duct _____

12. coiled tube above each testis; carries and stores sperm _____

13. male gonad; produces hormone and sperm cells _____

14. foreskin _____

D. *Match the term in Column I with its meaning in Column II:*

Column I		Column II
15. castration	_____	A. To tie off or bind.
16. purulent	_____	B. Removal of a piece of vas deferens.
17. ligation	_____	C. Orchiectomy.
18. circumcision	_____	D. Removal of the prepuce.
19. ejaculation	_____	E. Destruction of tissue by freezing.
20. cryosurgery	_____	F. Pus-filled.
21. vasectomy	_____	G. Test of fertility (reproductive ability).
22. semen analysis	_____	H. Ejection of sperm and fluid from the urethra.

E. Give medical terms for the following abnormal conditions:

23. STD; etiology is berry-shaped bacteria _____

24. opening of the urethra on the undersurface of the penis _____

25. enlarged, swollen veins near the testes _____

26. undescended testicles _____

27. STD; primary stage marked by a chancre _____

28. malignant tumor of the prostate gland _____

F. Give meanings for the following abbreviations:

29. TURP _____

30. PSA _____

31. BPH _____

G. Give the meaning of the following:

32. -sclerosis _____   37. oophor/o _____

33. -cele _____   38. colp/o _____

34. -rrhagia _____   39. balan/o _____

35. -phagia _____   40. salping/o _____

36. -genesis _____   41. -ptosis _____

H. Match the surgical procedures in Column I with the reasons they would be performed in Column II.

Column I

42. bilateral orchiectomy _____

43. TURP _____

44. vasectomy _____

45. orchiopexy _____

46. hydrocelectomy _____

47. circumcision _____

48. radical prostatectomy _____

49. vasovasostomy _____

50. varicocelectomy _____

Column II

A. Carcinoma of the prostate gland.

B. Cryptorchism.

C. Sterilization (hormones remain).

D. Benign prostatic hyperplasia.

E. Reversal of sterilization.

F. Removal of swollen, twisted veins near the testes.

G. Abnormal fluid collection in scrotum.

H. Seminoma.

I. Phimosis.

Chapter Nine

DICTATION AND COMPREHENSION QUIZ

Name: _____

A. *Dictation of Terms*

1. _____   11. _____
2. _____   12. _____
3. _____   13. _____
4. _____   14. _____
5. _____   15. _____
6. _____   16. _____
7. _____   17. _____
8. _____   18. _____
9. _____   19. _____
10. _____   20. _____

B. *Comprehension of Terms: Match the number of the above term with its meaning below.*

_____ Inflammation of the tube that carries sperm from the testicle to the vas deferens

_____ Hard ulcer that is a sign of a sexually transmitted disease

_____ Pus-filled

_____ A hormone that produces male secondary sex characteristics

_____ Inflammation of a testicle

_____ Fluid that contains sperm cells and secretions and is produced during ejaculation

_____ Hernia of fluid in the testicle

_____ Malignant tumor of the testes

_____ Foreskin

_____ Essential cells of the testes; seminiferous tubules

_____ Excision of the testicles or ovaries

_____ Increase in growth of cells of a gland below the urinary bladder in males

_____ Glands that secrete a fluid into the vas deferens

_____ Enlarged, dilated veins near the testicle

_____ Undescended testicle

_____ Condition of scanty sperm cell production

_____ Congenital opening of the male urethra on the undersurface of the penis

_____ Chronic STD caused by a type of bacteria (spirochete)

_____ Inflammation of the genital tract mucosa caused by infection with berry-shaped bacteria

_____ Infection of the skin and mucous membranes with HSV; small fluid-filled blisters occur

Chapter Nine
SPELLING QUIZ

Name: _____

A. *Circle the term that is spelled correctly and write its meaning in the space provided.*

1. Chyamydia   Chlamydia _____

2. impotance   impotence _____

3. chanker   chancre _____

4. seminoma   semenoma _____

5. scrotum   scrotim _____

6. parynchomal   parenchymal _____

7. purulent   puerluent _____

8. adenocarcinoma   adenocarsinoma _____

9. prostrate gland   prostate gland _____

10. prepus   prepuce _____

B. *Circle the term that is spelled correctly. The meaning of each term is given.*

11. absence of a testicle	anorhism	anorchism	anorkism
12. glands that secrete semen	bulbourethral	bulboureteral	bolboureteral
13. tubules that produce sperm	seminiferous	semeniferious	seminefarous
14. sexually transmitted infection	syphilis	syphillis	syfalus
15. carcinoma of the testes	embrional	embryonal	enbryomal
16. sperm cells and fluid	semin	seman	semen
17. scanty sperm production	olagospermia	oliospermia	oligospermia
18. pus-filled	purulent	poorulent	pureulent
19. male sex hormone	testostarone	testosterone	testosterome
20. male gonad	testus	testas	testis

Chapter Nine
PRONUNCIATION QUIZ

Name: _____

A. *Underline the accented syllable in the following terms:*

1. parenchymal   4. interstitial   7. seminoma   10. impotence
2. prepuce   5. flagellum   8. prostatectomy
3. varicocele   6. androgen   9. testosterone

B. *Match the term in Column I with its meaning in Column II:*

Column I   Column II

1. cryptorchism _____   A. Sac that holds the testes.

2. testosterone _____   B. Hormone produced by the testes.

3. spermolytic _____   C. Removal of the testes.

4. circumcision _____   D. Undescended testicle.

5. vasectomy _____   E. Sterilization; removal of part of the vas deferens.

6. scrotum _____   F. Congenital opening of the urethra on the underside of the penis.

7. gonorrhea _____   G. Pus-filled.

8. hypospadias _____   H. Venereal disease marked by urethral discharge.

9. orchiectomy _____   I. Removal of the foreskin around the glans penis.

10. purulent _____   J. Pertaining to destruction of sperm cells.

C. *Complete the following terms from their definitions:*

1. _____opexy   Fixation of a testicle in place.

2. oligo _____   Condition of scanty sperm production.

3. _____itis   Inflammation of the glans penis.

4. prostatic _____   Excessive development; enlargement of the prostate gland.

5. hydro_____   Hernia of fluid in the scrotal sac.

6. _____ itis   Inflammation of the epididymis.

7. vaso _____   New connection between two parts of the vas deferens.

8. spermato _____   Formation of sperm cells.

9. gono _____   Sexually transmitted infection.

10. _____ osis   Narrowing of the foreskin over the glans penis.

Chapter Nine
DIAGRAM QUIZ

Name: _____

Label the diagram below using the terms listed below:

Cowper (bulbourethral) gland
Ejaculatory duct
Epididymis
Glans penis
Penis
Perineum
Prepuce (foreskin)

Prostate gland
Scrotum
Seminal vesicle
Seminiferous tubules
Testis
Urethra
Vas deferens

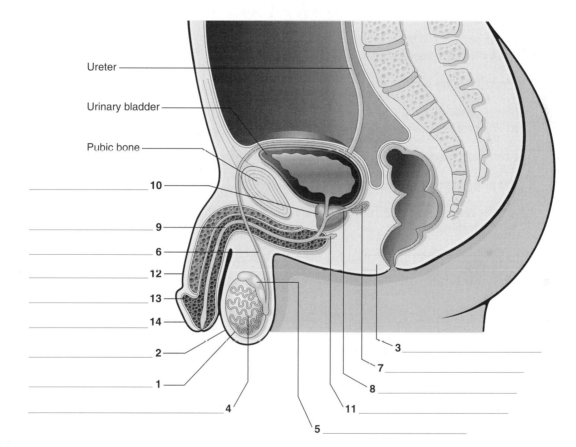

Ureter

Urinary bladder

Pubic bone

10

9

6

12

13

14

2

1

4

3 _____

7 _____

8 _____

11 _____

5 _____

Chapter Nine
VOCABULARY QUIZ

Name: _____

A. Match the following terms with their meanings below:

bulbourethral gland   fraternal twins   parenchyma
ejaculatory duct   identical twins   perineum
epididymis   impotence
flagellum   interstitial cells

1. Inability of an adult male to achieve an erection _____

2. External region between the anus and the scrotum _____

3. One of a pair of long, tightly coiled tubes lying on top of each testis _____

4. Two infants born of the same pregnancy from two separate ova _____
   fertilized by two different sperm

5. Tube through which semen enters the male urethra _____

6. Two infants resulting from division of one fertilized egg into two _____
   distinct embryos

7. Tissue composed of essential and functional cells of an organ _____

8. Hair-like projection on a sperm cell that makes it motile _____

9. Cells that lie between the seminiferous tubules and produce the _____
   hormone testosterone

10. One of a pair of exocrine glands near the male urethra _____

B. *Match the following terms with their meanings below:*

prepuce   seminal vesicle   testis
prostate gland   seminiferous tubules   vas deferens
scrotum   spermatozoon
semen   sterilization

1. Sperm cells and fluid _____

2. Narrow tube that carries sperm from the epididymis into the body and
    toward the urethra _____

3. Foreskin of the penis _____

4. External sac that contains the testes _____

5. Procedure that removes an individual's ability to produce or release
    reproductive cells _____

6. Male gonad _____

7. Exocrine gland in men at the base of the urinary bladder _____

8. Either of a paired sac-like male exocrine glands that secrete
    seminal fluid _____

9. A sperm cell _____

10. Narrow, coiled tubules that produce sperm cells _____

Chapter Nine
REVIEW SHEET QUIZ

Name: _____

A. *Give meanings for the following combining forms:*

1. balan/o _____

2. orchi/o _____

3. vas/o _____

4. zo/o _____

5. andr/o _____

6. crypt/o _____

7. cry/o _____

8. hydr/o _____

9. epididym/o _____

10. terat/o _____

B. *Give meanings for the following suffixes:*

1. -plasia _____

2. -lysis _____

3. -cele _____

4. -pexy _____

5. -stomy _____

6. -tomy _____

7. -trophy _____

8. -genesis _____

9. -ectomy _____

10. -rrhea _____

Chapter Nine
CROSSWORD PUZZLE

Name: _____

Fill in the crossword puzzle below using the clues listed underneath it.

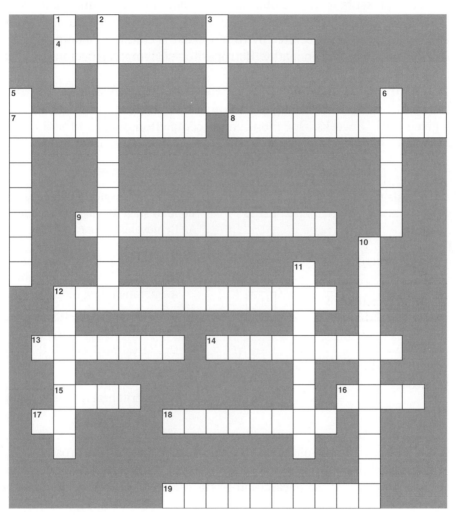

Across Clues

4. Sperm cell.
7. Sac of clear fluid in the testes.
8. Enlarged, swollen veins near the testicle.
9. Undescended testicle.
12. Procedure rendering an individual incapable of reproduction.
13. Foreskin.
14. Hair-like projection on a sperm cell that makes it motile.
15. Transurethral resection of the prostate (abbrev.).
16. Andr/o.
17. Genitourinary (abbrev.).
18. Chronic sexually transmitted infectious disease caused by spirochete bacterium.
19. Orchiectomy.

Down Clues

1. Herpes simplex virus (abbrev.).
2. Hormone secreted by the interstitial tissue of the testes.
3. Cry/o.
5. Narrowing of the opening of the foreskin over the glans penis.
6. Vas/o.
10. Ejection of sperm and fluid from the male urethra.
11. Skin covering the tip of the penis.
12. External sac that contains the testes.

Chapter Nine
PRACTICAL APPLICATIONS

Name: _____

A. Case Report

A 22-year-old male presents with a scrotal mass that does not transilluminate. An orchiectomy reveals embryonal carcinoma with teratoma. Chest x-rays and lung tomograms are normal. Serum AFP (alpha-fetoprotein, a protein secreted by tumor cells) is elevated. Abdominal CT scan reveals minimal retroperitoneal lymphadenopathy. Retroperitoneal lymphadenectomy indicates 4 of 42 nodes positive for embryonal carcinoma.

Six months after the node dissection, the patient remains asymptomatic but his chest x-ray reveals pulmonary metastases. AFP is slightly elevated. Chemotherapy, (cisplatin, vinblastine, and bleomycin) is given over 12 weeks. One month after completion of chemotherapy, a thoracotomy is done and residual lung lesions are removed. He remains free of disease 32 months after the start of chemotherapy.

1. What is the diagnosis for this patient? .... ☐
  A. Prostate cancer
  B. Testicular cancer
  C. Benign prostatic hyperplasia
  D. Lung cancer

2. What was the primary method of treatment? .... ☐
  A. Chemotherapy
  B. Radiation therapy
  C. Surgical removal of the prostate gland
  D. Surgical removal of a testis

3. What other surgical procedure was done to stage the patient's condition? .... ☐
  A. Removal of tumor from the lung
  B. Chest x-ray
  C. Removal of pelvic lymph nodes
  D. Removal of lymph nodes behind the membrane lining the abdominal cavity

4. What treatment was initially given for spread of the tumor to the lungs? .... ☐
  A. Drug treatment with AFP
  B. Thoracotomy
  C. Chemotherapy
  D. Retroperitoneal lymphadenectomy

B. Chart Note

History: The patient is a 55-year-old male with adenocarcinoma of the prostate. He had a TURP 1 year ago for presumed prostatic hyperplasia, but tissue fragments examined by a pathologist revealed a poorly differentiated adenocarcinoma. He received local irradiation to the prostate; however, PSA levels increased to 10 (normal is less than 4). A bone scan showed bony metastases. Bilateral orchiectomy was advised, but refused. Alternative hormonal treatment with Lupron and flutamide to decrease testosterone production will be offered.

1. What is the patient's diagnosis? .... ☐
  A. Prostate cancer
  B. Bone cancer
  C. Testicular cancer
  D. BPH

2. What procedure revealed the diagnosis? .... ☐
  A. Irradiation
  B. Removal of the testicles
  C. Bone scan
  D. Transurethral resection of the prostate

3. Poorly differentiated means: .... ☐
  A. Cells are mature
  B. Cells are very immature
  C. Cells have metastasized
  D. Cells are not malignant

4. What type of drug treatment was offered to the patient? .... ☐
  A. Standard chemotherapy with cytotoxic agents
  B. Androgens
  C. Antiandrogen drugs
  D. PSA treatment

Chapter Nine
ANSWERS TO THE QUIZZES

Multiple Choice Quiz

1. C	4. C	7. A	10. C	13. B	16. D	19. E	22. A	25. C
2. E	5. D	8. D	11. A	14. B	17. D	20. B	23. D	
3. A	6. C	9. E	12. D	15. A	18. A	21. C	24. E	

Exercise Quiz

A
1. orchitis
2. prostatectomy
3. oligospermia
4. spermatogenesis
5. orchiopexy

B
6. essential cells of an organ
7. male hormone
8. tumor of the testes (malignant)
9. connective tissue in an organ
10. condition of no sperm cells in semen

C
11. seminal vesicles
12. epididymis
13. testis
14. prepuce

D
15. C
16. F
17. A
18. D
19. H
20. E
21. B
22. G

E
23. gonorrhea
24. hypospadias
25. varicocele
26. cryptorchism
27. syphilis
28. prostatic adenocarcinoma

F
29. transurethral resection of the prostate
30. prostate specific antigen
31. benign prostatic hyperplasia

G
32. hardening
33. hernia
34. bursting forth of blood
35. eating, swallowing
36. formation
37. ovary
38. vagina
39. glans penis
40. fallopian tube
41. falling, sagging, prolapse

H
42. H
43. D
44. C
45. B
46. G
47. I
48. A
49. E
50. F

Dictation and Comprehension Quiz

A
1. androgen
2. castration
3. chancre
4. cryptorchism
5. epididymitis
6. gonorrhea
7. herpes genitalis
8. hydrocele
9. hypospadias
10. oligospermia
11. orchitis
12. parenchymal tissue
13. prepuce
14. prostatic hyperplasia
15. purulent
16. semen
17. seminal vesicles
18. seminoma
19. syphilis
20. varicocele

B
5   Inflammation of the tube that carries sperm from the testicle to the vas deferens

3   Hard ulcer that is a sign of a sexually transmitted disease

15   Pus-filled

1   A hormone that produces male secondary sex characteristics

11   Inflammation of a testicle

16   Fluid that contains sperm cells and secretions and is produced during ejaculation

8   Hernia of fluid in the testicle

18   Malignant tumor of the testes

13   Foreskin

12   Essential cells of the testes; seminiferous tubules

2   Excision of the testicles or ovaries

14   Increase in growth of cells of a gland below the urinary bladder in males

17   Glands that secrete a fluid into the vas deferens

20   Enlarged, dilated veins near the testicle

4   Undescended testicle

10   Condition of scanty sperm cell production

9   Congenital opening of the male urethra on the undersurface of the penis

19   Chronic STD caused by a type of bacteria (spirochete)

6   Inflammation of the genital tract mucosa caused by infection with berry-shaped bacteria

7   Infection of the skin and mucous membranes with HSV; small fluid-filled blisters occur

Spelling Quiz

A

1. Chlamydia—bacteria causing sexually transmitted infection
2. impotence—inability of an adult male to achieve an erection
3. chancre—ulcer associated with syphilis
4. seminoma—malignant tumor of the testes
5. scrotum—sac that holds the testes
6. parenchymal—pertaining to essential cells of an organ
7. purulent—pus-filled
8. adenocarcinoma—cancerous tumor of a gland
9. prostate gland—below the urinary bladder (males); secretes seminal fluid
10. prepuce—foreskin

B

11. anorchism
12. bulbourethral
13. seminiferous
14. syphilis
15. embryonal
16. semen
17. oligospermia
18. purulent
19. testosterone
20. testis

Pronunciation Quiz

A

1. parenchymal
2. prepuce
3. varicocele
4. interstitial
5. flagellum
6. androgen
7. seminoma
8. prostatectomy
9. testosterone
10. impotence

B

1. D
2. B
3. J
4. I
5. E
6. A
7. H
8. F
9. C
10. G

C

1. orchiopexy
2. oligospermia
3. balanitis
4. prostatic hyperplasia (or hypertrophy)
5. hydrocele
6. epididymitis
7. vasovasostomy
8. spermatogenesis
9. gonorrhea
10. phimosis

Diagram Quiz

1. Testis
2. Scrotum
3. Perineum
4. Seminiferous tubules
5. Epididymis
6. Vas deferens
7. Seminal vesicle
8. Ejaculatory duct
9. Urethra
10. Prostate gland
11. Cowper (bulbourethral) gland
12. Penis
13. Glans penis
14. Prepuce (foreskin)

Vocabulary Quiz

A

1. impotence
2. perineum
3. epididymis

4. fraternal twins
5. ejaculatory duct
6. identical twins
7. parenchyma
8. flagellum
9. interstitial cells
10. bulbourethral gland

B

1. semen
2. vas deferens
3. prepuce
4. scrotum
5. sterilization
6. testis
7. prostate gland
8. seminal vesicle
9. spermatozoon
10. seminiferous tubules

Review Sheet Quiz

A

1. glans penis
2. testis
3. vessel, duct; vas deferens
4. animal life
5. male
6. hidden
7. cold
8. water
9. epididymis
10. monster

B

1. formation
2. destruction; separation
3. hernia
4. fixation
5. new opening
6. incision
7. nourishment, development
8. formation
9. removal, excision, resection
10. flow, discharge

chapter 10

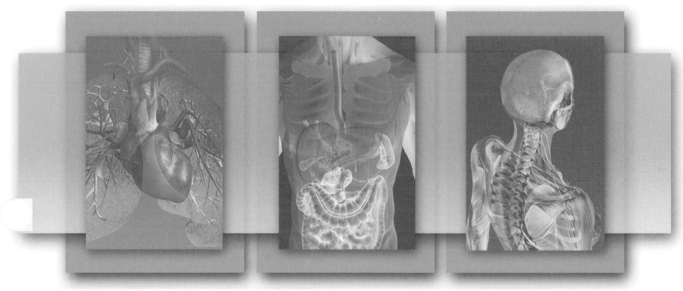

Chapter Ten

MULTIPLE CHOICE QUIZ

Name: _____

In the box write the letter of the choice that is the definition of the term or best answers the question. There is only one correct answer for each question.

1. **Part of the brain responsible for coordinating muscle movements and maintaining balance:**.......................... ☐
   A. Pons
   B. Cerebrum
   C. Thalamus
   D. Hypothalamus
   E. Cerebellum

2. **Pertaining to muscles and nerves:**....... ☐
   A. Myoneural
   B. Neuroanastomosis
   C. Myelogram
   D. Meningomyelocele
   E. Polyneuritis

3. **Neurotransmitter:**............................. ☐
   A. Cerebrospinal fluid
   B. Myelin
   C. Acetylcholine
   D. Lymph
   E. Sulcus

4. **Part of the nerve cell that first receives the nervous impulse is the:**.................. ☐
   A. Axon
   B. Cell body
   C. Neurilemma
   D. Convolution
   E. Dendrite

5. **Elevated portions of the cerebral cortex are called:** .... ☐
   A. Sulci
   B. Plexuses
   C. Gyri
   D. Ventricles
   E. Glial cells

6. **Burning sensation of pain:**.................. ☐
   A. Analgesia
   B. Cephalgia
   C. Anesthesia
   D. Causalgia
   E. Dysesthesia

7. **A network of interlacing nerve fibers in the peripheral nervous system:** .... ☐
   A. Microglia
   B. Astrocyte
   C. Plexus
   D. Synapse
   E. Receptor

8. **Portion of the brain that controls the pituitary gland, water balance, and body temperature:** .... ☐
   A. Medulla oblongata
   B. Cauda equina
   C. Cerebellum
   D. Thalamus
   E. Hypothalamus

9. **Glial cells:** .... ☐
   A. Neurons
   B. Astrocytes
   C. Meninges
   D. Parenchymal cells
   E. Nerve cells that conduct impulses

10. **Space between nerve cells is called the:** .... ☐
    A. Subdural space
    B. Subarachnoid space
    C. Ventricle
    D. Synapse
    E. Stimulus

11. **Part of the brain that controls breathing, heartbeat, and the size of blood vessels:** .... ☐
    A. Cerebellum
    B. Pons
    C. Cauda equina
    D. Medulla oblongata
    E. Thalamus

12. **Inability to speak:** .... ☐
    A. Apraxia
    B. Dysplasia
    C. Aphasia
    D. Aphagia
    E. Ataxia

13. **Collection of spinal nerves below the end of the spinal cord:** .... ☐
    A. Gyrus
    B. Dendrites
    C. Cauda equina
    D. Microglia
    E. Oligodendroglia

14. **X-ray record of the spinal cord:** .... ☐
    A. Electroencephalogram
    B. Electromyogram
    C. Cerebral angiogram
    D. Pneumoencephalogram
    E. Myelogram

15. **Collection of blood within the meningeal layers:** .... ☐
    A. Leptomeningitis
    B. Cerebromalacia
    C. Subdural hematoma
    D. Hydrocephalus
    E. Hemiparesis

16. **Abnormal sensation of tingling or prickling:** .... ☐
    A. Anesthesia
    B. Paresthesia
    C. Analgesia
    D. Neurasthenia
    E. Hyperkinesis

17. **Inflammation of a spinal nerve root:** ... ☐
    A. Encephalitis
    B. Meningitis
    C. Blepharitis
    D. Radiculitis
    E. Polyneuritis

18. **A highly malignant brain tumor:** .... ☐
    A. Meningioma
    B. Epidural hematoma
    C. Glioblastoma
    D. Subdural hematoma
    E. Teratoma

19. **Paralysis of four extremities:** .... ☐
    A. Hemiparesis
    B. Hemiplegia
    C. Paraplegia
    D. Quadriplegia
    E. Apraxia

20. **Cerebral aneurysm, thrombosis, or hemorrhage can be the cause of:** .... ☐
    A. Cerebrovascular accident
    B. Concussion
    C. Multiple sclerosis
    D. Myasthenia gravis
    E. Epilepsy

21. **Fainting:** .... ☐
    A. Shingles
    B. Hypesthesia
    C. Ataxia
    D. Syncope
    E. Palsy

22. **Spina bifida is associated with:** .... ☐
    A. Poliomyelitis
    B. Meningomyelocele
    C. Multiple myeloma
    D. Hyperkinesis
    E. Narcolepsy

23. **Parkinson disease is characterized by:** .... ☐
    A. Shuffling gait
    B. Cerebellar ataxia
    C. Bell palsy
    D. Herpes zoster infection
    E. Narcolepsy

24. **Disorder of reading, writing, and learning is:** .... ☐
    A. Epilepsy
    B. Apraxia
    C. Bradykinesis
    D. Neurasthenia
    E. Dyslexia

25. **Condition of no nervous sensation:** ..... ☐
    A. Analgesia
    B. Anencephaly
    C. Anesthesia
    D. Huntington disease
    E. Alzheimer disease

Chapter Ten
EXERCISE QUIZ

Name: _____

A. *Match the following neurologic structures with their meanings:*

axon	cerebral cortex	meninges	oligodendroglia
cauda equina	dendrite	myelin sheath	plexus

1. three protective membranes surrounding the brain and spinal cord _____

2. microscopic fiber that carries the nervous impulse along a nerve cell _____

3. a large, interlacing network of nerves _____

4. branching fiber that is the first part of a neuron to receive a nervous impulse _____

5. protective fatty tissue that surrounds the axon of a nerve cell _____

6. collection of spinal nerves below the end of the spinal cord _____

7. glial cell that produces myelin _____

8. outer region of the largest part of the brain; composed of gray matter _____

B. *Give meanings for the following terms:*

9. dura mater _____

10. synapse _____

11. medulla oblongata _____

12. hypothalamus _____

C. *Match the following terms with their meanings or associated terms below:*

gyri	parenchymal cell	sensory nerve
neurotransmitter	pia mater	subarachnoid space

13. carries messages toward the brain from receptors _____

14. essential cell of the nervous system; a neuron _____

15. innermost meningeal membrane _____

16. elevations in the cerebral cortex _____

17. acetylcholine is an example of this chemical released into a synapse _____

18. contains cerebrospinal fluid _____

D. *Give meanings for the following terms:*

19. intrathecal _____

20. glioma _____

21. myelogram _____

22. subdural hematoma _____

23. meningioma _____

24. paresthesias _____

E. *Match the following neurologic symptoms with their meanings below:*

apraxia	bradykinesia	hemiparesis	narcolepsy
ataxia	causalgia	hyperesthesia	syncope

25. slow movement _____

26. increased nervous sensation _____

27. seizure of sleep _____

28. movements and behavior are not purposeful _____

29. fainting _____

30. burning pain _____

31. no coordination _____

32. slight paralysis in half the body _____

F. *Match the following terms with their descriptions below:*

Alzheimer disease	epilepsy	myasthenia gravis
Bell palsy	multiple sclerosis	Parkinson disease

33. Destruction of myelin sheath; replacement by plaques of hard scar tissue _____

34. Sudden, transient disturbances of brain function marked by seizures _____

35. Loss of muscle strength; breakdown of acetylcholine, a neurotransmitter _____

36. Degeneration of nerves in the brain leading to tremors, shuffling
gait, and muscle stiffness (mask-like facial expression); dopamine
is deficient in the brain _____

37. Deterioration of mental capacity (dementia) beginning in middle age;
cerebral cortex atrophy, microscopic neurofibrillary tangles _____

38. Unilateral facial paralysis _____

G. *Give meanings for the following abnormal conditions:*

39. pyogenic meningitis _____

40. Tourette syndrome _____

41. shingles _____

42. cerebral embolus _____

H. *Match the term in Column I with its meaning in Column II:*

Column I

43. aura _____

44. palliative _____

45. transient ischemic attack _____

46. occlusion _____

47. dopamine _____

48. glioblastoma multiforme _____

49. absence seizure _____

50. tonic-clonic seizure _____

Column II

A. Relieving but not curing.

B. Major convulsive epileptic seizure.

C. Peculiar symptoms appearing before more definite symptoms.

D. Malignant brain tumor of immature glial cells.

E. Interruption of blood supply to the cerebrum.

F. Minor form of epileptic seizure.

G. Blockage.

H. Neurotransmitter.

Chapter Ten
DICTATION AND COMPREHENSION QUIZ: VOCABULARY AND TERMINOLOGY

Name: _____

A. Dictation of Terms

1. _____   11. _____

2. _____   12. _____

3. _____   13. _____

4. _____   14. _____

5. _____   15. _____

6. _____   16. _____

7. _____   17. _____

8. _____   18. _____

9. _____   19. _____

10. _____   20. _____

B. Comprehension of Terms: Match the number of the above term with its meaning below.

_____ The connective and framework tissue of any organ

_____ Fatty tissue that surrounds and protects the axon of a nerve cell

_____ Largest part of the brain

_____ Posterior part of the brain; responsible for maintaining balance

_____ A type of glial cell

_____ Neurotransmitter chemical released at the ends of nerve cells

_____ The space through which a nerve impulse passes from one nerve cell to another

_____ Inflammation of membranes around the brain and spinal cord

_____ Malignant brain tumor

_____ Slow movement

_____ Lack of muscle coordination

_____ Condition of absence of a brain (congenital anomaly)

_____ Pertaining to fainting

_____ Benign tumor of the membranes around the brain

_____ Part of the brain that controls the secretions of the pituitary gland

_____ Nervous exhaustion; "lack of nerve strength"

_____ Movements and behavior are not purposeful

_____ Paralysis of the lower part of the body

_____ State of unconsciousness from which a patient cannot be aroused

_____ Elevations on the surface of the cerebral cortex

Chapter Ten
DICTATION AND COMPREHENSION QUIZ: PATHOLOGY

Name: _____

A. Dictation of Terms

1. _____   10. _____

2. _____   11. _____

3. _____   12. _____

4. _____   13. _____

5. _____   14. _____

6. _____   15. _____

7. _____   16. _____

8. _____   17. _____

9. _____   18. _____

B. Comprehension of Terms: Match the number of the above term with its meaning below.

_____ A floating clot; mass of material suddenly blocks a blood vessel

_____ Relieving symptoms, but not curing

_____ Mini-stroke

_____ X-ray record of blood vessels within the brain

_____ Mental decline and deterioration

_____ Breakage of a blood vessel within the brain

_____ Demyelination of tissue around the axons of CNS neurons

_____ Paralysis and loss of muscular coordination caused by brain damage in the perinatal period

_____ Congenital defect of the spinal column with herniation of the spinal cord and meninges

_____ Major convulsive epileptic seizure

_____ Malignant brain tumor

_____ Relapsing weakness of skeletal muscles ("no muscle strength"); autoimmune condition

_____ Collection of fluid in the ventricles of the brain

_____ Degeneration of nerves in the brain; occurring in later life and leading to tremors and bradykinesia

_____ Manner of walking

_____ Type of neurotransmitter

_____ Peculiar sensation appearing before more definite symptoms

_____ Involuntary, spasmodic twitching movements; uncontrollable utterances

Chapter Ten
SPELLING QUIZ

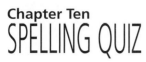

Name: _____

A. *Circle the term that is spelled correctly and write its meaning in the space provided:*

1. hypothalamus   hypothalmus _____
2. neurorrhapy   neurorrhaphy _____
3. motor nerve   moter nerve _____
4. myelin sheath   mylein sheath _____
5. acetylcholene   acetylcholine _____
6. meningoma   meningioma _____
7. hyperkinesis   hyperkenesis _____
8. neurasthenia   neurastenea _____
9. pareasis   paresis _____
10. demyleination   demyelination _____

B. *Circle the term that is spelled correctly. The meaning of each term is given.*

11. pertaining to fainting .... sincopal   syncopal   sinkaple
12. abnormal sensation .... paresthesia   parasthesia   parasthezia
13. relieving, but not curing .... pailiative   paliative   palliative
14. peculiar symptoms appearing
    before more definite symptoms .... aura   aurra   hora
15. loss of mental capacity .... demenshea   dementia   dementsha
16. within the meninges .... intrathecal   interthecal   intrathekal
17. essential cells of an organ .... parenchymal   parenchymel   parencyhmal
18. space between nerve cells.......................... sinapse   synnapse   synapse
19. part of the brain that controls
    muscular coordination............................ cerebellum   serabellum   serebellum
20. manner of walking................................... gate   gaite   gait

Chapter Ten
PRONUNCIATION QUIZ

Name: _____

A. Underline the accented syllable in the following terms:

1. angiography
2. encephalopathy
3. occlusion
4. meningomyelocele
5. syncope
6. dendrite
7. myelogram
8. glioma
9. hyperesthesia
10. narcolepsy

B. Match the term in Column I with its meaning in Column II:

Column I

1. axon _____
2. meninges _____
3. embolism _____
4. cauda equina _____
5. glial _____
6. thalamus _____
7. synapse _____
8. plexus _____
9. acetylcholine _____
10. neurasthenia _____

Column II

A. Pertaining to supportive cells of the nervous system.
B. Substance that helps transmit a nervous impulse.
C. Part of a nerve cell.
D. Obstruction of a blood vessel by a clot or foreign substance.
E. Network of nerve fibers.
F. Tail end of the spinal cord.
G. Three membranes surrounding the brain and spinal cord.
H. Space between nerve cells.
I. A part of the brain that serves as a relay station for impulses.
J. Lack of strength in nerves; sense of weakness and exhaustion.

C. Complete the following terms from their definitions:

1. dys_____   Difficult speech.
2. an _____   A condition of insensitivity to pain.
3. hemi _____   Slight paralysis of the right or left side of the body.
4. _____itis   Inflammation of a spinal nerve root.
5. neuro _____   Disease of a nerve.
6. vago _____   Incision of the vagus nerve.
7. a _____   Lack of coordination.
8. dys_____   Condition of painful nervous sensations.
9. glio _____   Tumor of immature brain cells (glia).
10. electro _____   Electrical record of the brain.

Chapter Ten
DIAGRAM QUIZ

Name: _____

Label the diagram below using the terms listed below:

Axon
Cell body
Cell nucleus
Dendrites
Myelin sheath
Synapse
Terminal end fibers

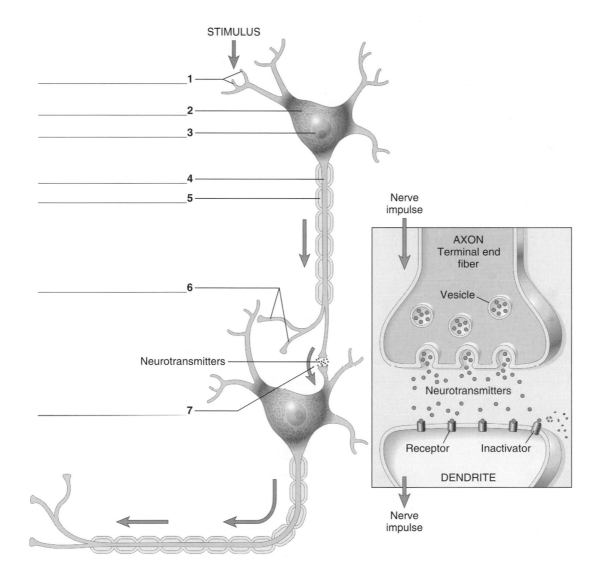

STIMULUS

1

2

3

4

5

Nerve impulse

AXON
Terminal end fiber

Vesicle

6

Neurotransmitters

Neurotransmitters

7

Receptor   Inactivator

DENDRITE

Nerve impulse

Chapter Ten
VOCABULARY QUIZ

Name: _____

A. *Match the following terms with their meanings below:*

arachnoid membrane	hypothalamus	pia mater
cerebellum	medulla oblongata	pons
cerebrum	neurotransmitter	thalamus
dura mater		

1. Main relay center of the brain _____

2. Chemical messenger released at the end of neurons _____

3. Outermost layer of meninges _____

4. Largest part of the brain _____

5. Part of the brain that coordinates muscle movement and maintains balance _____

6. Beneath the thalamus; controls appetite, sleep, and the pituitary gland_____

7. Thin, delicate inner membrane of meninges _____

8. Part of the brain that controls respiration, heartbeat, and
    the size of blood vessels _____

9. Middle meningeal membrane; spider-like _____

10. Lying between the medulla and the rest of the brain; bridge
    connecting various parts of the brain _____

B. *Match the following terms with their meanings below:*

acetylcholine	dendrite	parenchyma
autonomic nervous system	glial cell	sensory nerve
axon	myelin sheath	synapse
central nervous system		

1. Astrocyte is an example _____

2. Microscopic branching fiber of a nerve cell; first part
    of the neuron to receive the nervous impulse_____

3. Essential, distinguishing cells of an organ _____

4. Space through which a nervous impulse is transmitted _____

5. Neurotransmitter _____

6. Brain and the spinal cord

7. Carries messages to the brain and spinal cord _____

8. Microscopic nerve fiber that carries impulse from
    the cell body along the nerve cell _____

9. Sympathetic and parasympathetic nerves. _____

10. Fatty tissue surrounding and protecting the axon of a nerve cell. _____

C. Match the following terms with their meanings below:

blood-brain barrier	gyrus	stimulus
brain stem	receptor	sulcus
cauda equina	plexus	ventricles of the brain
ganglion		

1. Collection of spinal nerves below the end of the spinal cord _____

2. Canals in the interior of the brain containing cerebrospinal fluid _____

3. Collection of nerve cell bodies in the PNS _____

4. Capillaries that let certain substances enter the brain and
   keep other substances out of the brain _____

5. Organ that receives a nervous stimulation and passes it
   on to nerves within the body; ear and eye are examples_____

6. Any change in the internal or external environment that evokes a response _____

7. Elevation in the surface of the cerebral cortex _____

8. Depression or groove in the surface of the cerebral cortex _____

9. Large, interlacing network of nerves _____

10. Lower portion of the brain connecting the cerebrum with the spinal cord _____

Chapter Ten
REVIEW SHEET QUIZ

Name: _____

A. *Give meanings for the following combining forms:*

1. encephal/o _____

2. kines/o _____

3. mening/o _____

4. neur/o _____

5. my/o _____

6. vag/o _____

7. radicul/o _____

8. tax/o _____

9. myel/o _____

10. esthesi/o _____

B. *Give meanings for the following prefixes:*

1. quadri- _____

2. hypo- _____

3. hemi- _____

4. poly- _____

5. sub- _____

6. micro- _____

7. hyper- _____

8. dys- _____

9. epi- _____

10. para- _____

C. *Give meanings for the following suffixes:*

1. -algesia _____

2. -paresis _____

3. -phasia _____

4. - ptosis _____

5. -sclerosis _____

6. -plegia _____

7. -sthenia _____

8. -praxia _____

9. -blast _____

10. -cele _____

Chapter Ten
CROSSWORD PUZZLE

Name: _____

Fill in the crossword puzzle below using the clues listed underneath it.

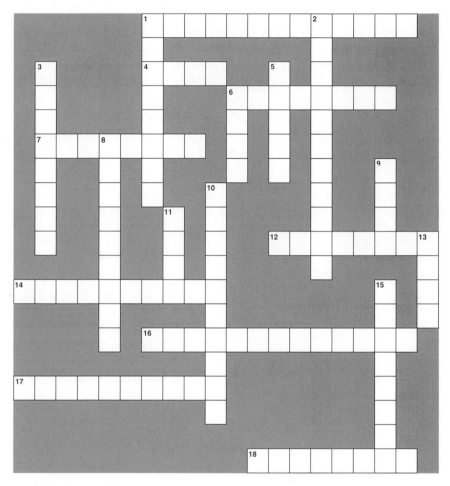

Across Clues

1. Destruction of myelin on the axons of nerves.
4. Part of the brain; means "bridge."
6. Abnormal widening of a blood vessel.
7. Mass of material travels through the bloodstream and suddenly blocks a vessel.
12. Mental decline and deterioration.
14. Relieving symptoms, but not curing.
16. Neurotransmitter released at the ends of some nerve cells.
17. Posterior part of the brain.
18. Three protective membranes that surround the brain and spinal cord.

Down Clues

1. Neurotransmitter that is deficient in Parkinson disease.
2. Malignant tumor of glial cells (astrocytes) in the brain.
3. Largest part of the brain.
5. Macroscopic structure consisting of axons and dendrites in bundle-like strands.
6. Peculiar sensation appearing before more definite symptoms.
8. Blockage.
9. Manner of walking.
10. Removal of the thymus gland; treatment for myasthenia gravis.
11. Sheets of nerve cells that produce elevation in the cerebral cortex, convolution.
13. Microscopic fiber that carries the nervous impulse along a nerve cell.
15. Microscopic branching fiber of a nerve cell that is the first part to receive the nervous impulse.

Chapter Ten
PRACTICAL APPLICATIONS

Name: _____

MRI Report

MRI was performed through the brain, cervical spine, and upper thoracic region. Scans were generated in the transaxial, sagittal, and coronal (frontal) planes.

Evaluation of the brain parenchyma demonstrates the presence of multiple areas of abnormal increased signal intensity scattered through the white matter of both cerebral hemispheres. These areas are periventricular in location. The pattern is most compatible with a demyelinative process. Scans through the cervical spine and spinal cord demonstrate no definite areas of abnormal increased or decreased signal within the cord. The disks are intact. Evaluation of the upper thoracic region demonstrates an appearance similar to that of the cervical region.

1. **What is MRI?** .... ☐
   A. Ultrasound images that show the structure of organs and tissues
   B. X-rays on a transverse plane
   C. Magnetic and radiowaves are used to create images
   D. Radioactive materials are injected, and images are recorded of their uptake in tissues

2. **What combining forms indicate the regions of the body imaged?** .... ☐
   A. Myel/o and my/o
   B. Encephal/o and myel/o
   C. My/o and encephal/o
   D. Encephal/o

3. **What is the brain parenchyma?** .... ☐
   A. Neuronal tissue of the brain
   B. Glial tissue of the brain
   C. Ventricles of the brain
   D. Connective tissue of the brain

4. **From the report, what is a likely diagnosis?** .... ☐
   A. Alzheimer disease
   B. Parkinson disease
   C. Amyotrophic bilateral sclerosis
   D. Multiple sclerosis

Chapter Ten
ANSWERS TO THE QUIZZES

Multiple Choice Quiz

1. E	4. E	7. C	10. D	13. C	16. B	19. D	22. B	25. C
2. A	5. C	8. E	11. D	14. E	17. D	20. A	23. A	
3. C	6. D	9. B	12. C	15. C	18. C	21. D	24. E	

Exercise Quiz

A

1. meninges
2. axon
3. plexus
4. dendrite
5. myelin sheath
6. cauda equina
7. oligodendroglia
8. cerebral cortex

B

9. outermost layer of the meninges
10. space between nerve cells
11. lower portion of the brain; controls blood pressure, heartbeat, and respiration
12. portion of the brain under thalamus; controls sleep, appetite, and pituitary gland

C

13. sensory nerve
14. parenchymal cell
15. pia mater
16. gyri
17. neurotransmitter
18. subarachnoid space

D

19. within the membranes around the brain and spinal cord
20. tumor of neuroglial cells in the brain
21. record (x-ray) of the spinal cord
22. mass of blood under the dura mater
23. tumor of the meninges
24. abnormal sensations

E

25. bradykinesia
26. hyperesthesia
27. narcolepsy
28. apraxia
29. syncope
30. causalgia
31. ataxia
32. hemiparesis

F

33. multiple sclerosis
34. epilepsy
35. myasthenia gravis
36. Parkinson disease
37. Alzheimer disease
38. Bell palsy

G

39. inflammation of meninges with pus formation
40. involuntary spasmodic twitching movements
41. herpes zoster infection with blisters in a band-like pattern on the body
42. blood clot that suddenly enters a blood vessel in the brain

H

43. C
44. A
45. E
46. G
47. H
48. D
49. F
50. B

Dictation and Comprehension Quiz: Vocabulary and Terminology

A

1. acetylcholine
2. anencephaly
3. apraxia
4. astrocyte
5. ataxia
6. bradykinesia
7. cerebellum
8. cerebrum
9. comatose
10. glioma
11. gyri
12. hypothalamus
13. leptomeningitis
14. meningioma
15. myelin sheath
16. neurasthenia
17. paraplegia
18. stroma
19. synapse
20. syncopal

B

18 The connective and framework tissue of any organ
15 Fatty tissue that surrounds and protects the axon of a nerve cell
8   Largest part of the brain
7   Posterior part of the brain; responsible for maintaining balance
4   A type of glial cell
1   Neurotransmitter chemical released at the ends of nerve cells
19 The space through which a nerve impulse passes from one nerve cell to another
13 Inflammation of membranes around the brain and spinal cord
10 Malignant brain tumor
6   Slow movement
5   Lack of muscle coordination
2   Condition of absence of a brain (congenital anomaly)
20 Pertaining to fainting
14 Benign tumor of the membranes around the brain
12 Part of the brain that controls the secretions of the pituitary gland
16 Nervous exhaustion; "lack of nerve strength"
3   Movements and behavior are not purposeful
17 Paralysis of the lower part of the body

9 State of unconsciousness from which a patient cannot be aroused

11 Elevations on the surface of the cerebral cortex

Dictation and Comprehension Quiz: Pathology

A

1. aura
2. cerebral angiography
3. cerebral hemorrhage
4. cerebral palsy
5. dementia
6. dopamine
7. embolus
8. gait
9. glioblastoma multiforme
10. hydrocephalus
11. multiple sclerosis
12. myasthenia gravis
13. palliative
14. Parkinson disease
15. spina bifida
16. tonic-clonic
17. Tourette syndrome
18. transient ischemic attack

B

7 A floating clot; mass of material suddenly blocks a blood vessel

13 Relieving symptoms, but not curing

18 Mini-stroke

2 X-ray record of blood vessels within the brain

5 Mental decline and deterioration

3 Breakage of a blood vessel within the brain

11 Demyelination of tissue around the axons of CNS neurons

4 Paralysis and loss of muscular coordination caused by brain damage in the perinatal period

15 Congenital defect of spinal column with herniation of the spinal cord and meninges

16 Major convulsive epileptic seizure

9 Malignant brain tumor

12 Relapsing weakness of skeletal muscles ("no muscle strength"); autoimmune condition

10 Collection of fluid in the ventricles of the brain

14 Degeneration of nerves in the brain; occurring in later life and leading to tremors and bradykinesia

8 Manner of walking

6 Type of neurotransmitter

1 Peculiar sensation appearing before more definite symptoms

17 Involuntary, spasmodic twitching movements; uncontrollable utterances

Spelling Quiz

A

1. hypothalamus—region of the brain below the thalamus
2. neurorrhaphy—suture of a nerve
3. motor nerve—takes messages to muscles from brain
4. myelin sheath—covering on nerve cell axon
5. acetylcholine—neurotransmitter
6. meningioma—tumor of the meninges
7. hyperkinesis—excessive movement
8. neurasthenia—lack of strength in nerves; irritability
9. paresis—slight paralysis
10. demyelination—lack of myelin

B

11. syncopal
12. paresthesia
13. palliative
14. aura
15. dementia
16. intrathecal
17. parenchymal
18. synapse
19. cerebellum
20. gait

Pronunciation Quiz

A

1. angi<u>o</u>graphy
2. encepha<u>lo</u>pathy
3. oc<u>clu</u>sion
4. mening<u>omy</u>elocele
5. <u>syn</u>cope
6. <u>den</u>drite
7. <u>my</u>elogram
8. gli<u>o</u>ma
9. hyperes<u>the</u>sia
10. <u>nar</u>colepsy

B

1. C
2. G
3. D
4. F
5. A
6. I
7. H
8. E
9. B
10. J

C

1. dysphasia
2. analgesia
3. hemiparesis
4. radiculitis
5. neuropathy
6. vagotomy
7. ataxia
8. dysesthesias
9. glioblastoma
10. electroencephalography

Diagram Quiz

1. Dendrites
2. Cell body
3. Cell nucleus
4. Axon
5. Myelin sheath
6. Terminal end fibers
7. Synapse

Vocabulary Quiz

A

1. thalamus
2. neurotransmitter
3. dura mater
4. cerebrum
5. cerebellum
6. hypothalamus
7. pia mater
8. medulla oblongata
9. arachnoid membrane
10. pons

B

1. glial cell
2. dendrite
3. parenchyma
4. synapse
5. acetylcholine
6. central nervous system
7. sensory nerve
8. axon
9. autonomic nervous system
10. myelin sheath

chapter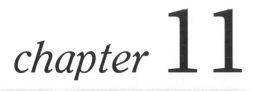

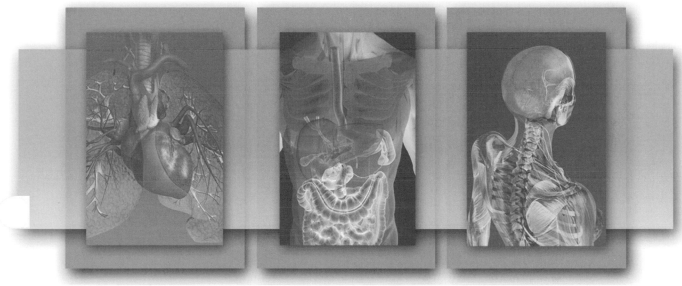

Chapter Eleven

MULTIPLE CHOICE QUIZ

Name: _____

In the box write the letter of the choice that is the definition of the term or best answers the question. There is only one correct answer for each question.

1. **A blood vessel that carries oxygen-poor blood from heart to lungs:** .... ☐
   A. Pulmonary vein
   B. Pulmonary artery
   C. Aorta
   D. Superior vena cava
   E. Inferior vena cava

2. **Contraction phase of the heartbeat:** ..... ☐
   A. Septum
   B. Diastole
   C. Tachycardia
   D. Systole
   E. Pacemaker

3. **Located between the left upper and lower chambers of the heart:** .... ☐
   A. Mitral valve
   B. Tricuspid valve
   C. Aortic valve
   D. Pulmonary valve
   E. Superior vena cava

4. **Saclike membrane surrounding the heart:** .... ☐
   A. Endocardium
   B. Bundle of His
   C. Interatrial septum
   D. Ventricle
   E. Pericardium

5. **Sensitive tissue in the right atrium wall that begins the heartbeat:** .... ☐
   A. Tricuspid valve
   B. Atrioventricular node
   C. Bundle of His
   D. Epicardium
   E. Sinoatrial node

6. **Blood vessels branching from the aorta to carry oxygen-rich blood to the heart muscle:** .... ☐
   A. Capillaries
   B. Venae cavae
   C. Coronary arteries
   D. Carotid arteries
   E. Renal arteries

7. **Disease of heart muscle:** .... ☐
   A. Cardiomegaly
   B. Endocarditis
   C. Arteriolitis
   D. Cardiomyopathy
   E. Aortic stenosis

8. **Phlebitis:** .... ☐
   A. Narrowing of a valve with inflammation
   B. Inflammation of a capillary
   C. Blockage of a heart valve
   D. Inflammation of a vein
   E. Narrowing of an artery

9. **Instrument to measure blood pressure:** .... ☐
   A. Sphygmomanometer
   B. Electrocardiogram
   C. Stress test
   D. Stethoscope
   E. Cardiac catheterization

10. **A local widening of an artery:** .... ☐
    A. Thrombosis
    B. Infarction
    C. Arterial anastomosis
    D. Aortic stenosis
    E. Aneurysm

11. **Cyanosis:** .... ☐
    A. Bluish coloration of the skin
    B. Yellow coloration of the skin
    C. Associated with a hemangioma
    D. A form of atherosclerosis
    E. Associated with increased oxygen in the blood

12. **Ischemia:** .... ☐
    A. Can lead to myocardial infarction
    B. Blood is held back from an area
    C. Can be caused by thrombotic occlusion of a blood vessel
    D. May be a result of coronary artery disease
    E. All of the above

13. **Angina is:** .... ☐
    A. Chest pain relieved with nitroglycerin
    B. An extra heart sound
    C. An abnormal heart rhythm
    D. Caused by rheumatic fever
    E. Associated with Raynaud disease

14. **Cardiac arrhythmia:** .... ☐
    A. Calcium channel blocker
    B. Beta-blocker
    C. Fibrillation
    D. Hypoxia
    E. Atheroma

15. **Petechiae:** .... ☐
    A. Small, pinpoint hemorrhages
    B. Vegetations
    C. Dilation of large vessels
    D. Defects, or holes in heart septa
    E. Hemorrhoids

16. **Blood clot forms in a large lower limb vessel:** .... ☐
    A. Aortic stenosis
    B. Mitral valve prolapse
    C. Deep-vein thrombosis
    D. Hypercholesterolemia
    E. Acute coronary syndromes

17. **Four separate congenital heart defects:** .... ☐
    A. Coarctation of the aorta
    B. Patent ductus arteriosus
    C. Raynaud disease
    D. Tetralogy of Fallot
    E. Peripheral vascular disease

18. **Patent means:** .... ☐
    A. Deoxygenated
    B. Oxygenated
    C. Open
    D. Closed
    E. Half closed

19. **The cause of essential hypertension is:** .... ☐
    A. Due to some secondary factor
    B. Pyelonephritis
    C. Glomerulonephritis
    D. Adrenal cortex adenoma
    E. Idiopathic

20. **Digoxin:** .... ☐
    A. Drug used to strengthen the heartbeat
    B. A calcium blocker
    C. Used to dissolve emboli
    D. Used to treat varicose veins
    E. A strong antibiotic

21. **CK, LD, and AST (SGOT) are:** .... ☐
    A. Lipids
    B. Lipoproteins
    C. Serum enzymes
    D. Fatty acids
    E. Nitrate-like drugs

22. **ECHO:** .... ☐
    A. Dye is injected into the blood and x-rays are taken of the heart
    B. Catheter is positioned in a vein and guided into the heart
    C. A stress test of cardiac function is performed
    D. High frequency sound waves are transmitted into the chest
    E. Electricity is measured as it flows through the heart

23. **Incision of a vein:** .... ☐
    A. Phebotomy
    B. Phlebitis
    C. Phlebotomy
    D. Vasoconstriction
    E. Ventriculotomy

24. **Removal of plaque from inner lining of an artery:** .... ☐
    A. Endarterectomy
    B. Arteriography
    C. Aneurysmectomy
    D. Ventriculotomy
    E. Valvuloplasty

25. **A Holter monitor is:** .... ☐
    A. An EEG test
    B. A stress test
    C. Part of a chest CT scan
    D. An EKG taken during daily activity
    E. Part of a cardiac catheterization

Chapter Eleven

EXERCISE QUIZ

Name: _____

A. Match the following terms with their meanings below:

aorta	capillary	pulmonary vein	ventricle
arteriole	mitral valve	superior vena cava	
atrium	pulmonary artery	tricuspid valve	

1. smallest blood vessel _____

2. largest artery in the body _____

3. lower chamber of the heart _____

4. valve between the right atrium and ventricle _____

5. carries blood from the lungs to the heart _____

6. brings blood to heart from upper parts of the body _____

7. upper chamber of the heart _____

8. valve between the left atrium and ventricle _____

9. carries blood to the lungs from the heart _____

10. small artery _____

B. Complete the following sentences:

11. The pacemaker of the heart is the _____

12. The saclike membrane surrounding the heart is the _____

13. The contractive phase of the heartbeat is called _____

14. The relaxation phase of the heartbeat is called _____

15. Abnormal heart sound caused by improper closure of heart valves is _____

C. Complete the following terms from their definitions:

16. hardening of arteries: arterio _____

17. enlargement of the heart: cardio _____

18. inflammation of a vein with a clot _____ itis

19. disease condition of heart muscle: cardio _____

20. condition of rapid heartbeat: _____ cardia

D. *Give meanings for the following terms:*

21. cyanosis _____

22. Raynaud disease _____

23. heart block _____

24. ischemia _____

25. atheroma _____

26. vasoconstriction _____

27. myocardial infarction _____

28. angina _____

29. thrombotic occlusion _____

E. *Match the following pathological conditions with their meanings below:*

coarctation of the aorta   flutter
congestive heart failure   hypertensive heart disease
coronary artery disease   mitral valve prolapse
fibrillation   tetralogy of Fallot

30. rapid but regular atrial or ventricular contractions _____

31. improper closure of the valve between the left atrium and ventricle during systole _____

32. blockage of the arteries surrounding the heart leading to ischemia _____

33. high blood pressure affecting the heart _____

34. congenital narrowing of large artery leading from the heart _____

35. rapid, random, ineffectual, and irregular contractions of the heart _____

36. inability of the heart to pump its required amount of blood _____

37. congenital malformation involving four separate heart defects _____

F. *Match the following terms with their descriptions:*

aneurysm   emboli   secondary hypertension
auscultation   essential hypertension   vegetations
claudication   petechiae

38. listening with a stethoscope _____

39. lesions that form on heart valves after damage by infection _____

40. small, pinpoint hemorrhages _____

41. high blood pressure due to kidney disease _____

42. high blood pressure with idiopathic etiology _____

43. local widening of an artery _____

44. pain, tension, and weakness in a limb after walking has begun _____

45. clots that travel to and suddenly block a blood vessel _____

G. *Give meanings for the following:*

46. HDL _____

47. thrombolytic therapy _____

48. cardiac catheterization _____

49. SA node _____

50. ECG _____

Chapter Eleven
DICTATION AND COMPREHENSION QUIZ: VOCABULARY AND TERMINOLOGY

Name: _____

A. Dictation of Terms

1. _____   11. _____
2. _____   12. _____
3. _____   13. _____
4. _____   14. _____
5. _____   15. _____
6. _____   16. _____
7. _____   17. _____
8. _____   18. _____
9. _____   19. _____
10. _____   20. _____

B. Comprehension of Terms: Match the number of the above term with its meaning below.

_____ Smallest blood vessel

_____ Instrument to measure blood pressure

_____ Incision of a vein

_____ Condition of deficient oxygen

_____ Largest vein in the body

_____ Pacemaker of the heart

_____ Largest artery in the body

_____ High levels of a fatty substance in the blood

_____ Wall between the upper chambers of the heart

_____ Widening of a blood vessel

_____ Vessel carrying blood to the arm

_____ Removal of fatty plaque (from a blood vessel)

_____ New connection between two arteries

_____ Inflammation of a valve on the left side of the heart

_____ Breakdown (destruction) of a blood clot

_____ Vessel carrying blood to the lungs

_____ Surgical repair of a valve

_____ Hardening of arteries

_____ Enlargement of the heart

_____ Surgical puncture to remove fluid between the membranes surrounding the heart

Chapter Eleven

DICTATION AND COMPREHENSION QUIZ: PATHOLOGY

Name: _____

A. *Dictation of Terms*

1. _____ 10. _____

2. _____ 11. _____

3. _____ 12. _____

4. _____ 13. _____

5. _____ 14. _____

6. _____ 15. _____

7. _____ 16. _____

8. _____ 17. _____

9. _____ 18. _____

B. *Comprehension of Terms: Match the number of the above term with its meaning below.*

_____ High blood pressure of idiopathic etiology

_____ Varicose veins near the anus

_____ Closure (blockage) of a blood vessel

_____ Collections of material (clots) that travel to and suddenly block a vessel

_____ Chest pain resulting from temporary difference between supply and demand of oxygen to the heart muscle

_____ Short episodes of pallor and numbness in fingers and toes due to temporary constriction of arterioles

_____ Examples are flutter, fibrillation, and heart block

_____ A small duct between the aorta and pulmonary artery, which normally closes soon after birth, remains open

_____ The heart is unable to pump its required amount of blood; pulmonary edema may result

_____ Congenital malformation of the heart involving four distinct defects

_____ An extra heart sound heard between normal beats

_____ Inflammation of the inner lining of the heart

_____ Local widening of an artery caused by weakness in the arterial wall

_____ Improper closure of a heart valve when the heart is pumping blood

_____ Drugs used to treat abnormal heart rhythms and high blood pressure

_____ Blockage of arteries in the lower extremities due to atherosclerosis

_____ Bluish discoloration of the skin

_____ Uncomfortable sensations in the chest

Chapter Eleven

SPELLING QUIZ

Name: _____

A. *Circle the term that is spelled correctly and write its meaning in the space provided.*

1. capillary   capilliary _____

2. ventricle   ventracle _____

3. carbon dyoxide   carbon dioxide _____

4. vien   vein _____

5. myocardium   myocardiam _____

6. arterosclerosis   arteriosclerosis _____

7. pulmunary   pulmonary _____

8. tricuspid valve   trikuspid valve _____

9. arterioles   arteroiles _____

10. aortia   aorta _____

B. *Circle the term that is spelled correctly. The meaning of each term is given.*

11. pertaining to the heart ....coronery   coronary   corenary

12. relaxation phase of the heartbeat ....diastole   diostole   dieastole

13. pain ....angina   anjena   anjina

14. abnormal rapid heart rhythm ....fibrilation   filbrilation   fibrillation

15. swollen blood vessels in the ....hemmorhoids   hemmorrhoids   hemorrhoids
    rectal region

16. incision of a vein ....phlebotomy   phebotomy   phliebotomy

17. widening of a vessel ....vasodialation   vassodialation vasodilation

18. bluish coloration of the skin ....cianosis   cyanosis   cyianosis

19. traveling clot that suddenly blocks ....embulus   embulos   embolus
    a blood vessel

20. contraction phase of the heartbeat ....systole   sistolle   sistole

Chapter Eleven

PRONUNCIATION QUIZ

Name: _____

A. *Underline the accented syllable in the following terms:*

1. diastole
2. arteriolitis
3. sphygmomanometer
4. pericarditis
5. coronary
6. capillary
7. anastomosis
8. phlebotomy
9. idiopathic
10. coarctation

B. *Match the term in Column I with its meaning in Column II:*

Column I

1. ventricle _____
2. petechiae _____
3. hemangioma _____
4. embolus _____
5. systole _____
6. septum _____
7. aorta _____
8. aneurysm _____
9. digoxin _____
10. hemorrhoids _____

Column II

A. Contraction phase of the heartbeat.

B. Small, pinpoint hemorrhages.

C. Largest artery in the body.

D. Tumor of blood vessels.

E. Widening or dilation of a blood vessel.

F. Lower chamber of the heart.

G. Swollen, twisted veins in the rectal region.

H. Wall or partition within the heart.

I. Floating blood clot or other material.

J. Drug used to reduce abnormal heart rhythms.

C. *Complete the following terms from their definitions:*

1. _____ itis   Inflammation of a vein.

2. _____ cardia   Fast heartbeat.

3. _____ ectomy   Removal of the inner lining of an artery.

4. _____ ia   Condition of abnormal heart rhythm.

5. _____ osis   Abnormal condition of blue coloration of the skin.

6. _____ emia   High levels of cholesterol in the bloodstream.

7. _____ ium   Muscle layer of the heart.

8. vaso _____   Widening of a blood vessel.

9. thrombo _____   Destruction of clots.

10. hyp _____   Decreased oxygen condition.

Chapter Eleven

ABBREVIATIONS QUIZ

Name: _____

Spell out the abbreviations in Column I and then match each abbreviation with an associated explanation in column II:

Column I

1. LVAD _____ _____
2. ACS _____ _____
3. ICD _____ _____
4. TEE _____ _____
5. HTN _____ _____
6. Tc _____ _____
7. PCI _____ _____
8. CCU _____ _____
9. PVC _____ _____
10. tPA _____ _____

Column II

A. Type of ultrasound imaging of the heart.

B. Includes unstable angina and myocardial infarction.

C. Radioactive element used in cardiac scans.

D. Drug used to present thrombosis.

E. Used as a "bridge to transplant."

F. High blood pressure.

G. Hospital area where acute heart conditions are treated.

H. This helps to correct heart arrhythmia.

I. Abnormal heart rhythm.

J. Surgical intervention with catheter, balloon, and stents.

Chapter Eleven
DIAGRAM QUIZ

Name: _____

Label the diagram below using the following terms:

Aorta
Aortic valve
Inferior vena cava
Left atrium
Left ventricle

Mitral valve
Pulmonary artery
Pulmonary valve
Pulmonary vein
Right atrium

Right ventricle
Superior vena cava
Tricuspid valve

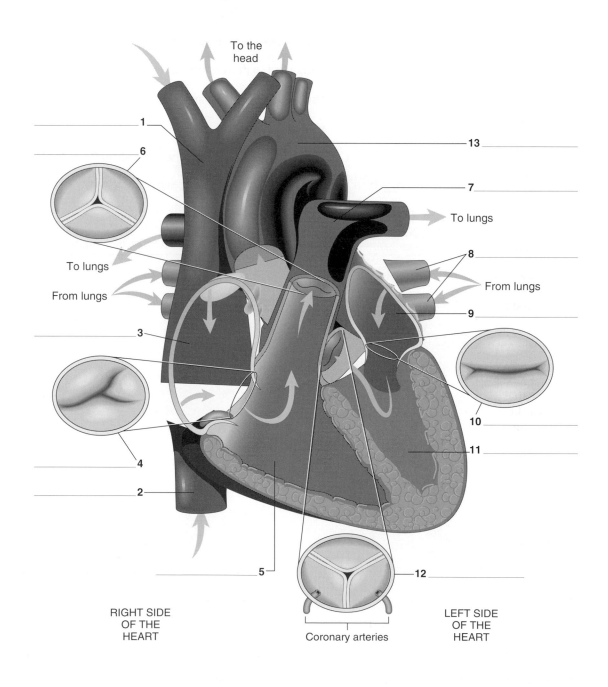

RIGHT SIDE
OF THE
HEART

Coronary arteries

LEFT SIDE
OF THE
HEART

Chapter Eleven

VOCABULARY QUIZ

Name: _____

A. *Match the following terms with their meanings below:*

aorta	capillary	endocardium
arteriole	carbon dioxide	oxygen
atrioventricular bundle	diastole	systole
atrium		

1. Gas that enters the blood through the lungs _____

2. Smallest blood vessel _____

3. Relaxation phase of the heartbeat _____

4. Upper chamber of the heart _____

5. Gas released by body cells; travels via blood to the lungs where it is exhaled _____

6. Small artery _____

7. nner lining of the heart _____

8. Specialized muscle fibers connecting the upper and lower heart
    chambers; bundle of His _____

9. Contraction phase of the heartbeat _____

10. Largest artery in the body _____

B. *Match the following terms with their meanings below:*

coronary arteries	mitral valve	normal sinus rhythm
deoxygenated blood	murmur	pacemaker
electrocardiogram	myocardium	pericardium
endothelium		

1. Double-layered membrane surrounding the heart _____

2. Muscular, middle layer of the heart _____

3. Positioned between the left upper and lower heart chambers _____

4. Innermost lining of blood vessels _____

5. Resting rate of 60–100 beats per minute _____

6. Blood lacking in oxygen _____

7. Blood vessels that carry oxygen-rich blood to the heart muscle _____

8. Abnormal heart sound _____

9. Specialized nervous tissue in the right atrium that begins the
    heartbeat; sinoatrial node _____

10. Record of the electricity flowing through the heart _____

C. Match the following terms with their meaning below:

pulmonary artery   septum   vena cava
pulmonary valve   sphygmomanometer   ventricle
pulmonary vein   tricuspid valve   venule
pulse

1. Small vein _____

2. Beat of the heart as felt through the wall of the arteries _____

3. Located between the upper and lower right heart chambers _____

4. Instrument to measure blood pressure _____

5. Partition or wall dividing the chambers of the heart _____

6. Located between the lower right chamber and the vessel carrying
    blood to the lungs _____

7. Lower chamber of the heart _____

8. One of two pairs of vessels carrying oxygenated blood from the lungs
    to the heart _____

9. Vessel that carries oxygen-poor blood from the heart to the lungs _____

10. Largest vein in the body _____

Chapter Eleven
REVIEW SHEET QUIZ

Name: _____

A. *Give meanings for the following combining forms:*

1. angi/o _____   6. aort/o _____

2. ather/o _____   7. axill/o _____

3. brachi/o _____   8. coron/o _____

4. my/o _____   9. pulmon/o _____

5. phleb/o _____   10. ox/o _____

B. *Give meanings for the following combining forms:*

1. cyan/o _____   6. vas/o _____

2. thromb/o _____   7. myx/o _____

3. atri/o _____   8. ventricul/o _____

4. valvul/o _____   9. ven/o _____

5. sphygm/o _____   10. vascul/o _____

C. *Give meanings for the following suffixes:*

1. -constriction _____   6. -sclerosis _____

2. -dilation _____   7. -stenosis _____

3. -graphy _____   8. -tomy _____

4. -megaly _____   9. -lysis _____

5. -plasty _____   10. -emia _____

D. *Give meanings for the following prefixes:*

1. brady- _____   6. inter- _____

2. hyper- _____   7. tri- _____

3. hypo- _____   8. tachy- _____

4. endo- _____   9. peri- _____

5. dys- _____   10. a-, an- _____

Chapter Eleven
CROSSWORD PUZZLE

Name: _____

Fill in the crossword puzzle below using the clues listed underneath it.

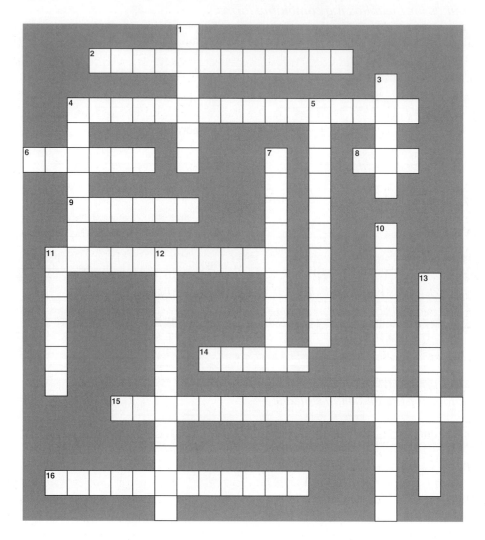

Across Clues

2. Listening with a stethoscope.
4. Instrument to measure blood pressure.
6. Angi/o.
8. Brachi/o.
9. Gas that enters the blood through the lungs.
11. Saclike membrane surrounding the heart.
14. Coron/o.
15. Process of using ultrasound to record images of the heart.
16. Inflammation of the inner lining of the heart; etiology is bacterial.

Down Clues

1. An abnormal heart sound.
3. Cardi/o.
4. Contraction phase of the heartbeat.
5. Muscle layer of the heart.
7. Sensitive tissue in the right atrium that begins the heartbeat; sinoatrial node.
10. Pain, tension, and weakness in a leg after walking has begun, but absence of pain at rest.
11. Open; as in ductus arteriosus.
12. Abnormal heart rhythms.
13. Small, pinpoint hemorrhages.

Chapter Eleven
PRACTICAL APPLICATIONS

Name: _____

A. Emergency Room—Patient Report

Mr. Smith was seen by the emergency medical technicians (EMTs) and found to have tachycardia. Lidocaine (a cardiac antiarrhythmic) was started, and by the time he reached the ER his heart rate was between 75 and 80 with a sinus rhythm. He had excellent ST segments and T waves. Blood pressure was 156/88. He had a good carotid pulse bilaterally. No cardiomegaly and no murmurs.

He was started on a cardiac monitor and observed for any ECG change. He had no episode of hypotension and no further arrhythmia. There was no evidence to do cardiac enzyme studies, and the patient was discharged to be followed by his regular physician.

1. What type of problem did the patient have before coming to the ER? .... ☐
   - A. Chest pain
   - B. Low blood pressure
   - C. High blood pressure
   - D. Rapid heartbeat

2. What did the EMTs do for the patient? ... ☐
   - A. They administered an electrocardiogram and put him on a heart monitor
   - B. They administered a drug to reverse his arrhythmia
   - C. They checked his cardiac enzymes and got him to the hospital
   - D. They shocked his heart into a normal rhythm

3. What is a sinus rhythm? .... ☐
   - A. A normal heart rhythm
   - B. A rapid heartbeat
   - C. A very slow heartbeat
   - D. An abnormal heartbeat caused by respiratory problems

4. ST and T waves are elements of: .... ☐
   - A. An EEG
   - B. An ECG
   - C. A cardiac scan
   - D. Echocardiography

B. Patient Assessment

The patient is a 58-year-old male who has had angina for a duration of 3 years. His symptom of substernal (stern/o means breastbone) tightness occurs with exertion and is relieved promptly by rest (typical of angina). A treadmill stress test showed definite ST segment abnormalities consistent with myocardial ischemia at stage 3 of the test. In addition, the patient has multiple risk factors including hypertension, hypercholesterolemia, and past history of smoking.

I have started the patient on Cardizem (a calcium channel blocker) as antianginal medication. If the patient has evidence of significant stenosis in the future, he should undergo coronary angiography and possibly PCI.

1. What is the patient's major symptom? ... ☐
   - A. Pain in his left arm
   - B. High blood pressure
   - C. High blood levels of cholesterol
   - D. Chest pain

2. What did the treadmill test show? .... ☐
   - A. Hypertension
   - B. Decrease in blood flow to heart muscle
   - C. Fracture of the breastbone
   - D. Past history of smoking

3. What is the effect of Cardizem? ☐
   - A. Increases blood pressure
   - B. Lowers blood cholesterol
   - C. Decreases myocardial ischemia
   - D. Promotes aortic stenosis

4. What procedures are recommended? ...... ☐
   - A. X-ray of heart blood vessels and balloon angioplasty with stent placement
   - B. Coronary artery bypass surgery
   - C. Thrombolytic therapy
   - D. Exercise tolerance test and radioactive scan

C. General Hospital Nuclear Cardiology Center Stress Test Imaging Report

Patient Name:	SALLY SMITH	Procedure Date:	14-APR-2004
Procedure:	MYOCARDIAL IMAGING, SPECT	Date of Birth:	21-OCT-1956
Ref Physician:	TOM JONES, MD		

CLINICAL HISTORY:
Family history of CAD. Ex-smoker, palpitations. Sudden onset of SSCP and shortness of breath with radiation to back and down both arms at rest.

INDICATION(S):
Diagnosis of ischemia.

MEDICATIONS:
ASA, Premarin.

PROCEDURE:
The patient underwent a 99mTc sestamibi exercise treadmill stress test using standard Bruce protocol (patient must get to 85% of maximum heart rate for age). Sestamibi at 8 AM.

302MBq (radioactive dose) 99mTc sestamibi were injected intravenously at peak exercise and tomographic imaging data acquired. Additional data were acquired following intravenous injection of another 893MBq 99mTc sestamibi at rest on the same day.

ENDPOINT(S):
Exercise was limited by fatigue. Chest pain did not occur.

REST ECG:
The baseline cardiac rhythm was normal sinus rhythm. The rest electrocardiogram revealed nonspecific ST segment and T-wave abnormalities.

STRESS ECG:
No ST segment changes were observed during this test.
Arrhythmias: None.

STRESS TEST COMMENTS:
Negative for ischemia.

CONCLUSIONS:
The patient has excellent exercise capacity. The ECG response to stress was negative for ischemia. The perfusion images show equivocal mild anterior ischemia.

1. **What type of test is the patient receiving?** .... ☐
   A. Cardiac MRI and stress test
   B. Radioactive scan to image blood flow to heart muscle with an exercise stress test
   C. Image of cardiac structures with ultrasound and exercise stress test
   D. Computed tomography after exercise stress test
   E. Holter monitor with stress test

2. **Why was the procedure indicated?** .... ☐
   A. History of previous MI
   B. Symptoms of intermittent claudication
   C. Congestive heart failure
   D. Substernal chest pain and SOB
   E. Family history of essential hypertension

3. **What are the results of the test?** .... ☐
   A. Patient experienced angina
   B. Patient experienced palpitations and tiredness
   C. Heart function is good, and ischemia is not clearly evident
   D. Abnormal heart rhythms were evident with ST and T wave abnormalities
   E. Heart block and ischemia occurred

Chapter Eleven
ANSWERS TO THE QUIZZES

Multiple Choice Quiz

1. B	4. E	7. D	10. E	13. A	16. C	19. E	22. D	25. D
2. D	5. E	8. D	11. A	14. C	17. D	20. A	23. C	
3. A	6. C	9. A	12. E	15. A	18. C	21. C	24. A	

Exercise Quiz

A

1. capillary
2. aorta
3. ventricle
4. tricuspid valve
5. pulmonary vein
6. superior vena cava
7. atrium
8. mitral valve
9. pulmonary artery
10. arteriole

B

11. sinoatrial node
12. pericardium
13. systole
14. diastole
15. murmur

C

16. arteriosclerosis
17. cardiomegaly
18. thrombophlebitis
19. cardiomyopathy
20. tachycardia

D

21. bluish coloration of the skin
22. recurrent episodes of cyanosis and pallor in fingers and toes
23. failure of conduction of impulses from the AV node to bundle of His
24. blood is held back from tissues
25. mass of plaque (cholesterol)
26. narrowing of a vessel
27. dead tissue in heart muscle
28. chest pain
29. blockage of a vessel due to a clot

E

30. flutter
31. mitral valve prolapse
32. coronary artery disease
33. hypertensive heart disease
34. coarctation of the aorta
35. fibrillation

36. congestive heart failure
37. tetralogy of Fallot

F

38. auscultation
39. vegetations
40. petechiae
41. secondary hypertension
42. essential hypertension
43. aneurysm
44. claudication
45. emboli

G

46. high-density lipoproteins
47. treatment to dissolve clots in blood vessels
48. tube is introduced into a vessel and guided into the heart to detect pressures and blood flow
49. sinoatrial node (pacemaker)
50. electrocardiogram

Dictation and Comprehension Quiz: Vocabulary and Terminology

A

1. aorta
2. arterial anastomosis
3. arteriosclerosis
4. atherectomy
5. brachial artery
6. capillary
7. cardiomegaly
8. hypercholesterolemia
9. hypoxia
10. interatrial septum
11. mitral valvulitis
12. pericardiocentesis
13. phlebotomy
14. pulmonary artery
15. sinoatrial node
16. sphygmomanometer
17. thrombolysis
18. valvuloplasty
19. vasodilation
20. vena cava

B

6   Smallest blood vessel
16 Instrument to measure blood pressure
13 Incision of a vein
9   Condition of deficient oxygen
20 Largest vein in the body
15 Pacemaker of the heart
1   Largest artery in the body
8   High levels of a fatty substance in the blood
10 Wall between the upper chambers of the heart
19 Widening of a blood vessel
5   Vessel carrying blood to the arm
4   Removal of fatty plaque (from a blood vessel)
2   New connection between two arteries
11 Inflammation of a valve on the left side of the heart
17 Breakdown (destruction) of a blood clot
14 Vessel carrying blood to the lungs
18 Surgical repair of a valve
3   Hardening of arteries
7   Enlargement of the heart
12 Surgical puncture to remove fluid between the membranes surrounding the heart

Dictation and Comprehension Quiz: Pathology

A

1. aneurysm
2. angina
3. arrhythmias
4. beta blockers
5. claudication
6. congestive heart failure
7. cyanosis
8. emboli
9. endocarditis
10. essential hypertension
11. hemorrhoids

12. mitral valve prolapse
13. murmur
14. occlusion
15. palpitations
16. patent ductus arteriosus
17. Raynaud phenomenon
18. Tetralogy of Fallot

B

10 High blood pressure of idiopathic etiology

11 Varicose veins near the anus

14 Closure (blockage) of a blood vessel

8 Collections of material (clots) that travel to and suddenly block a vessel

2 Chest pain resulting from temporary difference between supply and demand of oxygen to the heart muscle

17 Short episodes of pallor and numbness in fingers and toes due to temporary constriction of arterioles

3 Examples are flutter, fibrillation, and heart block

16 A small duct between the aorta and pulmonary artery, which normally closes soon after birth, remains open

6 The heart is unable to pump its required amount of blood; pulmonary edema may result

18 Congenital malformation of the heart involving four distinct defects

13 An extra heart sound heard between normal beats

9 Inflammation of the inner lining of the heart

1 Local widening of an artery caused by weakness in the arterial wall

12 Improper closure of a heart valve when the heart is pumping blood

4 Drugs used to treat abnormal heart rhythms and high blood pressure

5 Blockage of arteries in the lower extremities due to atherosclerosis

7 Bluish discoloration of the skin

15 Uncomfortable sensations in the chest

Spelling Quiz

A

1. capillary—smallest blood vessel
2. ventricle—lower heart chamber
3. carbon dioxide—gas released from lungs
4. vein—vessel carrying blood to the heart from tissues
5. myocardium—heart muscle
6. arteriosclerosis—hardening of arteries
7. pulmonary—pertaining to the lung
8. tricuspid valve—between the upper and lower right chambers of the heart
9. arterioles—small arteries
10. aorta—largest artery

B

11. coronary
12. diastole
13. angina
14. fibrillation
15. hemorrhoids
16. phlebotomy
17. vasodilation
18. cyanosis
19. embolus
20. systole

Pronunciation Quiz

A

1. di<u>a</u>stole
2. arterio<u>li</u>tis
3. sphygmoma<u>nome</u>ter
4. pericar<u>di</u>tis
5. <u>coro</u>nary
6. <u>capi</u>llary
7. anasto<u>mos</u>is
8. phle<u>bot</u>omy
9. idio<u>path</u>ic
10. coarc<u>ta</u>tion

B

1. F
2. B
3. D
4. I
5. A
6. H
7. C
8. E
9. J
10. G

C

1. phlebitis
2. tachycardia
3. endarterectomy
4. arrhythmia
5. cyanosis
6. hypercholesterolemia
7. myocardium
8. vasodilation
9. thrombolysis
10. hypoxia

Abbreviations Quiz

1. Left ventricular assist device <u>E</u>
2. Acute coronary syndromes <u>B</u>
3. Implantable cardiac defibrillator <u>H</u>
4. Transesophageal echocardiography <u>A</u>
5. Hypertension <u>F</u>
6. Technetium <u>C</u>
7. Percutaneous coronary intervention <u>J</u>
8. Coronary care unit <u>G</u>
9. Premature ventricular contraction <u>I</u>
10. Tissue plasminogen activator <u>D</u>

Diagram Quiz

1. Superior vena cava
2. Inferior vena cava
3. Right atrium
4. Tricuspid valve
5. Right ventricle
6. Pulmonary valve
7. Pulmonary artery
8. Pulmonary vein
9. Left atrium
10. Mitral valve
11. Left ventricle
12. Aortic valve
13. Aorta

Vocabulary Quiz

A

1. oxygen
2. capillary
3. diastole
4. atrium
5. carbon dioxide
6. arteriole
7. endocardium
8. atrioventricular bundle
9. systole
10. aorta

B

1. pericardium
2. myocardium
3. mitral valve
4. endothelium
5. normal sinus rhythm
6. deoxygenated blood
7. coronary arteries
8. murmur
9. pacemaker
10. electrocardiogram

C

1. venule
2. pulse
3. tricuspid valve
4. sphygmomanometer
5. septum
6. pulmonary valve
7. ventricle
8. pulmonary vein
9. pulmonary artery
10. vena cava

Review Sheet Quiz

A

1. vessel
2. yellowish plaque; fatty substance
3. arm
4. muscle
5. vein
6. aorta
7. armpit
8. heart
9. lung
10. oxygen

B

1. blue
2. clot
3. atrium; upper chamber of the heart
4. valve
5. pulse
6. vessel
7. mucus
8. ventricle; lower chamber of the heart
9. vein
10. vessel

C

1. to tighten or narrow
2. to widen or enlarge
3. process of recording
4. enlargement
5. surgical repair
6. hardening

7. narrowing
8. incision
9. separation; breakdown
10. blood condition

D

1. slow
2. too much; above
3. too little; below
4. within
5. painful, difficult, abnormal
6. between
7. three
8. fast
9. surrounding
10. no, not, without

Practical Applications

A

1. D
2. B
3. A
4. B

B

1. D
2. B
3. C
4. A

C

1. B
2. D
3. C

Crossword Puzzle

Chapter Twelve
MULTIPLE CHOICE QUIZ

Name: _____

In the box write the letter of the choice that is the definition of the term or best answers the question. There is only one correct answer for each question.

1. **Tubes that bifurcate from the windpipe:**.............. ☐
   A. Alveoli
   B. Bronchioles
   C. Sinuses
   D. Adenoids
   E. Bronchi

2. **Uppermost portion of the lung:**........... ☐
   A. Hilum
   B. Apex
   C. Base
   D. Lobe
   E. Diaphragm

3. **Space between the lungs in the chest:** ☐
   A. Pleura
   B. Peritoneum
   C. Mediastinum
   D. Trachea
   E. Bronchial tubes

4. **Nasopharyngeal lymphatic tissue:** .... ☐
   A. Mucosa
   B. Adenoids
   C. Visceral pleura
   D. Paranasal sinuses
   E. Epiglottis

5. **Pulmonary parenchyma:** .... ☐
   A. Trachea
   B. Pharynx
   C. Alveoli and bronchioles
   D. Red blood cells
   E. Cilia

6. **Removal of the voice box:** .... ☐
   A. Larnygectomy
   B. Pharnygectomy
   C. Laryngectomy
   D. Esophagectomy
   E. Pharyngectomy

7. **Phren/o means:** .... ☐
   A. Lung
   B. Chest
   C. Membrane around the lung
   D. Air sac
   E. Diaphragm

8. **Medical term for a condition of decreased oxygen in the blood:**............ ☐
   A. Hematemesis
   B. Paroxysmal
   C. Hypoxemia
   D. Hemorrhage
   E. Hemoptysis

9. **Type of pneumoconiosis:** .... ☐
   A. Asbestosis
   B. Pyothorax
   C. Atelectasis
   D. Pneumonia
   E. Epiglottis

10. **Breathing is easier in an upright position:**... ☐
    A. Dysphonia
    B. Hemothorax
    C. Dyspnea
    D. Orthopnea
    E. Anosmia

11. **Collection of pus in the pleural cavity:** .... ☐
    A. Cyanosis
    B. Pleuritis
    C. Hemoptysis
    D. Pyothorax
    E. Pneumothorax

12. **Sharp, short blows to the surface of the chest:** .... ☐
    A. Auscultation
    B. Percussion
    C. Stridor
    D. Rales
    E. Expectoration

13. **The "P" in DPT stands for:** .... ☐
    A. Pneumonia
    B. Pertussis
    C. Pleurisy
    D. Pneumothorax
    E. Pulmonary

14. **Stridor occurs in which upper respiratory disorder?**........................ ☐
   A. Croup
   B. Diphtheria
   C. Asthma
   D. Epistaxis
   E. Pneumonia

15. **Difficult breathing:**............................ ☐
   A. Anosmia
   B. Dyspnea
   C. Dysphonia
   D. Tachypnea
   E. Hypoxia

16. **Bronchial airway obstruction marked by paroxysmal dyspnea, wheezing, and cough:** .... ☐
   A. Pleurisy
   B. Epistaxis
   C. Cor pulmonale
   D. Diphtheria
   E. Asthma

17. **Collapsed lung:**................................ ☐
   A. Pneumonitis
   B. Endotracheal
   C. Thoracotomy
   D. Atelectasis
   E. Tracheoesophageal fistula

18. **Material is expelled from the lungs:** .... ☐
   A. Rhinorrhea
   B. Bronchiolitis
   C. Sinusitis
   D. Expiration
   E. Expectoration

19. **Localized area of pus formation in the lungs:**.................................. ☐
   A. Pulmonary edema
   B. Pulmonary embolism
   C. Pleural effusion
   D. Pulmonary abscess
   E. Pleurisy

20. **Spitting up blood from the lungs:** .... ☐
   A. Pleurodynia
   B. Hematemesis
   C. Hemothorax
   D. Hydrothorax
   E. Hemoptysis

21. **Tube is placed through the mouth to the trachea to establish an airway:**... ☐
   A. Endotracheal intubation
   B. Tracheostomy
   C. Tracheotomy
   D. Thoracentesis
   E. Laryngoscopy

22. **PPD:**... ☐
   A. Pulmonary function test
   B. Type of lung x-ray
   C. Drug used to treat pneumonia
   D. Tuberculin test
   E. None of the above

23. **Airway obstruction associated with emphysema and chronic bronchitis:** .... ☐
   A. RDS
   B. COPD
   C. CPR
   D. SOB
   E. IPPB

24. **Which of the following is an endoscopic examination?** .... ☐
   A. Tracheostomy
   B. Lung scan
   C. Thoracentesis
   D. Bronchoscopy
   E. Auscultation

25. **Hypercapnia:** .... ☐
   A. Increased oxygen to the tissues
   B. High blood pressure
   C. High carbon dioxide levels in the blood
   D. Decreased carbon dioxide in the blood
   E. Decreased oxygen in the blood

Chapter Twelve
EXERCISE QUIZ

Name: _____

A. *Select from the following anatomical structures to complete the sentences below:*

alveoli	larynx
bronchi	mediastinum
cilia	palatine tonsils
epiglottis	paranasal sinuses
hilum	parietal pleura

1. Branches of the windpipe that lead into the lungs are the _____

2. The region between the lungs in the chest cavity is the _____

3. Collections of lymph tissue in the oropharynx are the _____

4. Air sacs of the lung are called _____

5. The outer fold of pleura lying closest to the ribs is called _____

6. Thin hairs attached to the mucous membrane lining the respiratory tract are _____

7. The voice box is called the _____

8. Middle region where bronchi, blood vessels, and nerves enter and exit lungs is the _____

9. Air-containing cavities in the bones around the nose are the _____

10. The lid-like piece of cartilage that covers the voice box is the _____

B. *Complete the following sentences:*

11. The gas produced by cells and exhaled through the lungs is called _____

12. Divisions of the lungs are called _____

13. The essential cells of the lung; performing its main function are the pulmonary _____

14. Breathing in air is called _____

C. *Give meanings for the following medical terms:*

15. bronchiectasis _____

16. anosmia _____

17. phrenic _____

18. pneumothorax _____

D. *Complete the medical terms for the following respiratory symptoms:*

19. excessive carbon dioxide in the blood: hyper _____

20. spitting up blood: hemo _____

21. hoarseness; voice impairment: dys _____

22. breathing is possible only in an upright position: _____pnea

23. nosebleed: epi _____

E. *Give meanings for the following medical terms:*

24. purulent _____ _____

25. rales_____ _____

26. auscultation _____ _____

27. pulmonary infarction _____ _____

F. *Match the following terms with their descriptions:*

asbestosis   chronic bronchitis
asthma   cystic fibrosis
atelectasis   emphysema
bronchogenic carcinoma   pertussis

28. hyperinflation of air sacs with destruction of alveolar walls_____

29. inflammation of tubes leading from the trachea (over a long period of time)_____

30. spasm and narrowing of bronchi leading to airway obstruction _____

31. lung or portion of a lung is collapsed _____

32. malignant neoplasm originating in a bronchus _____

33. whooping cough; bacterial infection of the pharynx _____

34. inherited disease of exocrine glands leading to airway obstruction_____

35. type of pneumoconiosis; dust particles are inhaled _____

G. *Give meanings for the following medical terms:*

36. adenoid hypertrophy _____ _____

37. tachypnea _____ _____

38. pleurodynia_____ _____

39. pulmonary embolism _____ _____

40. pulmonary edema_____ _____

41. pulmonary abscess _____ _____

H. Match the clinical procedure or abbreviation with its description:

bronchioalveolar lavage   pulmonary angiography
endotracheal intubation   thoracentesis
lung scan (V/Q)   tracheostomy

42. Tube is placed through the mouth into the trachea to establish an airway_____

43. Radioactive material is injected or inhaled and images are recorded _____

44. After contrast is injected into blood vessels of the lungs, x-rays are taken _____

45. Opening into the trachea through the neck to establish an airway_____

46. Chest wall is punctured with a needle to obtain fluid from the pleural space_____

47. Fluid is injected into the bronchi and then removed for examination _____

I. Give meanings for the following abbreviations:

48. COPD _____

49. PFT _____

50. URI _____

Chapter Twelve

DICTATION AND COMPREHENSION QUIZ: VOCABULARY AND TERMINOLOGY

Name: _____

A. Dictation of Terms

1. _____   11. _____
2. _____   12. _____
3. _____   13. _____
4. _____   14. _____
5. _____   15. _____
6. _____   16. _____
7. _____   17. _____
8. _____   18. _____
9. _____   19. _____
10. _____   20. _____

B. Comprehension of Terms: Match the number of the above term with its meaning below.

_____ Condition of increased carbon dioxide in the blood
_____ Space in the chest between the lungs
_____ Essential tissue of the lung
_____ Surgical repair of the nose
_____ Drug that opens up (widens) the bronchial tubes
_____ Spitting up blood
_____ Instrument to measure breathing
_____ Incision of the chest
_____ Inflammation of the flap of cartilage over the windpipe
_____ Pertaining to the throat
_____ Resection of a lung
_____ Inflammation of the small bronchial tubes
_____ Pertaining to the voice box
_____ Inflammation of the membrane lining the lungs
_____ Widening of bronchial tubes
_____ Difficult, painful breathing
_____ Absence of a sense of smell
_____ Pus in the chest (between the membranes around the lung)
_____ Incision of the windpipe
_____ Muscle that aids in breathing and is located between the chest and the abdomen

Chapter Twelve

DICTATION AND COMPREHENSION QUIZ: PATHOLOGY

Name: _____

A. Dictation of Terms

1. _____   11. _____

2. _____   12. _____

3. _____   13. _____

4. _____   14. _____

5. _____   15. _____

6. _____   16. _____

7. _____   17. _____

8. _____   18. _____

9. _____   19. _____

10. _____ 20. _____

B. Comprehension of Terms: Match the number of the above term with its meaning below.

_____ Pertaining to containing pus

_____ Escape of fluid into the pleural cavity

_____ Visual examination of the voice box

_____ Adenocarcinoma and small cell carcinoma are examples

_____ Musical sounds heard during expiration

_____ Whooping cough

_____ Swelling and fluid in alveoli and bronchioles

_____ Spasm and narrowing of bronchi leading to airway obstruction

_____ Creation of an opening into the windpipe

_____ Coal dust accumulation in the lungs

_____ Malignant tumor arising in the pleura

_____ Collapsed lung

_____ Infectious disease of the lungs; caused by bacilli

_____ Nosebleed

_____ Strained, high-pitched noisy breathing

_____ Listening to sounds within the body

_____ Surgical puncture to remove fluid from the chest (pleural cavity)

_____ Hyperinflation of alveoli with damage to alveolar walls; type of COPD

_____ Pertaining to a sudden occurrence

_____ Injecting and retrieving fluid from the bronchial tubes

Chapter Twelve
SPELLING QUIZ

Name: _____

A. *Circle the term that is spelled correctly and write its meaning in the space provided:*

1. epiglottis   epiglottus _____

2. diaphrame   diaphragm _____

3. ascultation   auscultation _____

4. astmah   asthma _____

5. emphysema   emphyzema _____

6. cilia   cili _____

7. traychea   trachea _____

8. plural   pleural _____

9. pnuemonia   pneumonia _____

10. alveoli   alveroli _____

B. *Circle the term that is spelled correctly. The meaning of each term is given.*

11. incision of the chest .... thorocotomy   thorecotomy   thoracotomy

12. collapsed lung.. telactasis   atelectasis   atelelectisis

13. rod-shaped bacteria .... bacilli   basilli   basceilli

14. collection of pus .... absess   absecess   abscess

15. surgical repair of the nose......................... rhinoplasty   rrhinoplasty   rinoplasty

16. removal of the tonsils.............................. tonsilectomy   tonselectomy   tonsillectomy

17. whooping cough .... pertusis   pertussis   partussus

18. visual examination of the voice box.......... larnygoscopy   larnygoscipe   laryngoscopy

19. pain of the pleura (chest wall).................. phrenodynia   frenodynia   phrenodinia

20. incision of the windpipe........................... trachiotomy   tracheotomy   traycheotomy

Chapter Twelve
PRONUNCIATION QUIZ

Name: _____

A. *Underline the accented syllable in the following terms:*

1. dyspnea
2. bacilli
3. larynx

4. rhinoplasty
5. pleural effusion
6. adenoids

7. bronchoscopy
8. expectoration
9. hypoxia

10. tonsillectomy

B. *Match the term in Column I with its meaning in Column II:*

Column I

1. mediastinum   _____
2. empyema   _____
3. auscultation   _____
4. edema   _____
5. atelectasis   _____
6. pleura   _____
7. pharynx   _____
8. trachea   _____
9. cilia   _____
10. diphtheria   _____

Column II

A. Throat.

B. Collection of fluid in tissues.

C. Membranes surrounding the lungs.

D. Central cavity between the lungs in the chest.

E. The windpipe.

F. Condition of imperfect lung expansion; collapsed lung.

G. Thin hairs attached to the lining of the respiratory tract.

H. Pus in the pleural cavity.

I. Listening to the sounds in the chest.

J. Infectious disease of the throat and upper respiratory tract; caused by bacteria

C. *Complete the following terms using the definitions given:*

1. dys_____   Difficult breathing.

2. hemo_____   Spitting up blood.

3. _____itis   Inflammation of a small bronchial tube.

4. _____ osis   Abnormal condition of dust in the lung.

5. _____ otomy   Incision of the windpipe.

6. par_____   Essential cells of an organ.

7. pleuro_____   Pain of the pleura (chest wall).

8. _____itis   Inflammation of the nose and throat.

9. em_____   Lung disease marked by distention or swelling of the alveoli.

10. _____ pnea   Breathing is easier in an upright position.

Chapter Twelve

ABBREVIATIONS QUIZ

Name: _____

Spell out the abbreviation in Column I and then match each abbreviation to an associated explanation in Column II:

Column I

1. ARDS _____ _____

2. COPD _____ _____

3. CPAP _____ _____

4. RSV _____ _____

5. VATS _____ _____

6. RDS _____ _____

7. MDI _____ _____

8. DOE _____ _____

9. PFTs _____ _____

10. NSCLC _____ _____

Column II

A. This virus causes bronchiolitis and bronchopneumonia.

B. Difficult breathing with strenuous exercise.

C. Examples are FEV_1 and TLC.

D. Adenocarcinomas and squamous cell carcinomas are examples.

E. Tachypnea, dyspnea, cyanosis, tachycardia, and hypoxemia in an adult.

F. Chronic bronchitis and emphysema are examples.

G. Procedure to visually examine the chest via small incisions and video equipment.

H. Device to deliver aerosolized medication.

I. This device helps relieve obstructive sleep apnea.

J. Related to absence of surfactant, a substance that helps expansion of lungs in infants.

Chapter Twelve
DIAGRAM QUIZ

Name: _____

Label the diagram below using the following terms:

Adenoids	Erythrocytes	Nasal cavity	Parietal pleura
Alveoli	Esophagus	Nasopharynx	Terminal bronchiole
Bronchi	Laryngopharynx	Nose	Trachea
Capillary	Larynx	Oropharynx	Visceral pleura
Diaphragm	Lung	Palatine tonsils	
Epiglottis	Mediastinum	Paranasal sinuses	

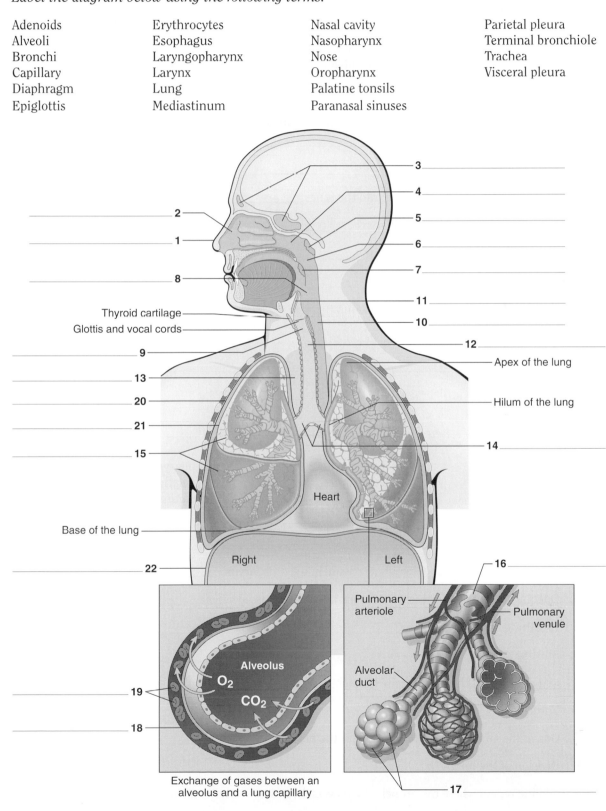

Thyroid cartilage
Glottis and vocal cords

Apex of the lung

Hilum of the lung

Heart

Base of the lung

Right   Left

Pulmonary arteriole
Pulmonary venule

Alveolar duct

Alveolus
O_2
CO_2

Exchange of gases between an
alveolus and a lung capillary

Chapter Twelve
VOCABULARY QUIZ

Name: _____

A. *Match the following terms with their meanings below:*

adenoids   bronchi   diaphragm
alveolus   bronchioles   epiglottis
apex of the lung   cilia   expiration
base of the lung

1. Thin hairs attached to the mucous membrane epithelium
   lining the respiratory tract _____

2. Lower portion of the lung _____

3. Branches of the trachea leading into the lungs _____

4. Lymphatic tissue in the nasopharynx _____

5. Tip or uppermost portion of the lung _____

6. Breathing out (exhalation) _____

7. Small branches of the tubes leading into the lungs _____

8. Muscle separating the chest and abdomen _____

9. Air sac in the lung _____

10. Lid-like piece of cartilage covering the larynx _____

B. *Match the following terms with their meanings below:*

glottis   lobe of the lung   pharynx
hilum of the lung   mediastinum   palatine tonsil
inspiration   nares   paranasal sinus
larynx

1. Voice box _____

2. One of a pair of masses of lymphatic tissue in the oropharynx _____

3. Openings through the nose carrying air into the air passageways _____

4. Breathing in _____

5. Slit-like opening to the voice box _____

6. Region between the lungs in the thoracic cavity _____

7. Throat _____

8. One of the air cavities in the bones near the nose _____

9. Division of the lung _____

10. Midline region where the bronchi, blood vessels, and nerves enter and exit the lungs _____

C. Match the following terms with their meaning below:

carbon dioxide   pleural cavity   trachea
oxygen   pulmonary parenchyma   visceral pleura
parietal pleura   respiration

1. Gas that passes into the bloodstream at the lungs and travels to all body cells _____

2. Space between the double-folded membrane surrounding each lung _____

3. Inner fold of membrane surrounding each lung and closest to the lung tissue _____

4. Windpipe _____

5. Essential parts of the lung responsible for respiration; bronchioles and alveoli _____

6. Gas that is exhaled through the lungs _____

7. Process of moving air into and out of the lungs; breathing _____

8. Outer fold of membrane surround each lung and lying closest to the ribs _____

Chapter Twelve
REVIEW SHEET QUIZ

Name: _____

A. *Give meanings for the following combining forms:*

1. adenoid/o _____

2. alveol/o _____

3. bronch/o _____

4. bronchiol/o _____

5. pulmon/o _____

6. nas/o _____

7. or/o _____

8. ox/o _____

9. pector/o _____

10. orth/o _____

B. *Give combining forms for the following meanings:*

1. voice box _____

2. throat _____

3. blue _____

4. voice _____

5. diaphragm _____

6. dust _____

7. pus _____

8. complete _____

9. windpipe _____

10. tonsils _____

C. *Give meanings for the following suffixes and prefixes:*

1. -centesis _____

2. -osmia _____

3. -pnea _____

4. -stenosis _____

5. -ectasis _____

6. -ptysis _____

7. brady- _____

8. per- _____

9. hypo- _____

10. para- _____

Chapter Twelve
CROSSWORD PUZZLE

Name: _____

Fill in the crossword puzzle below using the clues listed underneath it.

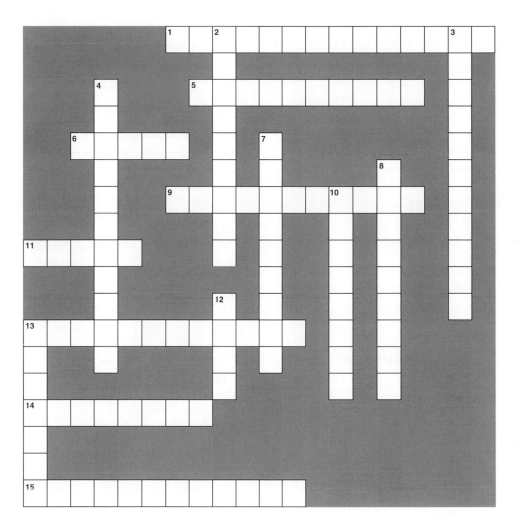

Across Clues

1. Abnormal condition caused by dust in the lungs.
5. Lid-like piece of cartilage that covers the larynx.
6. Phon/o means sound or _____.
9. Collapsed lung; or incomplete expansion of lung.
11. Thin hairs attached to the mucous membranes.
13. An infectious disease caused by bacilli and treated with INH (Isoniazid).
14. Tel/o means _____, as in atelectasis.
15. Listening to sounds within the body.

Down Clues

2. Air is trapped in lungs, and bronchioles are plugged with mucus; a type of COPD.
3. Breathing in.
4. Smallest branches of the bronchi.
7. Acute inflammation and infection of the lung caused by bacteria (pneumococci), viruses, or fungi.
8. Muscle separating the chest and abdomen.
10. Collection of lymph tissue in the nasopharynx.
12. Rhin/o means _____.
13. Windpipe.

Chapter Twelve
PRACTICAL APPLICATIONS

Name: _____

A. Questions for the Case Report on page 464 of the text

1. What did the initial chest x-ray show? .... ☐
   A. Collapsed lung
   B. Shallow respirations
   C. Pleurodynia
   D. Collection of fluid between the pleura

2. What term indicates that the condition was caused by fractured ribs? .... ☐
   A. Secondary
   B. Comatose
   C. Heroin
   D. Effusion

3. What procedure was used to relieve the condition? .... ☐
   A. Chest x-ray
   B. Thoracotomy and tube insertion
   C. Paracentesis
   D. Pericardiocentesis

4. What is the lesson from this case report? .... ☐
   A. Get a chest x-ray immediately upon entering the ER.
   B. Removal of fluid from the pleural space showed no blood was present.
   C. Be sure that a chest x-ray is read correctly.
   D. Be careful when injecting heroin.

B. Two Chart Notes

Bill Smith: The patient is being treated palliatively with irradiation to the left ilium for metastatic lung cancer.

1. Where is the treatment being given? ...... ☐
   A. To the lungs
   B. To the whole chest
   C. To the hip
   D. To the abdomen (small intestine)

2. What does palliative mean? .... ☐
   A. Strong treatment is given.
   B. Treatment will relieve but not cure.
   C. Treatment is given often.
   D. Treatment is weak so that the patient does not suffer.

3. What type of physician gives this treatment? .... ☐
   A. Radiologist
   B. Medical oncologist
   C. Radiation oncologist
   D. Pulmonologist

Mary Jones: Recurrent episodes of dyspnea, coughing, and wheezing. She has never been hospitalized, but she requires daily therapy with a bronchodilator.

4. What do you think the patient's condition might be? .... ☐
   A. Small cell lung cancer
   B. Epistaxis
   C. Sinusitis
   D. Asthma

C. Pathology Report

Date:	November 16, 2005	Pathology No. 450231
Patient:	Carolyn Jones	Room No. 422
Physician:	Howard T. Waxman, MD	Hospital No. 550330
Specimen:	Biopsy of left bronchus	

GROSS DESCRIPTION: The specimen consisted of a very tiny, wispy portion of soft, whitish-pink tissue measuring $3 \times 2 \times 1$ mm in toto. The entire specimen is submitted.

MICROSCOPIC DESCRIPTION: The sections of the bronchial biopsy show approximately half of the mucosa to be composed of pseudostratified, ciliated, respiratory-type epithelium, and the second half to be composed of respiratory epithelium that has undergone squamous metaplasia. There is one small area of cells that has become detached from the mucosa, which is composed of rather pleomorphic and hyperchromatic cells with loss of polarity. This small area of tissue would be classified as the squamous carcinoma. However, I see no evidence of (the) infiltration through the basement membrane in this section. Additional tissue may show more extensive involvement with the carcinoma.

DIAGNOSIS: Small fragment of squamous carcinoma without evidence of infiltration into the underlying submucosa, left bronchus, biopsy (see description).

Pathologist _____
Mark M. Mosley, MD

New Terms:

hyperchromatic	Pertaining to cells that stain intensely (chrom/o = color).
loss of polarity	Cells lose normal sense of organization (characteristic of malignancy).
pleomorphic	Pertaining to cells with many (ple/o = more) different shapes (and a form characteristic of malignancy).
pseudostratified	Type of layered epithelium in which nuclei of adjacent cells are at different levels.
squamous metaplasia	Reversible conversion of normal cells into another, less specialized cell type. Often, these cells can transform into cancerous cells.

Chapter Twelve
ANSWERS TO THE QUIZZES

Multiple Choice Quiz

1. E	4. B	7. E	10. D	13. B	16. E	19. D	22. D	25. C
2. B	5. C	8. C	11. D	14. A	17. D	20. E	23. B	
3. C	6. C	9. A	12. B	15. B	18. E	21. A	24. D	

Exercise Quiz

A
1. bronchi
2. mediastinum
3. palatine tonsils
4. alveoli
5. parietal pleura
6. cilia
7. larynx
8. hilum
9. paranasal sinuses
10. epiglottis

B
11. carbon dioxide
12. lobes
13. parenchyma
14. inspiration

C
15. dilation of bronchi
16. lack of sense of smell
17. pertaining to the diaphragm
18. collection of air in the pleural space (chest)

D
19. hypercapnia
20. hemoptysis
21. dysphonia
22. orthopnea
23. epistaxis

E
24. pus-filled
25. abnormal crackling sounds during inspiration
26. listening with a stethoscope
27. dead tissue in the lung

F
28. emphysema
29. chronic bronchitis
30. asthma
31. atelectasis
32. bronchogenic carcinoma
33. pertussis
34. cystic fibrosis
35. asbestosis

G
36. enlargement of adenoids
37. rapid breathing
38. pain in the chest wall (pleura)
39. blood clot suddenly blocks a vessel in the lungs
40. swelling, collection of fluid in the lungs
41. collection of pus (infection in the lungs)

H
42. endotracheal intubation
43. lung scan (V/Q)
44. pulmonary angiography
45. tracheostomy
46. thoracentesis
47. bronchioalveolar lavage

I
48. chronic obstructive pulmonary disease
49. pulmonary function test
50. upper respiratory infection

Dictation and Comprehension Quiz: Vocabulary

A
1. anosmia
2. bronchiectasis
3. bronchiolitis
4. bronchodilator
5. diaphragm
6. dyspnea
7. epiglottitis
8. hemoptysis
9. hypercapnia
10. laryngeal
11. mediastinum
12. pharyngeal
13. pleuritis
14. pneumonectomy
15. pulmonary parenchyma
16. pyothorax
17. rhinoplasty
18. spirometer
19. thoracotomy
20. tracheotomy

B
9 Condition of increased carbon dioxide in the blood
11 Space in the chest between the lungs
15 Essential tissue of the lung
17 Surgical repair of the nose
4 Drug that opens up (widens) the bronchial tubes
8 Spitting up blood
18 Instrument to measure breathing
19 Incision of the chest
7 Inflammation of the flap of cartilage over the windpipe
12 Pertaining to the throat
14 Resection of a lung
3 Inflammation of the small bronchial tubes
10 Pertaining to the voice box
13 Inflammation of the membrane lining the lungs
2 Widening of bronchial tubes
6 Difficult, painful breathing
1 Absence of a sense of smell
16 Pus in the chest (between the membranes around the lung)
20 Incision of the windpipe
5 Muscle that aids in breathing and is located between the chest and the abdomen

Dictation and Comprehension Quiz: Pathology

A
1. anthracosis
2. asthma
3. atelectasis
4. auscultation
5. bronchial alveolar lavage
6. bronchogenic carcinoma
7. emphysema
8. epistaxis
9. laryngoscopy

10. mesothelioma
11. paroxysmal
12. pertussis
13. pleural effusion
14. pulmonary edema
15. purulent
16. stridor
17. thoracentesis
18. tracheostomy
19. tuberculosis
20. wheezes

B

15   Pertaining to containing pus
13   Escape of fluid into the pleural cavity
9   Visual examination of the voice box
6   Adenocarcinoma and small cell carcinoma are examples
20   Musical sounds heard during expiration
12   Whooping cough
14   Swelling and fluid in alveoli and bronchioles
2   Spasm and narrowing of bronchi leading to airway obstruction
18   Creation of an opening into the windpipe
1   Coal dust accumulation in the lungs
10   Malignant tumor arising in the pleura
3   Collapsed lung
19   Infectious disease of the lungs; caused by bacilli
8   Nosebleed
16   Strained, high-pitched noisy breathing
4   Listening to sounds within the body
17   Surgical puncture to remove fluid from the chest (pleural cavity)
7   Hyperinflation of alveoli with damage to alveolar walls; type of COPD
11   Pertaining to a sudden occurrence
5   Injecting and retrieving fluid from the bronchial tubes

Spelling Quiz

A

1. epiglottis—flap of cartilage over the windpipe
2. diaphragm—muscle between the chest and abdomen
3. auscultation—listening with a stethoscope
4. asthma—spasm and narrowing of bronchi
5. emphysema—hyperinflation of air sacs; destruction of alveoli
6. cilia—tiny hairs in the respiratory tract
7. trachea—windpipe
8. pleural—pertaining to the membrane around the lungs
9. pneumonia—acute inflammation and infection of air sacs
10. alveoli—air sacs

B

11. thoracotomy
12. atelectasis
13. bacilli
14. abscess
15. rhinoplasty
16. tonsillectomy
17. pertussis
18. laryngoscopy
19. phrenodynia
20. tracheotomy

Pronunciation Quiz

A

1. dyspnea
2. bacilli
3. larynx
4. rhinoplasty
5. pleural effusion
6. adenoids
7. bronchoscopy
8. expectoration
9. hypoxia
10. tonsillectomy

B

1. D
2. H
3. I
4. B
5. F
6. C
7. A
8. E
9. G
10. J

C

1. dyspnea
2. hemoptysis
3. bronchiolitis
4. pneumoconiosis
5. tracheotomy
6. parenchyma

7. pleurodynia
8. nasopharyngitis
9. emphysema
10. orthopnea

Abbreviations Quiz

1. adult respiratory distress syndrome E
2. chronic obstructive pulmonary disease F
3. continuous positive airway pressure I
4. respiratory syncytial virus A
5. video-assisted thoracic surgery (thoracoscopy) G
6. respiratory distress syndrome J
7. metered dose inhaler H
8. dyspnea on exertion B
9. pulmonary function tests C
10. non-small cell lung cancer D

Diagram Quiz

1. Nose
2. Nasal cavity
3. Paranasal sinuses
4. Nasopharynx
5. Adenoids
6. Oropharynx
7. Palatine tonsils
8. Laryngopharynx
9. Larynx
10. Esophagus
11. Epiglottis
12. Trachea
13. Mediastinum
14. Bronchi
15. Lung
16. Terminal bronchiole
17. Alveoli
18. Capillary
19. Erythrocytes
20. Parietal pleura
21. Visceral pleura
22. Diaphragm

Vocabulary Quiz

A

1. cilia
2. base of the lung
3. bronchi
4. adenoids
5. apex of the lung
6. expiration
7. bronchioles
8. diaphragm
9. alveolus

10. epiglottis

B

1. larynx
2. palatine tonsil
3. nares
4. inspiration
5. glottis
6. mediastinum
7. pharynx
8. paranasal sinus
9. lobe of the lung
10. hilum of the lung

C

1. oxygen
2. pleural cavity
3. visceral pleura
4. trachea
5. pulmonary parenchyma
6. carbon dioxide
7. respiration
8. parietal pleura

Review Sheet Quiz

A

1. adenoids
2. alveolus (air sac)
3. bronchial tube
4. bronchiole
5. lung
6. nose
7. mouth
8. oxygen
9. chest
10. straight

B

1. laryng/o
2. pharyng/o
3. cyan/o
4. phon/o
5. phren/o
6. coni/o
7. py/o
8. tel/o
9. trache/o

10. tonsill/o

C

1. surgical puncture to remove fluid
2. smell
3. breathing
4. narrowing, tightening
5. widening, expansion
6. spitting
7. slow
8. through
9. under, below; less than
10. near

Practical Applications

A

1. D
2. A
3. B
4. C

B

1. C
2. B
3. C
4. D

Crossword Puzzle

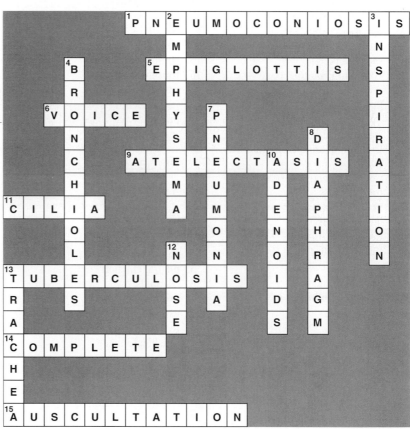

chapter 13

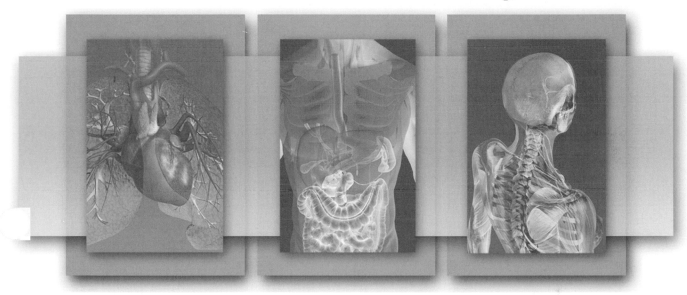

Chapter Thirteen

MULTIPLE CHOICE QUIZ

Name: _____

In the box write the letter of the choice that is the definition of the term or best answers the question. There is only one correct answer for each question.

1. **White blood cell with reddish granules; numbers increase in allergic reactions:** ....
   A. Lymphocyte
   B. Eosinophil
   C. Neutrophil
   D. Erythrocyte
   E. Basophil

2. **Protein threads that form the basis of a clot:** ....
   A. Fibrinogen
   B. Globulin
   C. Hemoglobin
   D. Thrombin
   E. Fibrin

3. **Method of separating out plasma proteins by electrical charge:** ....
   A. Plasmapheresis
   B. Hemolysis
   C. Electrophoresis
   D. Coagulation time
   E. Leukapheresis

4. **Foreign material that invades the body:** ....
   A. Neutrophils
   B. Macrophages
   C. Antibodies
   D. Antigens
   E. Granulocytes

5. **Pigment produced from hemoglobin when red blood cells are destroyed:** ......
   A. Serum
   B. Albumin
   C. Globulin
   D. Plasma
   E. Bilirubin

6. **An undifferentiated blood cell is called a(an):** ....
   A. Granulocyte
   B. Segmented cell
   C. Hematopoietic stem cell
   D. Thrombocyte
   E. Lymphocyte

7. **Anticoagulant found in the blood:** ....
   A. Heparin
   B. Prothrombin
   C. Thrombin
   D. Gamma globulin
   E. Vitamin B_{12}

8. **A disorder of red blood cell morphology is:** ....
   A. Multiple myeloma
   B. Poikilocytosis
   C. Monocytosis
   D. Acute myelocytic leukemia
   E. Hemochromatosis

9. **Deficiency in numbers of white blood cells:** ....
   A. Neutropenia
   B. Hypochromia
   C. Leukocytosis
   D. Chronic lymphocytic leukemia
   E. Spherocytosis

10. **Immature red blood cell:** ....
    A. Thrombocyte
    B. Monoblast
    C. Segmented
    D. Erythroblast
    E. Megakaryoblast

11. **Derived from bone marrow:** ....
    A. Myeloid
    B. Thrombocytopenic
    C. Granulocytopenic
    D. Polymorphonuclear
    E. Phagocytic

12. **Breakdown of recipient's red blood cells when incompatible bloods are mixed:** ....
    A. Erythrocytosis
    B. Hemolysis
    C. Embolism
    D. Anticoagulation
    E. Erythropoiesis

13. **Sideropenia occurs causing deficient production of hemoglobin:**................ ☐
    A. Pernicious anemia
    B. Iron-deficiency anemia
    C. Aplastic anemia
    D. Hemolytic anemia
    E. Thalassemia

14. **Reduction in red blood cells due to excessive cell destruction:**................ ☐
    A. Pernicious anemia
    B. Iron-deficiency anemia
    C. Aplastic anemia
    D. Hemolytic anemia
    E. Thalassemia

15. **Failure of blood cell production due to absence of formation of cells in the bone marrow:** .... ☐
    A. Pernicious anemia
    B. Iron-deficiency anemia
    C. Aplastic anemia
    D. Hemolytic anemia
    E. Thalassemia

16. **Inherited defect in ability to produce hemoglobin:** .... ☐
    A. Pernicious anemia
    B. Iron-deficiency anemia
    C. Aplastic anemia
    D. Hemolytic anemia
    E. Thalassemia

17. **Lack of mature red blood cells due to inability to absorb vitamin B_{12} into the body:**...................... ☐
    A. Pernicious anemia
    B. Iron-deficiency anemia
    C. Aplastic anemia
    D. Hemolytic anemia
    E. Thalassemia

18. **Excessive deposits of iron throughout the body:** .... ☐
    A. Polycythemia vera
    B. Cooley anemia
    C. Purpura
    D. Hemochromatosis
    E. Thrombocytopenia

19. **Symptoms of pallor, shortness of breath, infection, bleeding gums, predominance of immature and abnormally functioning leukocytes, and low numbers of mature neutrophils in a young child may indicate a likely diagnosis of:** .... ☐
    A. Sickle-cell anemia
    B. Hemostasis
    C. Acute lymphocytic leukemia
    D. Chronic lymphocytic leukemia
    E. Hemoglobinopathy

20. **Excessive bleeding caused by congenital lack of Factor VIII or IX:**.... ☐
    A. Autoimmune thrombocytopenic purpura
    B. Granulocytosis
    C. Polycythemia vera
    D. Erythremia
    E. Hemophilia

21. **Venous blood is clotted in a test tube:** ☐
    A. Hematocrit
    B. White blood cell differential
    C. Erythrocyte sedimentation rate
    D. Coagulation time
    E. Red blood cell morphology

22. **Sample of blood is spun in a test tube so that red blood cells fall to the bottom and percentage of RBCs is taken:** .... ☐
    A. Hematocrit
    B. White blood cell differential
    C. Erythrocyte sedimentation rate
    D. Coagulation time
    E. Red blood cell morphology

23. **Blood smear is examined to determine the shape or form of cells:** .... ☐
    A. Hematocrit
    B. White blood cell differential
    C. Erythrocyte sedimentation rate
    D. Coagulation time
    E. Red blood cell morphology

24. **Leukocytes are stained and counted under a microscope to see numbers of mature and immature forms:** ....
    A. Hematocrit
    B. White blood cell differential
    C. Erythrocyte sedimentation rate
    D. Coagulation time
    E. Red blood cell morphology

25. **Venous blood is collected; anti-coagulant added and the distance cells fall in a period of time is determined:** ....
    A. Hematocrit
    B. White blood cell differential
    C. Erythrocyte sedimentation rate
    D. Coagulation time
    E. Red blood cell morphology

26. **Blood protein that maintains the proper proportion and concentration of water in blood:** ....
    A. Bilirubin
    B. Prothrombin
    C. Fibrinogen
    D. Albumin
    E. Globulin

27. **Swelling; fluid leaks out into tissue spaces:** ....
    A. Petechiae
    B. Edema
    C. Ecchymoses
    D. Dyscrasia
    E. Autologous transfusion

28. **IgM, IgG, IgA, IgD, IgE:** ....
    A. Megakaryocytes
    B. Eosinophils
    C. Neutrophils
    D. Stem cells
    E. Immunoglobulins

29. **Symptoms of disease return:** ....
    A. Palliative
    B. Relapse
    C. Hemoglobinopathy
    D. Remission
    E. Spherocytosis

30. **Relieving symptoms, but not curing disease:** ....
    A. Coagulopathy
    B. Hemostasis
    C. Hemolysis
    D. Palliative
    E. Myelopoiesis

Chapter Thirteen
EXERCISE QUIZ

Name: _____

A. *Match the following cells with their meanings below:*

basophil	erythrocyte	lymphocyte	neutrophil
eosinophil	hematopoietic stem cell	monocyte	platelet

1. red blood cell _____

2. white blood cell; phagocyte and precursor of a macrophage _____

3. thrombocyte _____

4. bone marrow cell; gives rise to many types of blood cells _____

5. leukocyte formed in lymph tissue; produces antibodies_____

6. leukocyte with dense, reddish granules; associated with allergic reactions _____

7. leukocyte (poly) formed in bone marrow and having neutral-staining granules _____

8. leukocyte whose granules have an affinity for basic stain; releases histamine and heparin _____

B. *Give medical terms for the following descriptions:*

9. liquid portion of blood _____

10. hormone secreted by the kidney to stimulate erythrocyte production in bone marrow_____

11. proteins in plasma; can be separated into alpha, beta, and gamma types _____

12. plasma protein that maintains the proper amount of water in blood _____

13. proteins made by lymphocytes in response to antigens in the blood_____

C. *Divide the following terms into component parts and give the meaning of the term:*

14. leukocytopenia _____

15. myelopoiesis _____

16. anticoagulant _____

17. thrombolytic_____

D. *Match the following terms concerning red blood cells with their meanings:*

erythropoiesis   erythrocytopenia   poikilocytosis   macrocytosis
hemolysis   hypochromia   polycythemia vera   microcytosis

18. irregularity in shape _____

19. deficiency in numbers _____

20. reduction of hemoglobin ("color") _____

21. increase in numbers of small cells _____

22. erythremia _____

23. increase in numbers of large cells _____

24. formation of red cells _____

25. destruction of red cells _____

E. *Describe the problem in the following forms of anemia:*

26. sickle cell anemia _____

27. aplastic anemia _____

28. thalassemia _____

F. *Give the meanings for the following abbreviations and blood dyscrasias:*

29. CLL _____

30. AML _____

31. autoimmune thrombocytopenic purpura _____

32. hemophilia _____

G. *Match the term in Column I with its meaning in Column II:*

Column I

Column II

33. relapse _____

A. Relieving, but not curing.

34. remission _____

B. Deficiency of all blood cells.

35. purpura

C. Increase in numbers of granulocytes;
    seen in allergic conditions.

36. pancytopenia _____

D. Symptoms of disease return.

37. palliative _____

E. Multiple pinpoint hemorrhages; blood
   accumulates under the skin.

38. eosinophilia _____

F. Separation of blood into its components.

39. apheresis _____

G. Symptoms of disease disappear.

H. Match the following laboratory test or clinical procedure with its description:

autologous transfusion	Coombs test	platelet count
bleeding time	erythrocyte sedimentation rate	red blood cell morphology
bone marrow biopsy	hematocrit	WBC differential
coagulation time	hematopoietic stem cell transplant	

40. A stained blood smear is examined to determine the shape of individual red blood cells_____

41. Measures the percentage of red blood cells in a volume of blood _____

42. Determines the number of clotting cells per cubic millimeter _____

43. Ability of venous blood to clot in a test tube_____

44. Measures the speed at which erythrocytes settle out of plasma_____

45. Determines the numbers of different types of WBCs _____

46. Determines the presence of antibodies in infants of Rh-negative women or patients with autoimmune hemolytic anemia_____

47. Undifferentiated blood cells from a donor are infused into a patient being treated for leukemia or aplastic anemia_____

48. Time it takes for a small puncture wound to stop bleeding _____

49. Needle is introduced into the bone marrow cavity, and a small amount of marrow is aspirated and then examined under the microscope _____

50. Blood is collected from and later reinfused into the same patient_____

Chapter Thirteen
DICTATION AND COMPREHENSION QUIZ: VOCABULARY

Name: _____

A. Dictation of Terms

1. _____   11. _____

2. _____   12. _____

3. _____   13. _____

4. _____   14. _____

5. _____   15. _____

6. _____   16. _____

7. _____   17. _____

8. _____   18. _____

9. _____   19. _____

10. _____   20. _____

B. Comprehension of Terms: Match the number of the above term with its meaning below.

_____ Abnormal condition of blood clotting

_____ Change in structure and function of a cell as it matures; specialization

_____ Platelet precursor found in bone marrow

_____ Protein found in blood; maintains the proper amount of water in blood

_____ Deficiency of iron

_____ Immature bone marrow cell that develops into a white blood cell

_____ Deficiency of a type of white blood cell

_____ Protein threads that form the basis of a blood clot

_____ White blood cell with dense, reddish granules (associated with allergic reactions)

_____ A large cell that engulfs and destroys foreign material

_____ Separation of white blood cells from the rest of the blood (using a centrifuge)

_____ Plasma proteins that contain antibodies

_____ Blood protein found in red blood cells

_____ Plasma minus clotting proteins and cells

_____ Condition of irregularly shaped cells (red blood cells)

_____ Condition of cells of unequal size (red blood cells)

_____ A substance that prevents clotting of blood

_____ Breakdown of recipient's red blood cells when incompatible bloods are mixed

_____ Separation of clotting cells from the rest of the blood (using a centrifuge)

_____ Formation of red blood cells

Chapter Thirteen

DICTATION AND COMPREHENSION QUIZ: PATHOLOGY AND TESTS

Name: _____

A. Dictation of Terms

1 _____   11. _____

2. _____   12. _____

3. _____   13. _____

4. _____   14. _____

5. _____   15. _____

6. _____   16. _____

7. _____   17. _____

8. _____   18. _____

9. _____   19. _____

10. _____   20. _____

B. Comprehension of Terms: Match the number of the above term with its meaning below.

_____ Determines the numbers of different types of leukocytes

_____ Determines the shape or form of erythrocytes

_____ Percentage of erythrocytes in a volume of blood

_____ Any abnormal or pathological condition of the blood

_____ Inherited defect in the ability to produce hemoglobin

_____ Multiple pinpoint hemorrhages; thrombocytopenia

_____ Erythremia

_____ Excessive bleeding caused by lack of Factor VIII or IX

_____ Lymphoblasts predominate in the blood; most often seen in children

_____ Malignant tumor of bone marrow

_____ Separation of blood into its parts

_____ Time required for venous blood to clot in a test tube

_____ Small amount of bone marrow is aspirated and examined under a microscope

_____ Relieving pain, but not curing an illness

_____ Lack of mature erythrocytes owing to inability to absorb vitamin B_{12}

_____ Both mature and immature granulocytes are present in bone marrow and blood

_____ Total amount of a blood protein is measured in a sample of blood

_____ Symptoms of disease return

_____ Symptoms of disease disappear

_____ Speed at which red blood cells settle out of plasma

Chapter Thirteen
SPELLING QUIZ

Name: _____

A. Circle the term that is spelled correctly, and write its meaning in the space provided:

1. myeloma   myleoma _____
2. erythropoeisis   erythropoiesis _____
3. billirubin   bilirubin _____
4. fibrinogen   fibrinogin _____
5. platlet   platelet _____
6. poykilocytosis   poikilocytosis _____
7. leukopheresis   leukapheresis _____
8. heparin   heparine _____
9. electropheresis   electrophoresis _____
10. thallassemia   thalassemia _____

B. Circle the term that is spelled correctly. The meaning of each term is given.

11. deficiency of clotting cells .... thrombositopenea   thrombocytopenia   thrombocitopenia

12. process of clotting .... coagulation   coagglulation   coaglulation

13. large cell that engulfs foreign
material and worn out red blood cells ... macrophage   macropage   makrophage

14. white blood cell that destroys
foreign material by phagocytosis .... neutrophil   neutrophill   nuetrophil

15. blood protein .... allbumen   albumen   albumin

16. lack of mature red blood cells owing to
inability to absorb vitamin B_{12} .... pernicious anemia   perniscious anemia   panescius anemia

17. relieving symptoms but not
curing .... palliative   pallitive   paliative

18. produced in bone marrow .... myleogenous   myleoginus   myelogenous

19. a protein with antibody activity .... immunoglobulen   immunoglobulin   inmunoglobulen

20. increase in red blood cells .... polycythemia vera   polycytemia vera   polysithemia vera

Chapter Thirteen
PRONUNCIATION QUIZ

Name: _____

A. Underline the accented syllable in the following terms:

1. hemolysis
2. anisocytosis
3. erythropoietin
4. purpura
5. anticoagulant
6. eosinophil
7. albumin
8. differentiation
9. myelodysplasia
10. leukocytopenia

B. Match the term in Column I with its meaning in Column II:

Column I

1. megakaryocyte   _____
2. reticulocyte   _____
3. myeloid   _____
4. fibrin   _____
5. electrophoresis   _____
6. plateletpheresis   _____
7. bilirubin   _____
8. heparin   _____
9. hematocrit   _____
10. serum   _____

Column II

A. Orange-yellow pigment formed from destruction of hemoglobin.

B. Separation of clotting cells from rest of the blood.

C. Plasma minus clotting proteins and cells.

D. Derived from bone marrow.

E. An anticoagulant substance.

F. An immature red blood cell.

G. Percentage of red blood cells in a volume of blood.

H. Separation of plasma proteins using electricity.

I. An immature clotting cell.

J. Protein threads that form the essence of a blood clot.

C. Complete the following terms using the definitions given:

1. hemo_____   Stoppage or control of blood flow.

2. dys_____   Any blood disorder.

3. re_____   Symptoms of disease return.

4. _____ ology   Study of the shape of cells.

5. anti _____   A foreign substance that stimulates the formation of antibodies.

6. anti _____   Protein substances formed in the blood to destroy foreign substances.

7. _____ cyte   A cell that engulfs another cell.

8. _____emia   A type of inherited anemia marked by defective type of hemoglobin in people of Mediterranean background.

Chapter Thirteen
DIAGRAM QUIZ

Name: _____

Label the diagram below using the terms listed below:

Band cell	Hematopoietic stem cell	Monocyte	Platelets
Erythroblast	Lymphocyte	Myeloblast	
Erythrocytes	Megakaryocyte	Neutrophil	

1. _____

2. _____   4. _____   Monoblast   Lymphoblast   Mega-karyoblast

Bone marrow

Normoblast

Basophilic   Neutrophilic   Eosinophilic
metamyelocyte metamyelocyte metamyelocyte

Circulating in bloodstream

Reticulocyte

5. _____

Segmented

7. _____   8. _____

9. _____

Mature cells

3. _____   **Basophilic** granulocyte   6. _____   **Eosinophilic** granulocyte   **Mononuclear** agranulocytes   10. _____

Chapter Thirteen
VOCABULARY QUIZ

Name: _____

A. *Match the following terms with their meanings below:*

albumin	bilirubin	electrophoresis
antibody	differentiation	eosinophil
antigen	coagulation	
basophil	colony-stimulating factor	

1. Orange-yellow pigment in bile; formed by the breakdown of hemoglobin when red blood cells die _____

2. Protein that stimulates the growth and proliferation of white blood cells (granulocytes) _____

3. Protein in blood; maintains the proper amount of water in the blood _____

4. Granulocytic white blood cell; granules turn blue with basic stain_____

5. Blood clotting _____

6. Substance (usually foreign) that stimulates the production of antibodies _____

7. Change in structure and function of a cell as it matures; specialization_____

8. Protein produced by lymphocytes in response to antigens _____

9. Method of separating serum proteins by electrical charge_____

10. Granulocytic white blood cell associated with allergic reactions; granules turn red with acidic stain _____

B. *Match the following terms with their meanings below:*

erythrocyte	globulins	heparin
erythropoietin	granulocyte	immune reaction
fibrin	hemoglobin	hemolysis
fibrinogen		

1. Destruction or breakdown of blood (red blood cells) _____

2. Protein threads that form the basis of a blood clot_____

3. Blood protein that contains iron and carries oxygen in red blood cells_____

4. Red blood cell _____

5. White blood cell; eosinophil, basophil, and neutrophil _____

6. Plasma protein that is converted to fibrin in the clotting process_____

7. Anticoagulant found in blood and tissues _____

8. Hormone secreted by the kidneys; stimulates formation of red blood cells _____

9. Response of the immune system to invasion by foreign substances (antigens) _____

10. Part of the blood containing plasma proteins; alpha, beta, and gamma are examples _____

C. *Match the following terms with their meanings below:*

immunoglobulin	megakaryocyte	prothrombin
leukocyte	**plasma**	reticulocyte
lymphocyte	plasmapheresis	
macrophage	platelet	

1. Removal of plasma from blood _____

2. Mononuclear white blood cell that produces antibodies _____

3. Immature red blood cell _____

4. White blood cell _____

5. Large immature clotting cell _____

6. Plasma protein converted to thrombin in the clotting process _____

7. Protein with antibody activity; IgG, IgM, IgA, IgE, IgD are examples _____

8. Thrombocyte _____

9. Monocyte that is a large phagocyte _____

10. Liquid portion of blood; contains water, proteins, salts, nutrients, hormones,
   and vitamins _____

D.

1. What is serum? _____

2. What is a hematopoietic stem cell? _____

3. What is a neutrophil? _____

Chapter Thirteen
REVIEW SHEET QUIZ

Name: _____

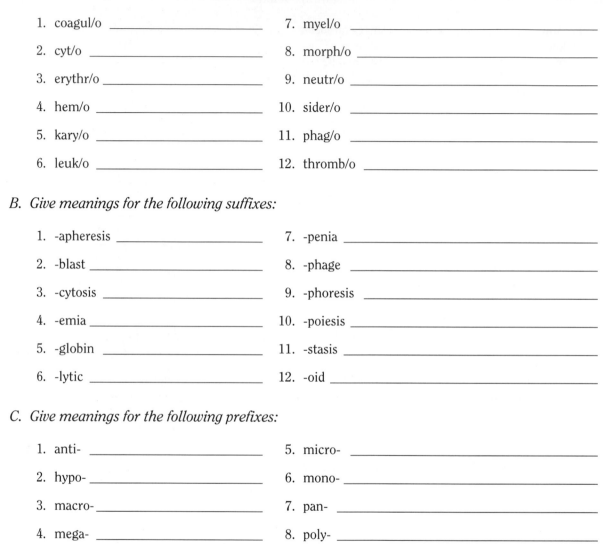

A. Give meanings for the following combining forms:

1. coagul/o _____   7. myel/o _____

2. cyt/o _____   8. morph/o _____

3. erythr/o _____   9. neutr/o _____

4. hem/o _____   10. sider/o _____

5. kary/o _____   11. phag/o _____

6. leuk/o _____   12. thromb/o _____

B. Give meanings for the following suffixes:

1. -apheresis _____   7. -penia _____

2. -blast _____   8. -phage _____

3. -cytosis _____   9. -phoresis _____

4. -emia _____   10. -poiesis _____

5. -globin _____   11. -stasis _____

6. -lytic _____   12. -oid _____

C. Give meanings for the following prefixes:

1. anti- _____   5. micro- _____

2. hypo- _____   6. mono- _____

3. macro- _____   7. pan- _____

4. mega- _____   8. poly- _____

Chapter Thirteen

CROSSWORD PUZZLE

Name: _____

Fill in the crossword puzzle below using the clues listed underneath it.

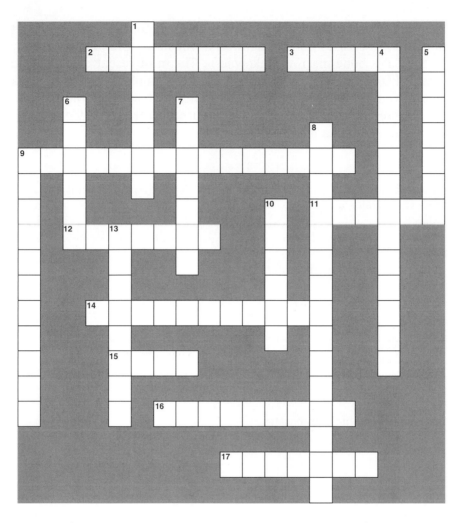

Across Clues

2. Excessive increase in white blood cells with immature forms.
3. Plasma minus clotting proteins and blood cells.
9. Method of separating plasma proteins by electrical charge.
11. Protein threads that form the base of a clot.
12. Protein found in blood.
14. Process of blood clotting.
15. Iron-containing nonprotein portion of the hemoglobin molecule.
16. White blood cell.
17. Derived from bone marrow.

Down Clues

1. Multiple pinpoint hemorrhages and accumulation of blood under the skin.
4. Platelet precursor formed in the bone marrow.
5. -globulin means_____.
6. Deficiency in erythrocytes or hemoglobin.
7. An anticoagulant produced by liver cells and found in blood and tissues.
8. Change in structure and function of a cell as it matures.
9. Red blood cell.
10. The protein part of hemoglobin.
13. White blood cell with large, dark-staining granules.

Chapter Thirteen

PRACTICAL APPLICATIONS

Name: _____

A. Research Report

Colony-stimulating factors are hormones that regulate hematopoiesis. Erythropoietin (Epogen), secreted by the kidney, increases bone marrow erythropoiesis. Granulocyte colony-stimulating factor (G-CSF) stimulates bone marrow leukopoiesis. The most recent colony-stimulating factor is thrombopoietin (TPO), which acts on bone marrow to promote the growth of platelets. These hormones are now produced biosynthetically by recombinant DNA techniques and have shown some impact in the prevention of chemotherapy-induced neutropenia, treatment of cytopenias associated with myelodysplasias, and aplastic anemia.

1. **What is erythropoietin?.......................** ☐
   A. A drug that causes bone marrow suppression
   B. A chemical that promotes white cell production
   C. A recombinant product that stimulates platelet growth
   D. A renal hormone that stimulates growth of RBCs

2. **G-CSF is helpful in:...........................** ☐
   A. Preventing decrease in WBCs during drug treatment for cancer
   B. Replacing red blood cells after hemorrhage
   C. Stimulating formation of thrombocytes
   D. Stimulating lymphocytes

3. **Myelodysplasia means:........................** ☐
   A. The spleen is not functioning.
   B. Liver formation is impaired.
   C. Blood cells are not made.
   D. The bone marrow is not forming blood cells properly.

4. **TPO is: ....** ☐
   A. A neutrophil growth factor
   B. An erythrocyte growth factor
   C. A clotting cell growth factor useful in the treatment of thrombocytopenia
   D. Useful in the treatment of hemophilia

B. Case Report

A 17-year-old white female was admitted to the ER for melena. A CBC showed the hemoglobin to be 9.0 g%, hematocrit 27%, WBC 32,000/mm³ with 21% polys, 7% bands, 70% lymphocytes, and 2% monocytes. Platelet count was 20,000/mm³. Bone marrow aspiration and smear shows evidence of lymphoblasts.

1. **What was the patient's admitting symptom?...** ☐
   A. Diarrhea
   B. Blood in her stool
   C. Vomiting blood
   D. Spitting up blood

2. **What do the lab data tell about RBCs?** ☐
   A. None of the tests reflect information about RBCs.
   B. RBCs are normal.
   C. RBCs are elevated.
   D. RBCs are decreased as evidenced by low hematocrit and hemoglobin.

3. **What is a likely diagnosis for the patient?...** ☐
   A. Sickle-cell anemia
   B. Hemophilia
   C. Acute lymphoblastic leukemia
   D. Chronic myelocytic leukemia

4. **The bone marrow was filled with:........** ☐
   A. Immature white blood cells
   B. Mature neutrophils
   C. Platelets
   D. Immature red blood cells

Chapter Thirteen
ANSWERS TO THE QUIZZES

Multiple Choice Quiz

1. B	5. E	9. A	13. B	17. A	21. D	25. C	29. B
2. E	6. C	10. D	14. D	18. D	22. A	26. D	30. D
3. C	7. A	11. A	15. C	19. C	23. E	27. B	
4. D	8. B	12. B	16. E	20. E	24. B	28. E	

Exercise Quiz

A

1. erythrocyte
2. monocyte
3. platelet
4. stem cell
5. lymphocyte
6. eosinophil
7. neutrophil
8. basophil

B

9. plasma
10. erythropoietin
11. globulin
12. albumin
13. immunoglobulins (antibodies)

C

14. deficiency of white blood cells
15. formation of bone marrow
16. substance that stops clotting
17. pertaining to destruction of clots

D

18. poikilocytosis
19. erythrocytopenia
20. hypochromia
21. microcytosis
22. polycythemia vera
23. macrocytosis
24. erythropoiesis
25. hemolysis

E

26. abnormally shaped red blood cells cause hemolysis (hereditary condition)
27. blood cells are not formed or produced in the bone marrow
28. inherited defect in ability to produce hemoglobin

F

29. chronic lymphocytic leukemia
30. acute myelogenous leukemia

31. deficiency of platelets with hemorrhages into the skin; no known cause
32. excessive bleeding caused by hereditary lack of clotting factor VIII or IX

G

33. D
34. G
35. E
36. B
37. A
38. C
39. F

H

40. red blood cell morphology
41. hematocrit
42. platelet count
43. coagulation time
44. erythrocyte sedimentation rate
45. WBC differential
46. Coombs test
47. bone marrow transplant
48. bleeding time
49. bone marrow biopsy
50. autologous transfusion

Dictation and Comprehension Quiz: Vocabulary and Terminology

A

1. hemolysis
2. albumin
3. anisocytosis
4. anticoagulant
5. differentiation
6. eosinophil
7. erythropoiesis
8. fibrin
9. gamma globulins
10. hemoglobin
11. leukapheresis
12. macrophage
13. megakaryocyte
14. myeloblast
15. neutropenia
16. plateletpheresis
17. poikilocytosis
18. serum
19. sideropenia
20. thrombosis

B

20 Abnormal condition of blood clotting
5 Change in structure and function of a cell as it matures; specialization
13 Platelet precursor found in bone marrow
2 Protein found in blood; maintains the proper amount of water in blood
19 Deficiency of iron
14 Immature bone marrow cell that develops into a white blood cell
15 Deficiency of a type of white blood cell
8 Protein threads that form the basis of a blood clot
6 White blood cell with dense, reddish granules (associated with allergic reactions)
12 A large cell that engulfs and destroys foreign material
11 Separation of white blood cells from the rest of the blood (using a centrifuge)
9 Plasma proteins that contain antibodies
10 Blood protein found in red blood cells
18 Plasma minus clotting proteins and cells
17 Condition of irregularly shaped cells (red blood cells)
3 Condition of cells of unequal size (red blood cells)
4 A substance that prevents clotting of blood

1 Breakdown of recipient's red blood cells when incompatible bloods are mixed
16 Separation of clotting cells from the rest of the blood (using a centrifuge)
7 Formation of red blood cells

Dictation and Comprehension Quiz: Pathology and Tests

A

1. acute lymphocytic leukemia
2. apheresis
3. bone marrow biopsy
4. chronic myelogenous leukemia
5. coagulation time
6. dyscrasia
7. erythrocyte sedimentation rate
8. hematocrit
9. hemoglobin test
10. hemophilia
11. multiple myeloma
12. palliative
13. pernicious anemia
14. polycythemia vera
15. purpura
16. red blood cell morphology
17. relapse
18. remission
19. thalassemia
20. white blood cell differential

B

20 Determines the numbers of different types of leukocytes
16 Determines the shape or form of erythrocytes
8 Percentage of erythrocytes in a volume of blood
6 Any abnormal or pathological condition of the blood
19 Inherited defect in the ability to produce hemoglobin
15 Multiple pinpoint hemorrhages; thrombocytopenia
14 Erythremia
10 Excessive bleeding caused by lack of Factor VIII or IX
1 Lymphoblasts predominate in the blood; most often seen in children
11 Malignant tumor of bone marrow
2 Separation of blood into its parts
5 Time required for venous blood to clot in a test tube
3 Small amount of bone marrow is aspirated and examined under a microscope

12 Relieving pain, but not curing an illness
13 Lack of mature erythrocytes owing to inability to absorb vitamin B_{12}
4 Both mature and immature granulocytes are present in bone marrow and blood
9 Total amount of a blood protein is measured in a sample of blood
17 Symptoms of disease return
18 Symptoms of disease disappear
7 Speed at which red cells settle out of plasma

Spelling Quiz

A

1. myeloma—tumor of bone marrow
2. erythropoiesis—formation of red blood cells
3. bilirubin—pigment released with RBC destruction
4. fibrinogen—clotting protein in blood
5. platelet—clotting cell
6. poikilocytosis—abnormal shape of RBCs
7. leukapheresis—separation of WBCs
8. heparin—anticoagulant found in tissues
9. electrophoresis—separation of proteins by electrical charge
10. thalassemia—deficiency of hemoglobin (hereditary)

B

11. thrombocytopenia
12. coagulation
13. macrophage
14. neutrophil
15. albumin
16. pernicious anemia
17. palliative
18. myelogenous
19. immunoglobulin
20. polycythemia vera

Pronunciation Quiz

A

1. he<u>mol</u>ysis
2. anisocy<u>tosis</u>
3. erythro<u>poi</u>etin
4. <u>pur</u>pura
5. anticoa<u>gul</u>ant

6. eo<u>sin</u>ophil
7. al<u>bu</u>min
8. differenti<u>ation</u>
9. myelodys<u>plasia</u>
10. leukocyto<u>penia</u>

B

1. I
2. F
3. D
4. J
5. H
6. B
7. A
8. E
9. G
10. C

C

1. hemostasis
2. dyscrasia
3. relapse
4. morphology
5. antigen
6. antibodies
7. phagocyte
8. thalassemia

Diagram Quiz

1. hematopoietic stem cell
2. erythroblast
3. erythrocytes
4. myeloblast
5. band cell
6. neutrophil
7. monocyte
8. lymphocyte
9. megakaryocyte
10. platelets

Vocabulary Quiz

A

1. bilirubin
2. colony-stimulating factor (CSF)
3. albumin
4. basophil
5. coagulation
6. antigen
7. differentiation
8. antibody
9. electrophoresis
10. eosinophil

B

1. hemolysis
2. fibrin
3. hemoglobin
4. erythrocyte
5. granulocyte

6. fibrinogen
7. heparin
8. erythropoietin
9. immune reaction
10. globulins

C

1. plasmapheresis
2. lymphocyte
3. reticulocyte
4. leukocyte
5. megakaryocyte
6. prothrombin
7. immunoglobulin
8. platelet
9. macrophage
10. plasma

D

1. Serum is plasma (clear, yellowish fluid) minus the clotting proteins and cells.
2. A hematopoietic stem cell is a stem cell in the bone marrow that gives rise to all the different types of blood cells.
3. A neutrophil is a granulocytic white blood cell that fights disease by phagocytosis. Also called a polymorphonuclear leukocyte ("poly") or a segmented cell ("seg").

Review Sheet Quiz

A

1. clotting
2. cell
3. red
4. blood
5. nucleus
6. white
7. bone marrow
8. shape, form
9. neutral (neutrophils)
10. iron
11. eat, swallow
12. clot

B

1. removal, carry away
2. immature cell, embryonic
3. abnormal condition of cells
4. blood condition
5. protein
6. pertaining to destruction
7. deficiency
8. eat, swallow
9. carrying, transmission
10. formation
11. stop, control
12. derived from

C

1. against
2. under, deficiency
3. large
4. large
5. small
6. one
7. all
8. many, much

Practical Applications

A

1. D
2. A
3. D
4. C

B

1. B
2. D
3. C
4. A

Crossword Puzzle

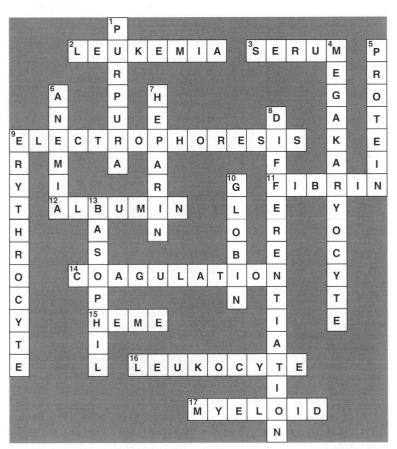

Chapter Thirteen
Answers to Combining Forms and Terminology Sections

Terminology	Meaning
basophil	White blood cell with dark-staining granules that have an affinity for basic dyes.
hypochromic	Pertaining to deficiency of color (reduction of hemoglobin in red blood cells).
anticoagulant	A substance that works against coagulation (blood clotting).
coagulopathy	Disease of the clotting process.
cytology	Study of cells.
eosinophil	White blood cell with dark-staining granules that have an affinity for acid dyes; granules turn red (eosin) in the presence of dye.
erythrocytopenia	Deficiency of red blood cells.
granulocyte	White blood cell with large, dark-staining granules in its cytoplasm.
hemolysis	Destruction of blood cells.
hematocrit	Separation of blood; percentage of red blood cells in a given volume of blood.
hemoglobinopathy	Disease of abnormal hemoglobins (sickle-cell anemia, thalassemia).
anisocytosis	Abnormal condition of unequal size of cells (erythrocytes).
megakaryocyte	Cell with multiple large nuclei; immature platelet.
leukocytopenia	Deficiency of white blood cells.
monocyte	White blood cell with one large nucleus; an agranulocyte and phagocyte.
morphology	Study of shape or form (of blood cells).
myeloblast	Bone marrow cell that develops into a myelocyte and then a leukocyte.
myelogenous	Pertaining to formed in the bone marrow.
neutropenia	Deficiency in neutrophils.
mononuclear	Pertaining to a white blood cell with one large nucleus (monocyte or lymphocyte).
polymorphonuclear	Pertaining to a white blood cell with a multilobed nucleus (neutrophil).
phagocyte	Cell that ingests other cells or microorganisms.
poikilocytosis	Irregularity in the shape of red blood cells.
sideropenia	Deficiency in iron in serum.
spherocytosis	Condition (abnormal) in which erythrocytes assume a spheroidal (rounded) shape.
thrombocytopenia	Deficiency of clotting cells.

Suffixes

plasmapheresis	Removal of plasma from the rest of the blood by mechanical means (centrifuge).
leukapheresis	Removal of white blood cells from the rest of the blood by centrifugation.
plateletpheresis	Removal of platelets from the rest of the blood by centrifugation.
monoblast	Immature white blood cell (monocyte).
erythroblast	Immature red blood cell.
macrocytosis	Abnormal condition (slight increase in numbers) of macrocytes (red blood cells that are larger than normal).
microcytosis	Abnormal condition (slight increase in numbers) of microcytes (red blood cells that are smaller than normal).
leukemia	Abnormal condition of white blood cells (increase in numbers of malignant cells).
hemoglobin	Blood protein in erythrocytes; enables the cell to carry oxygen.
immunoglobulin	Protein (antibody produced by plasma cells) that acts to protect the body by destroying antigens.
thrombolytic therapy	Treatment that destroys blood clots.

myeloid	Derived from bone marrow.
thrombosis	Abnormal condition of clotting.
granulocytopenia	Deficiency of granulocytes (white blood cells).
pancytopenia	Deficiency of all (blood) cells.
macrophage	Large cell (in blood and tissues) that eats (engulfs) other cells; derived from a monocyte.
eosinophilia	Increase in numbers of eosinophils.
neutrophilia	Increase in numbers of neutrophils.
electrophoresis	Separation of proteins in a solution by using an electric current (used to separate protein fractions of serum, urine, or cerebrospinal fluid).
hematopoiesis	Formation of blood cells.
erythropoiesis	Formation of erythrocytes.
myelopoiesis	Formation of bone marrow.
hemostasis	Stoppage of the flow of blood.

chapter 14

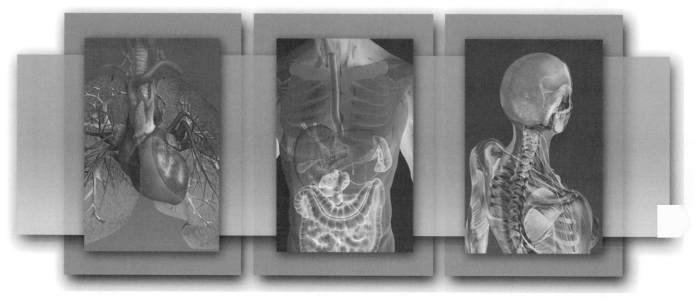

Chapter Fourteen
MULTIPLE CHOICE QUIZ
Name: _____

In the box write the letter of the choice that is the definition of the term or best answers the question. There is only one correct answer for each question.

1. **Formation of lymph:** .... ☐
   A. Lymphocytopenia
   B. Lymphadenitis
   C. Lymphedema
   D. Lymphopoiesis
   E. Lymphoid

2. **Interstitial fluid contains or is:** .... ☐
   A. Antibodies produced by white blood cells
   B. Red and white blood cells
   C. Found in the spaces between cells and becomes lymph when it enters lymph capillaries
   D. Connective tissue
   E. Blood clotting factors

3. **All of the following are part of the immune system EXCEPT:** .... ☐
   A. Lymphocytes
   B. Platelets
   C. Monocytes
   D. Phagocytes
   E. Antibodies

4. **All of the following describe areas of lymph node concentration EXCEPT:** ... ☐
   A. inguinal
   B. axillary
   C. bone marrow
   D. mediastinal
   E. cervical

5. **B cells, plasma cells, and antibodies are part of:** .... ☐
   A. Lymphocytosis
   B. Cytotoxic immunity
   C. Growth factor biology
   D. Cell-mediated immunity
   E. Humoral immunity

6. **Helper or suppressor cells are types of:** .... ☐
   A. B cells
   B. T cells
   C. Platelets
   D. Antigens
   E. Antibiotics

7. **Examples of immunoglobulins:** .... ☐
   A. IgA, IgG, IgE
   B. Monocytes
   C. Lymphocytes
   D. Hepatocytes
   E. Clotting factors

8. **Oropharyngeal lymph tissue:** .... ☐
   A. Spleen
   B. Thymus
   C. Bone marrow
   D. Tonsils
   E. Adenoids

9. **Mediastinal T cell producer:** .... ☐
   A. Spleen
   B. Thymus
   C. Bone marrow
   D. Tonsils
   E. Adenoids

10. **Nasopharyngeal lymph tissue:** .... ☐
    A. Spleen
    B. Thymus
    C. Bone marrow
    D. Tonsils
    E. Adenoids

11. **Abdominal organ that filters erythrocytes and activates lymphocytes:** .... ☐
    A. Spleen
    B. Thymus
    C. Bone marrow
    D. Tonsils
    E. Adenoids

12. **Produces lymphocytes and monocytes and all other blood cells:** .... ☐
    A. Spleen
    B. Thymus
    C. Bone marrow
    D. Tonsils
    E. Adenoids

13. **Cytotoxic cells are:** .... ☐
    A. B cell lymphocytes
    B. T cell lymphocytes
    C. Platelets
    D. Thrombocytes
    E. Eosinophils

14. **Interferons and interleukins are:** .... ☐
    A. Gamma globulins
    B. Interstitial fluid
    C. Antiviral proteins produced by T cell
       lymphocytes
    D. Produced by B cell lymphocytes
    E. Helper cells

15. **Slight increase in numbers of**
    lymphocytes: .... ☐
    A. Lymphocytopenia
    B. Lymphopoiesis
    C. Lymphoid
    D. Lymphocytosis
    E. Lymphedema

16. **Pertaining to poison:** .... ☐
    A. Necrotic
    B. Hypoxic
    C. Cyanotic
    D. Toxic
    E. Stenotic

17. **Computerized x-ray imaging in the**
    transverse plane: .... ☐
    A. CT scan
    B. Lymphangiogram
    C. Ultrasonography
    D. MRI
    E. Lymphadenectomy

18. **HIV is:** .... ☐
    A. A malignancy associated with AIDS
    B. A drug used to treat AIDS
    C. The virus that causes AIDS
    D. The test used to detect AIDS
    E. A type of lymphoma

19. **Malignant tumor of lymph nodes:** .... ☐
    A. Sarcoidosis
    B. Lymphedema
    C. Hodgkin disease
    D. Hypersplenism
    E. Lymphocytopenia

20. **Viral infection causing blisters on**
    skin of lips, nose, or genitals: .... ☐
    A. Kaposi sarcoma
    B. Herpes simplex
    C. Cryptococcus
    D. Toxoplasmosis
    E. *Pneumocystis carinii* pneumonia

21. **Cancer arising from the lining cells**
    of capillaries, producing bluish-red
    skin nodules: .... ☐
    A. Kaposi sarcoma
    B. Herpes simplex
    C. Cryptococcus
    D. Toxoplasmosis
    E. *Pneumocystis carinii* pneumonia

22. **Major lung infection with fever, cough,**
    chest pain, and sputum. Treatment is
    with Bactrim: .... ☐
    A. Kaposi sarcoma
    B. Herpes simplex
    C. Cryptococcus
    D. Toxoplasmosis
    E. *Pneumocystis carinii* pneumonia

23. **Protozoan (parasitic) infection**
    associated with AIDS. Produces
    pneumonitis, hepatitis, and
    encephalitis: .... ☐
    A. Kaposi sarcoma
    B. Herpes simplex
    C. Cryptococcosis
    D. Toxoplasmosis
    E. *Pneumocystis carinii* pneumonia

24. **Fungal infection associated with**
    AIDS. Involves brain and meninges,
    lungs, and skin: .... ☐
    A. Kaposi sarcoma
    B. Herpes simplex
    C. Cryptococcosis
    D. Toxoplasmosis
    E. *Pneumocystis carinii* pneumonia

25. **Atopy is:** .... ☐
    A. An early stage of AIDS
    B. A hypersensitivity or allergic state
    C. A type of lymphoma
    D. A disease found in tropical areas
    E. Acute infectious disease caused by
       Epstein-Barr virus

Chapter Fourteen
EXERCISE QUIZ

Name: _____

The questions on this quiz have all been taken from the exercises at the end of this chapter.

A. Give the name of the structure or fluid from its meaning below:

1. Stationary lymph tissue along the path of lymph vessels _____

2. Large thoracic lymph vessel draining lymph from lower and left side of the body _____

3. Organ near the stomach that produces, stores, and eliminates blood cells _____

4. Mass of lymph tissue in the nasopharynx _____

5. Organ in the mediastinum that produces T cell lymphocytes _____

6. Tiniest of lymph vessels _____

7. Large lymph vessel in the chest that drains lymph from right upper part of the body _____

8. Fluid that lies between cells and becomes lymph as it enters lymph capillaries _____

B. Give the locations of the following lymph nodes:

9. inguinal nodes _____   11. cervical nodes _____

10. axillary nodes _____   12. mediastinal nodes _____

C. Match the term in Column I with its description in Column II

Column I		Column II
13. immunoglobulins	_____	A. T-cell lymphocytes that inhibit the activity of B cell lymphocytes.
14. toxins	_____	B. Antibodies—IgG, IgE, IgM, IgD.
15. helper T cells	_____	C. T-cell lymphocytes; aid B cells and antibody production; T4 cells.
16. cytotoxic cells	_____	D. Poisons (antigens).
17. interferons	_____	E. T-cell lymphocytes that directly kill foreign cells; T8 cells.
18. plasma cells	_____	F. Anti-viral proteins secreted by T cells.
19. suppressor T cells	_____	G. Transformed B cells that secrete antibodies.

D. Build medical terms:

20. removal of the spleen _____

21. inflammation of lymph glands (nodes) _____

22. tumor of the thymus gland _____

23. disease of lymph glands (nodes) _____

24. formation of lymph _____

25. deficiency of lymph cells _____

26. pertaining to poison _____

27. enlargement of the spleen _____

E. Match the following terms with their meanings below:

AIDS   Hodgkin disease   lymphoid organs
allergen   hypersplenism   thymectomy
anaphylaxis   lymphedema

28. syndrome marked by enlargement of the spleen and associated
    with anemia, leukopenia, and anemia _____

29. an extraordinary hypersensitivity to a foreign protein; marked
    by hypotension, shock, respiratory distress _____

30. an antigen capable of causing allergy (hypersensitivity) _____

31. disorder in which the immune system is suppressed by exposure to HIV _____

32. removal of a mediastinal organ _____

33. malignant tumor of lymph nodes and spleen marked by
    Reed-Sternberg cell identified in lymph nodes _____

34. tissues that produce lymphocytes—spleen, thymus, tonsils, and adenoids _____

35. swelling of tissues due to interstitial fluid accumulation _____

F. Give meanings for the following terms or abbreviations:

36. HIV _____

37. Histo _____

38. KS _____

39. PCP _____

40. CT scan _____

41. Toxo _____

G. Circle the correct answer in the following sentences:

42. An immune response in which B cells transform into plasma cells and secrete antibodies is known as **(cell-mediated, humoral)** immunity.

43. Lymphocytes, formed in the thymus gland, that act on antigens are **(B cells, T cells, macrophages)**.

44. An immune response in which T cells destroy antigens is called **(cell-mediated, humoral)** immunity.

45. Lymphocytes that transform into plasma cells and secrete antibodies are called **(B cells, T cells)**.

H. Match the following terms with their meanings below:

ELISA   helper T cells
immunoelectrophoresis   zidovudine
opportunistic infections

46. white blood cells that are destroyed by HIV _____

47. test to separate immunoglobulins _____

48. drug used to treat AIDS by blocking the growth of AIDS virus _____

49. test used to detect anti-HIV antibodies _____

50. group of infectious diseases associated with AIDS _____

Chapter Fourteen
DICTATION AND COMPREHENSION QUIZ

Name: _____

A. Dictation of Terms

1. _____   11. _____
2. _____   12. _____
3. _____   13. _____
4. _____   14. _____
5. _____   15. _____
6. _____   16. _____
7. _____   17. _____
8. _____   18. _____
9. _____   19. _____
10. _____   20. _____

B. Comprehension of Terms: Match the number of the above term with its meaning below.

_____ Malignant tumor associated with AIDS; appears as bluish-red skin nodules

_____ Hypersensitive or allergic state involving hereditary predisposition

_____ Disease condition of lymph nodes

_____ Enlargement of the spleen

_____ Collection of lymph tissue in the groin

_____ Substance capable of causing a specific hypersensitivity reaction in the body

_____ A drug that is used to treat AIDS by blocking the production of an enzyme

_____ An exaggerated or unusual hypersensitivity to a foreign protein

_____ Immune response in which B cells transform into plasma cells and secrete antibodies

_____ Antiviral proteins secreted by T cells

_____ Malignant tumor of a gland in the chest

_____ Found within lymphatic vessels and surrounding tissues throughout the body

_____ Lymphatic tissue in the oropharynx

_____ Collection of lymph tissue under the arm (armpit)

_____ Immune response involving T-cell lymphocytes

_____ Malignant tumor of lymph nodes and tissue

_____ Antibodies such as IgG, IgA, IgD that are secreted by plasma cells

_____ Introduction of altered antigens to produce an immune response

_____ Repression of the immune response

_____ Fluid collects within the spaces between cells secondary to lymph vessel obstruction

Chapter Fourteen
SPELLING QUIZ

Name: _____

A. Circle the term that is spelled correctly and write its meaning:

1. mackrophage   macrophage _____

2. lypmh   lymph _____

3. immunoglobulins   immunoglobins _____

4. alergy   allergy _____

5. inguinal nodes   ingiunal nodes _____

6. anaphylaxis   anaphilaxis _____

7. Hogdkin disease   Hodgkin disease _____

8. axilliary nodes   axillary nodes _____

9. lymphosytopenia   lymphocytopenia _____

10. splenectomy   spleenectomy _____

B. Circle the term that is spelled correctly. The meaning of each term is given.

11. organ in the chest that produces
    T cells .... thymus gland   thymis gland   thimus gland

12. fluid in the spaces between cells .... intrastitial fluid   interstitial fluid   interstitiel fluid

13. collection of fluid in tissues .... lymphaedmea   lypmhfedema   lymphedema

14. proteins that stimulate the growth of
    T cells .... interleukins   interleukens   interluekins

15. masses of lymph tissue in the
    nasopharynx .... adneoidz   adeniods   adenoids

16. introduction of altered antigens
    to produce an immune response .... vaccination   vacination   vakcination

17. inflammation of tonsils .... tonsilitis   toncilitis   tonsillitis

18. formation of lymph .... lymphopoesis   lymphopoiesis   lymphopeosis.

Chapter Fourteen
PRONUNCIATION QUIZ

Name: _____

A. *Underline the accented syllables in the following terms:*

1. immunology
2. hypersensitivity
3. inguinal nodes
4. lymphedema
5. interstitial fluid
6. Kaposi sarcoma
7. macrophage
8. anaphylaxis
9. thoracic duct
10. lymphadenopathy

B. *Match the term in Column I with its meaning in Column II:*

Column I

1. anaphylaxis _____
2. AIDS _____
3. cervical nodes _____
4. adenoids _____
5. interferons _____
6. macrophage _____
7. Hodgkin disease _____
8. hypersplenism _____
9. atopy _____
10. immunoglobulins _____

Column II

A. Mass of lymph tissue in the nasopharynx.

B. Syndrome marked by enlargement of the spleen.

C. Suppression or deficiency of the immune response caused by exposure to HIV.

D. A hypersensitivity or allergic state involving an inherited predisposition.

E. Exaggerated hypersensitivity reaction.

F. Antibodies secreted by plasma cells.

G. Antiviral proteins secreted by T cells.

H. Lymph nodes in the neck.

I. Malignancy of lymph nodes.

J. Large phagocyte found in lymph nodes.

C. *Complete the following terms using the definitions given:*

1. _____ ectomy   Removal of the spleen.

2. _____ oma   Tumor of the thymus gland.

3. _____ gram   Record (x-ray) of lymph vessels.

4. _____ infections   Infectious diseases associated with AIDS.

5. lympho _____   Formation of lymph.

6. _____ ic   Pertaining to poison.

7. _____ immunity   Immune response in which B cells transform into plasma cells and secrete antibodies.

8. _____ immunity   Immune response involving T-cell lymphocytes.

Chapter Fourteen
ABBREVIATIONS QUIZ

Name: _____

Spell out the abbreviation in Column I and then match each abbreviation with an associated explanation in Column II:

Column I

1. HD _____ _____

2. HIV _____ _____

3. MOAB _____ _____

4. RTI _____ _____

5. NK cells _____ _____

6. HSV _____ _____

7. HAART _____ _____

8. IgE _____ _____

9. IL 1–15 _____ _____

10. KS _____ _____

Column II

A. Combination of drugs effective against AIDS.

B. Lymphocytes that recognize and destroy foreign antigens.

C. Causes small blisters on skin, lips, and genitals and is an opportunistic infection associated with AIDS.

D. Malignancy associated with AIDS.

E. Malignancy of lymph nodes and spleen; Reed-Sternberg cell is identified in bone marrow.

F. Proteins (cytokines) that stimulate growth of B- or T-cell lymphocytes.

G. Virus that causes AIDS.

H. Drug that destroys an enzyme necessary for the AIDS virus to replicate.

I. Proteins produced in a laboratory by cloning techniques; can be toxic to tumor cells.

J. Proteins produced naturally by B-cell lymphocytes in response to antigen stimulation.

Chapter Fourteen
DIAGRAM QUIZ

Name: _____

Label the diagram below using the terms listed below:

Axillary region
Cervical region
Inguinal region
Large veins in the neck
Lymph capillaries
Lymph nodes
Lymph vessels
Mediastinal region
Right lymphatic duct
Thoracic duct

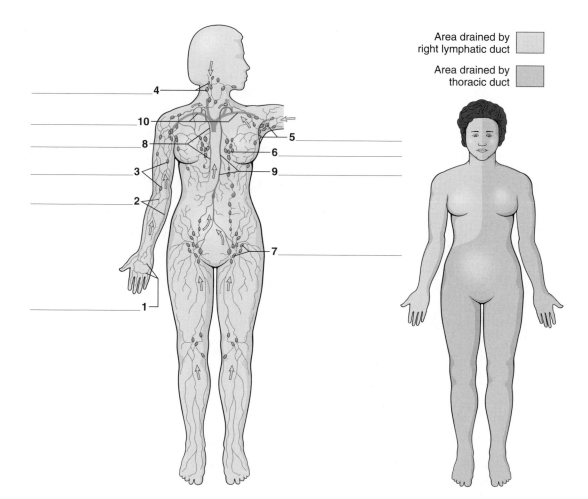

Area drained by
right lymphatic duct

Area drained by
thoracic duct

Chapter Fourteen
VOCABULARY QUIZ

Name: _____

A. *Match the following terms with their meanings below:*

acquired immunity	axillary node	cytokine
adenoids	B cell	cytotoxic cell
antibody	cell-mediated immunity	cervical node
antigen		

1. Lymph node in the neck region _____

2. Masses of lymphatic tissue in the nasopharynx _____

3. Lymph node in the armpit (underarm) _____

4. Immune response involving T-cell lymphocytes _____

5. Formation of antibodies and lymphocytes after exposure to an antigen; type of immunity _____

6. T-cell lymphocyte that directly kills foreign cells _____

7. Substance that the body recognizes as foreign; evokes an immune response _____

8. Protein made by T-cell lymphocytes to destroy foreign substances; interleukins
   and interferons _____

9. Lymphocyte that originates in bone marrow and transforms into a plasma
   cell to secrete antibodies _____

10. Protein produced by B-cell lymphocytes to destroy antigens _____

B. *Match the following terms with their meanings below:*

dendritic cell	immunoglobulins	interstitial fluid
helper T cell	immunotherapy	lymph capillaries
humoral immunity	inguinal node	interferons
immune response		

1. Body's capacity to resist foreign organisms and toxins; humoral
   and cell-mediated immunity are examples _____

2. Found in spaces between cells; forms lymph _____

3. Antibodies such as IgA, IgM, IgG, IgE, IgD _____

4. Use of immunologic knowledge and techniques to treat disease; vaccines
   and monoclonal antibodies _____

5. Cell that ingests antigens and presents them to other cells; specialized
   macrophage _____

6. Antiviral proteins (cytokines) secreted by T cells _____

7. Lymph node in the groin region _____

8. Immune response in which B cells transform into plasma cells
   and secrete antibodies _____

9. Tiniest lymphatic vessels _____

10. Lymphocyte that aids B cells in recognizing antigens and
    stimulating antibody production _____

C. *Match the following terms with their meanings below:*

macrophage	natural killer (NK) cell	T cell
mediastinal node	plasma cell	thoracic duct
monoclonal antibody	spleen	thymus gland
natural immunity		

1. Lymphocyte formed in the thymus gland; acts directly on antigens or
   produces chemicals that destroy antigens _____

2. Large phagocyte found in lymph nodes and
   other tissues of the body _____

3. Lymphocyte that recognizes and destroys foreign cells by releasing cytotoxins _____

4. An individual's own genetic ability to fight off disease _____

5. Organ that produces, stores, and eliminates blood cells _____

6. Lymphoid cell that secretes an antibody and originates from
   B-cell lymphocytes _____

7. Large lymphatic vessel in the chest; empties lymph into veins
   in the upper chest _____

8. Lymph node in the area between the lungs in the chest _____

9. Organ in the mediastinum that produces T-cell lymphocytes and aids
   in the immune response _____

10. Antibody produced in a laboratory to attack antigens; used in cancer treatment and
    immunotherapy _____

Chapter Fourteen
REVIEW SHEET QUIZ

Name: _____

A. *Give meanings for the following combining forms:*

1. inguin/o _____   5. tox/o _____

2. thym/o _____   6. immun/o _____

3. axill/o _____   7. splen/o _____

4. cervic/o _____   8. lymphaden/o _____

B. *Give meanings for the following suffixes and prefixes:*

1. -edema _____   6. -oid _____

2. -megaly _____   7. -pathy _____

3. -poiesis _____   8. inter- _____

4. -penia _____   9. hyper- _____

5. -phylaxis _____   10. retro- _____

Chapter Fourteen

OPPORTUNISTIC INFECTIONS QUIZ **Name:** _____

A. *Match the following opportunistic infections associated with AIDS with their descriptions below:*

Candidiasis	Cryptococcus
Cryptosporidiosis	Cytomegalovirus
Herpes simplex	Histoplasmosis
Mycobacterium avium intracellulare	*Pneumocystis carinii* pneumonia
Toxoplasmosis	Tuberculosis

1. _____ Viral infection causing small blisters on the lips, nose, or genitals; (HSV).

2. _____ Yeast-like fungal infection overgrows in the mouth (thrush), respiratory tract, and skin.

3. _____ Bacterial disease predominant in the lungs. Symptoms include fever, weight loss, anorexia, and low energy; (TB).

4. _____ Yeast-like fungal infection causes lung, brain, and blood infections; found in pigeon droppings, air, water, soil; (Crypto).

5. _____ Fungal infection caused by inhalation of dust contaminated with *histoplasma capsulatum*; symptoms include fever, chills and lung infection; (Histo).

6. _____ One-celled organism causes lung infection with fever, cough, and chest pain; (PCP).

7. _____ Parasitic infection involving the CNS and causing fever, chills, confusion, hemiparesis, and seizures; parasite is found in uncooked pork, raw eggs, and vegetables; (Toxo).

8. _____ One-celled parasitic infection of the gastrointestinal tract, brain, and spinal cord.

9. _____ Bacterial disease with fever, malaise, night sweats, diarrhea, lung, and blood infections; (MAI).

10. _____ Virus causes enteritis and retinitis; found in semen, saliva, urine, feces, blood, and breast milk; (CMV).

Chapter Fourteen
CROSSWORD PUZZLE

Name: _____

Fill in the crossword puzzle below using the clues listed underneath it.

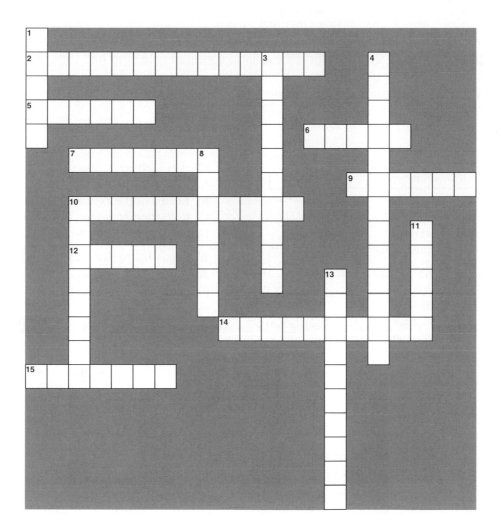

Across Clues

2. Record of lymph vessels after contrast is injected in the foot, and x-rays are taken to show the path of lymph.
5. Organ near the stomach that produces, stores, and eliminates blood cells.
6. Hypersensitivity or allergic state with an inherited predisposition. From a Greek word meaning "strangeness."
7. Malignant tumor of the thymus gland.
9. Tox/o means _____.
10. An exaggerated or unusual hypersensitivity to foreign protein or other substance.
12. Fluid found within lymphatic vessels.
14. Immun/o means _____.
15. Masses of lymph tissue in the oropharynx.

Down Clues

1. Enzyme-linked immunosorbent assay (abbrev.).
3. An RNA virus that makes copies of itself by using the host cell's DNA.
4. Formation of lymph.
8. A state of abnormal hypersensitivity acquired through exposure to a particular allergen.
10. Substance capable of causing specific hypersensitivity in the body; pollen, dust.
11. A poison; a protein produced by certain bacteria, animals, and plants.
13. A large phagocyte found in lymph nodes and other tissues of the body.

Chapter Fourteen
PRACTICAL APPLICATIONS

Name: _____

A. Case Report

This 48-year-old woman had an unexplained anemia with low-grade fever 4 years before her death. Six months before, bronchopneumonia developed, followed by return of severe anemia and continued pyrexia (fever). She was febrile (feverish), appeared pale, and had slight hepatomegaly and splenomegaly. Lymph nodes were palpated in the axillary and inguinal areas, and ascites developed. The chronic anemia did not respond to iron therapy. There was no evidence of blood loss or hemolysis. Diagnosis of lymphoma was confirmed by autopsy.

1. **What two organs were enlarged in the patient?** ....
   A. Liver and lungs
   B. Lungs and spleen
   C. Liver and spleen
   D. Spleen and bone marrow

2. **Where were lymph nodes felt?** ....
   A. Groin and armpit
   B. Armpit and chest
   C. Groin and abdomen
   D. Abdomen and armpit

3. **What is ascites?** ....
   A. Blockage of the intestine
   B. Edema in the extremities
   C. Collection of fluid in the chest
   D. Collection of fluid in the abdomen

4. **What was the probable cause of the patient's anemia?** ....
   A. Chronic blood loss
   B. Destruction of blood
   C. Malignant tumor of lymph nodes
   D. Iron deficiency

B. Symptoms of Hodgkin Disease

The most common initial feature of Hodgkin disease is painless, asymmetrical enlargement of cervical lymph nodes. Symptoms may also originate from compression of neighboring structures by growing tumor masses. For example, cough, dyspnea, dysphagia, and upper extremity edema may result from a mediastinal mass impinging on the tracheobronchial tree, esophagus, or superior vena cava. Edema of lower extremities and urinary or gastrointestinal disturbances may result from retroperitoneal lymphatic involvement. Splenomegaly is present in about half the cases.

1. **How do most patients present with Hodgkin disease?** ....
   A. Lymph nodes enlarged under the arm
   B. Enlargement of the spleen
   C. Compression of the trachea
   D. Lymphadenopathy in the neck

2. **How could upper extremity edema occur?** ....
   A. Tumor pressing on the esophagus
   B. Tumor blocking the main vein bringing blood to the heart
   C. Because of dysphagia
   D. Because of dyspnea

3. **What could cause bladder problems?** ....
   A. Tumor behind the abdomen
   B. Tumor pressing on the bronchial tubes
   C. Enlargement of the spleen
   D. Upper extremity edema

Chapter Fourteen
ANSWERS TO THE QUIZZES

Multiple Choice Quiz

1. D	4. C	7. A	10. E	13. B	16. D	19. C	22. E	25. B
2. C	5. E	8. D	11. A	14. C	17. A	20. B	23. D	
3. B	6. B	9. B	12. C	15. D	18. C	21. A	24. C	

Exercise Quiz

A

1. lymph nodes
2. thoracic duct
3. spleen
4. adenoids
5. thymus
6. lymph capillaries
7. right lymphatic duct
8. interstitial fluid

B

9. groin
10. armpit
11. neck
12. chest

C

13. B
14. D
15. C
16. E
17. F
18. G
19. A

D

20. splenectomy
21. lymphadenitis
22. thymoma
23. lymphadenopathy
24. lymphopoiesis
25. lymphocytopenia
26. toxic
27. splenomegaly

E

28. hypersplenism
29. anaphylaxis
30. allergen
31. AIDS
32. thymectomy
33. Hodgkin disease
34. lymphoid organs
35. lymphedema

F

36. human immunodeficiency virus
37. histoplasmosis
38. Kaposi sarcoma
39. *Pneumocystis carinii* pneumonia
40. computed tomography
41. toxoplasmosis

G

42. humoral
43. T cells
44. cell-mediated
45. B cells

H

46. helper T cells
47. immunoelectrophoresis
48. zidovudine
49. ELISA
50. opportunistic infections

Dictation and Comprehension Quiz

A

1. allergen
2. anaphylaxis
3. atopy
4. axillary nodes
5. cell-mediated immunity
6. humoral immunity
7. immunoglobulins
8. immunosuppression
9. inguinal nodes
10. interferons
11. interstitial fluid
12. Kaposi sarcoma
13. lymphadenopathy
14. lymphedema
15. lymphoma
16. protease inhibitor
17. splenomegaly
18. thymoma
19. tonsils
20. vaccination

B

12 Malignant tumor associated with AIDS; appears as bluish-red skin nodules

3 Hypersensitive or allergic state involving hereditary predisposition

13 Disease condition of lymph nodes

17 Enlargement of the spleen

9 Collection of lymph tissue in the groin

1 Substance capable of causing a specific hypersensitivity reaction in the body

16 A drug that is used to treat AIDS by blocking the production of an enzyme

2 An exaggerated or unusual hypersensitivity to a foreign protein

6 Immune response in which B cells transform into plasma cells and secrete antibodies

10 Antiviral proteins secreted by T cells

18 Malignant tumor of a gland in the chest

11 Found within lymphatic vessels and surrounding tissues throughout the body

19 Lymphatic tissue in the oropharynx

4 Collection of lymph tissue under the arm (armpit)

5 Immune response involving T-cell lymphocytes

15 Malignant tumor of lymph nodes and tissue

7 Antibodies such as IgG, IgA, IgD that are secreted by plasma cells

20 Introduction of altered antigens to produce an immune response

8 Repression of the immune response

14 Fluid collects within the spaces between cells secondary to lymph vessel obstruction

Spelling Quiz

A

1. macrophage—large phagocyte found in lymph nodes and other tissue
2. lymph—fluid found in lymph vessels
3. immunoglobulin—antibody secreted by plasma cells
4. allergy—hypersensitivity reaction
5. inguinal nodes—lymph nodes in the groin
6. anaphylaxis—extraordinary hypersensitivity reaction
7. Hodgkin disease—malignant tumor of lymph nodes
8. axillary nodes—lymph nodes in the armpit
9. lymphocytopenia—decrease in lymphocytes
10. splenectomy—removal of the spleen

B

11. thymus gland
12. interstitial fluid
13. lymphedema
14. interleukins
15. adenoids
16. vaccination
17. tonsillitis
18. lymphopoiesis

Pronunciation Quiz

A

1. immu<u>no</u>logy
2. hypersensi<u>tiv</u>ity
3. <u>in</u>guinal nodes
4. lymph<u>e</u>dema
5. inter<u>sti</u>tial <u>fluid</u>
6. <u>Ka</u>posi sar<u>co</u>ma
7. <u>mac</u>rophage
8. anaphy<u>lax</u>is
9. tho<u>ra</u>cic duct
10. lymphade<u>no</u>pathy

B

1. E
2. C
3. H
4. A
5. G
6. J
7. I
8. B
9. D
10. F

C

1. splenectomy
2. thymoma
3. lymphangiogram
4. opportunistic
5. lymphopoiesis
6. toxic
7. humoral
8. cell-mediated

Abbreviations Quiz

1. Hodgkin disease <u>E</u>
2. Human immunodeficiency virus <u>G</u>
3. Monoclonal antibody <u>I</u>
4. Reverse transcriptase inhibitor <u>H</u>
5. Natural killer cells <u>B</u>
6. Herpes simplex virus <u>C</u>
7. Highly active antiretroviral therapy <u>A</u>
8. Immunoglobulin E <u>J</u>
9. Interleukins 1–15 <u>F</u>
10. Kaposi sarcoma <u>D</u>

Diagram Quiz

1. Lymph capillaries
2. Lymph vessels
3. Lymph nodes
4. Cervical region
5. Axillary region
6. Mediastinal region
7. Inguinal region
8. Right lymphatic duct
9. Thoracic duct
10. Large veins in the neck

Vocabulary Quiz

A

1. cervical node
2. adenoids
3. axillary node
4. cell-mediated immunity
5. acquired immunity
6. cytotoxic cell
7. antigen
8. cytokine
9. B cell
10. antibody

B

1. immune response
2. interstitial fluid
3. immunoglobulins
4. immunotherapy
5. dendritic cell
6. interferons
7. inguinal node

8. humoral immunity
9. lymph capillaries
10. helper T cell

C

1. T cell
2. macrophage
3. natural killer (NK) cell
4. natural immunity
5. spleen
6. plasma cell
7. thoracic duct
8. mediastinal node
9. thymus gland
10. monoclonal antibody

Review Sheet Quiz

A

1. groin
2. thymus gland
3. armpit
4. neck
5. poison
6. protection
7. spleen
8. lymph node (gland)

B

1. swelling
2. enlargement
3. formation
4. deficiency
5. protection
6. resembling, derived from
7. disease
8. between
9. excessive
10. backward

Opportunistic Infections Quiz

A

1. herpes simplex
2. candidiasis
3. tuberculosis
4. cryptococcus
5. histoplasmosis
6. *Pneumocystis carinii* pneumonia
7. toxoplasmosis
8. cryptosporidiosis
9. *Mycobacterlum avium intracellulare*
10. cytomegalovirus

Crossword Puzzle

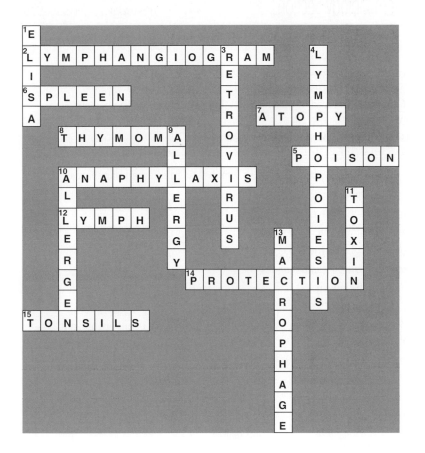

Practical Applications

A
1. C
2. A
3. D
4. C

B
1. D
2. B
3. A

Chapter Fourteen
Answers to Combining Forms and Terminology Sections

Terminology	Meaning
autoimmune disease	Chronic, disabling disease in which the body produces antibodies against its own tissues. Examples are rheumatoid arthritis and lupus erythematosus.
immunoglobulin	Protein (antibody produced by plasma cells) that acts to protect the body by destroying antigens.
immunosuppression	Suppression (stopping) of the immune response.
lymphopoiesis	Formation of lymph.
lymphedema	Swelling of tissue due to accumulation of lymph fluid in intercellular spaces.
lymphocytopenia	Deficiency of lymphocytes in the blood.
lymphocytosis	Abnormal condition of increase in lymphocytes.
lymphoid	Derived from lymph tissue.
lymphadenopathy	Disease of lymph glands (nodes).
lymphadenitis	Inflammation of lymph glands (nodes).
splenomegaly	Enlargement of the spleen.
splenectomy	Removal of the spleen.
hypersplenism	A syndrome marked by splenomegaly (associated with anemia, leukopenia, and thrombocytopenia).
thymoma	Tumor (malignant) of the thymus gland.
thymectomy	Removal of the thymus gland.
toxic	Pertaining to poison.

Prefix

anaphylaxis	An exaggerated hypersensitivity reaction to foreign proteins.
interstitial fluid	Pertaining to fluid that lies between body cells and eventually becomes lymph fluid.

chapter 15

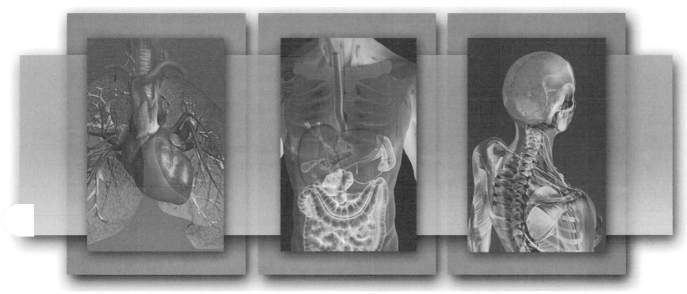

Chapter Fifteen
MULTIPLE CHOICE QUIZ

Name: _____

In the box write the letter of the choice that is the definition of the term or best answers the question. There is only one correct answer for each question.

1. **Spongy, porous bone tissue is also called:** .... ☐
   A. Yellow bone marrow
   B. Bone fissure
   C. Compact bone
   D. Bone sinus
   E. Cancellous bone

2. **Outward extension of the shoulder bone is the:** .... ☐
   A. Xiphoid process
   B. Acetabulum
   C. Acromion
   D. Vertebral arch
   E. Patella

3. **An opening or passage in bones where blood vessels and nerves enter and leave is a:** .... ☐
   A. Fissure
   B. Sulcus
   C. Tuberosity
   D. Foramen
   E. Fossa

4. **The projection of the temporal bone is the:** .... ☐
   A. Malleolus
   B. Epiphysis
   C. Xiphoid process
   D. Mastoid process
   E. Tubercle

5. **Knuckle-like process at the end of a bone is called a:** .... ☐
   A. Fontanelle
   B. Tuberosity
   C. Trochanter
   D. Xiphoid process
   E. Condyle

6. **Mandible, vomer, maxilla, and zygomatic are all bones of the:** .... ☐
   A. Face
   B. Cranium
   C. Spine
   D. Pelvis
   E. Thorax

7. **Occipital, sphenoid, frontal, temporal, and ethmoid are bones of the:** .... ☐
   A. Face
   B. Cranium
   C. Spine
   D. Pelvis
   E. Thorax

8. **The shaft of a long bone is called a(an):** .... ☐
   A. Olecranon
   B. Periosteum
   C. Osteoclast
   D. Epiphysis
   E. Diaphysis

9. **Poor formation of bone:** .... ☐
   A. Osteolysis
   B. Osteodystrophy
   C. Decalcification
   D. Myelopoiesis
   E. Osteoclasis

10. **Slipping or subluxation of a vertebra:** .... ☐
    A. Spondylitis
    B. Rachitis
    C. Kyphosis
    D. Spondylolisthesis
    E. Lordosis

11. **Operation performed to relieve the symptoms of a slipped disk:** .... ☐
    A. Patellapexy
    B. Arthroscopy
    C. Osteoclasis
    D. Laminectomy
    E. Metacarpectomy

12. **Lateral curvature of the spinal column:** .... ☐
    A. Lordosis
    B. Scoliosis
    C. Kyphosis
    D. Spina bifida
    E. Pubic symphysis

13. **Vitamin D deficiency leads to softening of bone, which is known as:** ....
    A. Osteomalacia
    B. Lumbago
    C. Osteogenesis imperfecta
    D. Osteoporosis
    E. Hypercalcemia

14. **Pertaining to the upper arm bone:** ......
    A. Humeral
    B. Tibial
    C. Radial
    D. Ulnar
    E. Carpal

15. **The shoulder bone is the:** ....
    A. Patella
    B. Sternum
    C. Scapula
    D. Clavicle
    E. Vertebra

16. **The smaller of the two lower leg bones is the:** ....
    A. Calcaneus
    B. Tibia
    C. Fibula
    D. Tarsal bone
    E. Malleolus

17. **Inflammation of bone and bone marrow:** ....
    A. Osteitis fibrosa cystica
    B. Multiple myeloma
    C. Osteomyelitis
    D. Osteoporosis
    E. Osteochondroma

18. **Clubfoot:** ....
    A. Exostosis
    B. Osteogenic sarcoma
    C. Bunion
    D. Talipes
    E. Bursitis

19. **A splintered or crushed bone:** ....
    A. Comminuted fracture
    B. Greenstick fracture
    C. Crepitation
    D. Compression fracture
    E. Impacted fracture

20. **Surgical repair of a joint:** ....
    A. Arthroplasty
    B. Fasciectomy
    C. Achondroplasia
    D. Tenorrhaphy
    E. Arthrosis

21. **Condition of stiffening and immobility of a joint:** ....
    A. Hemarthrosis
    B. Fibrositis
    C. Bursitis
    D. Kyphosis
    E. Ankylosis

22. **Chronic inflammation of bones and joints due to degenerative changes in cartilage:** ....
    A. Ankylosing spondylitis
    B. Rheumatoid arthritis
    C. Chondromalacia
    D. Osteoarthritis
    E. Systemic lupus erythematosus

23. **Inflammation of joints caused by excessive uric acid accumulation:** ....
    A. Bunion
    B. Bursitis
    C. Gouty arthritis
    D. Sciatica
    E. Myositis

24. **Malignant tumor of smooth muscle:** ...
    A. Rhabdomyosarcoma
    B. Leiomyosarcoma
    C. Rhabdomyoma
    D. Leiomyoma
    E. Myorrhaphy

25. **Wasting away (no development) of muscle:** ....
    A. Myasthenia
    B. Myalgia
    C. Hypertrophy
    D. Atrophy
    E. Myositis

Chapter Fifteen
EXERCISE QUIZ

Name: _____

PART I: BONES

A. Complete the following sentences:

1. Two mineral substances necessary for proper development of bones are _____

    and _____.

2. The shaft of a long bone is called the _____.

3. The ends of a long bone are called the _____.

4. The bones of a fetus are mainly composed of _____ tissue.

5. During bone development, immature bone cells called _____ produce bony tissue.

6. Red bone marrow is found in spongy or _____ bone.

7. The strong membrane surrounding the surface of a bone is the _____.

8. Hard, dense bone tissue lying under the periosteum is called _____.

9. The physician who treats bones and bone diseases is a(an) _____.

10. Series of bone canals containing blood vessels are the _____.

B. Give meanings for the following terms:

11. condyle _____   14. trochanter _____

12. fossa _____   15. foramen _____

13. tubercle _____   16. fissure _____

C. Match the following cranial and facial bones with their meanings:

frontal bone   mandible   occipital bone   temporal bone
lacrimal bone   maxilla   parietal bone   zygomatic bone

17. forms the forehead _____

18. cheek bone _____

19. upper jaw bone _____

20. forms the back and base of the skull _____

21. lower jaw bone _____

22. forms the roof and upper side of the skull _____

23. two paired bones at the corner of each eye _____

24. bone near the ear; connected to the lower jaw _____

D. Give the medical names for the following bones:

25. shoulder bone _____

26. upper arm bone _____

27. breastbone _____

28. thigh bone _____

29. finger bones _____

30. collar bone _____

31. wrist bones _____

32. kneecap _____

33. foot bones _____

34. backbone _____

E. Give the meanings for the following terms associated with bones:

35. calcaneus _____

36. acetabulum _____

37. acromion _____

38. malleolus _____

39. lamina _____

40. olecranon _____

41. pubic symphysis _____

42. osteoporosis _____

43. osteogenic sarcoma _____

F. Match the following terms with their descriptions:

exostoses   kyphosis
talipes   spondylolisthesis
myelopoiesis   scoliosis
lordosis

44. lateral curvature of the spine _____

45. formation of bone marrow _____

46. abnormal anterior curvature of the spine _____

47. benign tumors arising from the bone surface _____

48. humpback _____

49. clubfoot _____

50. subluxation of a vertebra _____

Chapter Fifteen
EXERCISE QUIZ

Name: _____

PART II: JOINTS AND MUSCLES

A. *Complete the following sentences:*

1. Connective tissue that binds bones to other bones is a(an) _____.

2. Connective tissue that binds muscles to bones is a(an) _____.

3. Fluid found within the joint is called _____.

4. A sac of fluid near a joint is a(an) _____.

5. Smooth cartilage that surrounds the surface of bones at joints is _____.

6. Surgical repair of a joint is called _____.

B. *Complete the medical term from its meaning and word parts given:*

7. inflammation of a tendon: _____ itis

8. doctor specializing in joint disorders: _____ logist

9. tumor (benign) of cartilage: _____ oma

10. incision of a joint: arthr _____

11. stiffened, immobile joint: _____ osis

12. suture of a tendon: ten _____

13. softening of cartilage: chondro _____

14. tumor (malignant) of cartilage: _____ oma

15. inflammation of a sac of fluid near a joint: _____ itis

C. *Give meanings for the following terms:*

16. subluxation _____

17. arthrodesis _____

18. podagra _____

19. pyrexia _____

20. sciatica _____

D. *Select the term that best fits the definition given:*

21. fibrous membrane separating muscles: **(fascia, flexion)**

22. movement away from the midline: **(abduction, adduction)**

23. pertaining to heart muscle: **(myasthenia, myocardial)**

24. pain of many muscles: **(myositis, polymyalgia)**

25. act of turning the palm forward or upward: **(supination, pronation)**

26. muscle connected to internal organs: **(skeletal, visceral)**

27. connection of muscle to the bone that moves: **(origin, insertion)**

28. connection of muscle to a stationary bone: **(origin, insertion)**

E. *Select from the following terms to name the abnormal conditions described below:*

achondroplasia	dislocation	osteoarthritis
ankylosing spondylitis	ganglion	rheumatoid arthritis
bunion	gouty arthritis	systemic lupus erythematosus
carpal tunnel syndrome	Lyme disease	

29. an inherited condition in which bones of the arms and legs fail to grow normally because of a

    defect in cartilage and bone formation _____

30. cystic mass arising from a tendon in the wrist _____

31. inflammation of joints caused by accumulation of uric acid _____

32. degenerative joint disease; chronic inflammation of bones and joints _____

33. chronic, progressive arthritis with stiffening of joints, especially of the spine _____

34. compression of the median nerve in the wrist _____

35. abnormal swelling of a metatarsophalangeal joint _____

36. tick-borne bacterium causes this type of arthritis _____

37. chronic joint disease with inflamed and painful joints;

    marked by swollen and thickened synovial membranes _____

38. chronic inflammatory disease affecting skin (red rash on the face),

    kidneys, heart, and lungs as well as joints _____

39. displacement of a bone from its joint _____

F. Give the meanings for the following abnormal conditions affecting muscles:

40. fibromyalgia _____

41. leiomyosarcoma _____

42. muscular dystrophy _____

43. polymyositis _____

44. fasciitis _____

G. Match the term in Column I with its meaning in Column II:

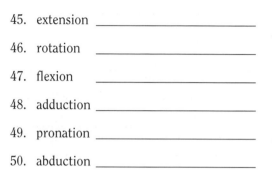

Column I

45. extension _____

46. rotation _____

47. flexion _____

48. adduction _____

49. pronation _____

50. abduction _____

Column II

A.   Bending a limb.

B.   Movement away from the midline.

C.   Movement toward the midline.

D.   Circular movement around an axis.

E.   Straightening out a limb.

F.   Turning the palm backward.

Chapter Fifteen

DICTATION AND COMPREHENSION QUIZ: BONES

Name: _____

A. Dictation of Terms

1. _____
2. _____
3. _____
4. _____
5. _____
6. _____
7. _____
8. _____
9. _____
10. _____

11. _____
12. _____
13. _____
14. _____
15. _____
16. _____
17. _____
18. _____
19. _____
20. _____

B. Comprehension of Terms: Match the number of the above term with its meaning below.

_____ Lateral curvature of the spinal column

_____ Bat-shaped cranial bone behind the eyes

_____ Large process below the neck of the femur

_____ End of a long bone

_____ Flexible connective tissue at joints

_____ Bone break at the wrist

_____ Round process on both sides of ankle

_____ Forms the back and base of the skull

_____ Poor development of bone

_____ Pertaining to the smaller lower leg bone

_____ Hip socket

_____ Thin, delicate cranial bone; supports the nasal cavity

_____ Formation of bone marrow

_____ Malignant bone tumor

_____ Upper part of the hip bone

_____ Forward vertebral subluxation

_____ Bone is splintered or crushed

_____ Heel bone

_____ Elbow bone

_____ Club foot

Chapter Fifteen

DICTATION AND COMPREHENSION QUIZ: JOINTS AND MUSCLES

Name: _____

A. Dictation of Terms

1. _____
2. _____
3. _____
4. _____
5. _____
6. _____
7. _____
8. _____
9. _____
10. _____

11. _____
12. _____
13. _____
14. _____
15. _____
16. _____
17. _____
18. _____
19. _____
20. _____

B. Comprehension of Terms: Match the number of the above term with its meaning below.

_____ Process of recording the electrical activity of muscles

_____ Chronic, progressive arthritis with stiffening of joints (primarily the spine)

_____ Bones are fused across the joint space

_____ Inflammation of the tissue connecting bones and muscles

_____ Bones of the arms and legs fail to grow to normal size (defect in cartilage formation)

_____ Bending of the foot backward (upward)

_____ Act of turning the palm forward

_____ Movement away from the midline of the body

_____ Inflammation of the membrane lining the joint

_____ Malignant tumor of smooth muscle

_____ Trauma to a muscle from violent contraction or excessive stretching

_____ Inflammation of many muscles

_____ Trauma to a joint due to injury to ligaments

_____ Fever

_____ Blood condition found in gouty arthritis

_____ Malignant tumor of skeletal muscle

_____ Chronic disease of joint inflammation (primarily the small joints of the hands and feet); an autoimmune reaction

_____ Abnormal swelling of the metatarsophalangeal joint

_____ Sac of fluid near a joint

_____ Extreme pain of the big toe associated with gouty arthritis

Chapter Fifteen
SPELLING QUIZ

Name: _____

A. *Circle the term that is spelled correctly and write its meaning in the space provided:*

1. arthrocentesis   arthrosentesis _____

2. osteoperosis   osteoporosis _____

3. cartiledge   cartilage _____

4. atropy   atrophy _____

5. chondrocostal   chrondrocostal _____

6. scoliosis   scoleosis _____

7. Uwing sarcoma   Ewing sarcoma _____

8. osteomyleitis   osteomyelitis _____

9. ascetabulum   acetabulum _____

10. osteodystrophy   osteodystropy _____

B. *Circle the term that is spelled correctly. The meaning of each term is given.*

11. upper arm bone	humerus	humerous	humorous
12. thigh bone	femor	femur	femmur
13. end of a long bone	epiphysis	epiphisis	epiphifisis
14. humpback	kyphiosis	kiphosis	kyphosis
15. heel bone	calcaneus	calcaneous	calcaineus
16. finger or toe bones	phalanges	pharynges	plalanges
17. collar bone	clavical	klavicle	clavicle
18. kneecap	patella	petella	patela
19. larger lower leg bone	tibbia	tibea	tibia
20. mineral substance in bone	phosphorus	phosphorous	phospherus

Chapter Fifteen
PRONUNCIATION QUIZ

Name: _____

A. *Underline the accented syllables in the following terms:*

1. acetabulum
2. osteodystrophy
3. epiphysis
4. scapular
5. kyphosis
6. malleolus
7. fibromyalgia
8. phalanges
9. podagra
10. rheumatologist

B. *Match the term in Column I with its meaning in Column II:*

Column I

1. ulna   _____
2. ilium   _____
3. diaphysis   _____
4. clavicle   _____
5. bursa   _____
6. lordosis   _____
7. fibula   _____
8. tibia   _____
9. olecranon   _____
10. metatarsal   _____

Column II

A. Collarbone.

B. Larger of the two lower leg bones.

C. Upper part of the hip bone.

D. Lower arm bone.

E. Condition of anterior curvature of the spine.

F. The elbow.

G. Sac of fluid near joints.

H. The shaft of a long bone.

I. A foot bone.

J. Smaller of the two leg bones.

C. *Complete the following terms using the definitions given:*

1. teno_____   Suture of a tendon.

2. _____ pexy   Fixation of the kneecap.

3. _____ al   Pertaining to the heel bone.

4. _____ oma   Tumor (benign) of smooth, visceral muscle.

5. _____emia   High levels of blood calcium.

6. _____ itis   Inflammation of bone and bone marrow.

7. _____ osis   Lateral curvature of the spine.

8. osteo _____   Malignant bone tumor.

9. _____ ing   Inflammation of the backbone with stiffness in the joints (two words).

   _____itis

Chapter Fifteen
ABBREVIATIONS QUIZ

Name: _____

Give the meanings for the following abbreviations in Column I and match each with an associated explanation in Column II:

<table>
<tr><td align="center">Column I</td><td align="center">Column II</td></tr>
<tr><td>1. ACL _____ _____</td><td>A. The articulation between a bone on the side of the cranium and the lower jaw bone.</td></tr>
<tr><td>2. RA _____ _____</td><td>B. A condition affecting the wrist and caused by pressure on a nerve.</td></tr>
<tr><td>3. SLE _____ _____</td><td>C. Bone density test.</td></tr>
<tr><td>4. TMJ _____ _____</td><td>D. Medication that treats inflammatory conditions.</td></tr>
<tr><td>5. DEXA _____ _____</td><td>E. Autoimmune condition marked by a wolf-like facial rash and joint pain.</td></tr>
<tr><td>6. EMG _____ _____</td><td>F. Bones in the back that are connected to ribs.</td></tr>
<tr><td>7. IM _____ _____</td><td>G. Process of recording muscle contractions.</td></tr>
<tr><td>8. T1-T12 _____ _____</td><td>H. Chronic inflammatory joint condition marked by damage to articular cartilage and ankylosis in smaller joints of the hands and feet.</td></tr>
<tr><td>9. NSAID _____ _____</td><td>I. Type of parenteral injection.</td></tr>
<tr><td>10. CTS _____ _____</td><td>J. Connective tissue joining bones in the anterior portion of the knee.</td></tr>
</table>

Chapter Fifteen
DIAGRAM QUIZ

Name: _____

Label the diagram below using the terms listed below:

Articular cartilage
Cancellous bone
Compact cortical bone
Diaphysis
Epiphyseal plate (line)
Epiphysis
Haversian canals
Medullary cavity
Metaphysis
Periosteum

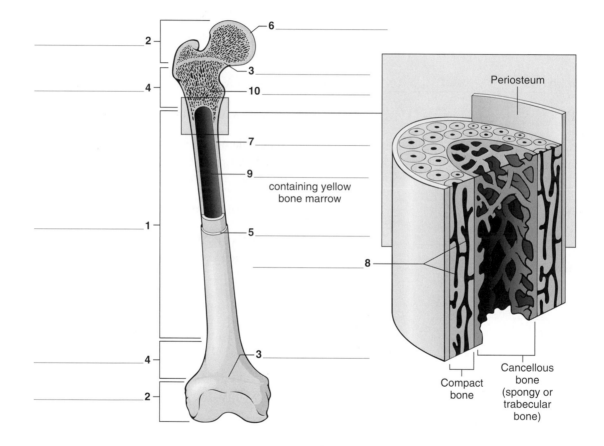

containing yellow
bone marrow

Periosteum

Compact
bone

Cancellous
bone
(spongy or
trabecular
bone)

Chapter Fifteen
VOCABULARY QUIZ

Name: _____

A. BONES

I. Match the following terms with their meanings below:

acetabulum   cancellous bone   compact bone
acromion   cartilage   condyle
articular cartilage collagen   cranial bones
calcium

1. Flexible connective tissue found in the immature skeleton, epiphyseal plate,
   and on joint surfaces _____

2. Skull bones; ethmoid, frontal, occipital, parietal,sphenoid, and temporal _____

3. Mineral constituent of bone _____

4. Outward extension of the shoulder bone _____

5. Spongy, porous bone tissue in the inner part of bone _____

6. Rounded depression or socket in the pelvis; forms the hip joint_____

7. Dense, connective tissue protein strands found in bone _____

8. Knuckle-like process at the end of a bone near a joint _____

9. Thin layer of cartilage surrounding the bones in a joint space _____

10. Hard, dense bone tissue usually found around the outer portion
    of a bone _____

II. Match the following terms with their meanings below:

diaphysis   fissure   fossa
disk (disc)   fontanelle   haversian canals
epiphysis   foramen   malleolus
facial bones

1. Shallow cavity in a bone _____

2. Shaft, or mid-portion of a long bone_____

3. Flat, round plate-like structure between two vertebrae _____

4. Soft spot between the skull bones of an infant _____

5. Narrow, slit-like opening in or between bones _____

6. Bones of the face; lacrimal, mandibular, maxillary, nasal, vomer
   and zygomatic bones. _____

7. Minute spaces filled with blood vessels; found in compact bone _____

8. Each end of a long bone _____

9. Opening or passage in bones where blood vessels and nerves enter and leave _____

10. Rounded process on both sides of the ankle joint_____

III. Match the following terms with their meanings below:

manubrium	olecranon	osteoblast
mastoid process	osseous tissue	osteoclast
medullary cavity	ossification	periosteum
metaphysis		

1. Process of bone formation _____

2. Bone cell that absorbs and removes unwanted bone tissue _____

3. Round projection on the temporal bone behind the ear_____

4. Central hollowed-out area in the shaft of a long bone _____

5. Upper portion of the sternum _____

6. Bone cell that helps form bone tissue _____

7. Membrane surrounding bones _____

8. Bone tissue _____

9. Flared portion of a long bone between the diaphysis and the epiphyseal plate _____

10. Large process on the proximal end of the ulna; part of the elbow joint _____

IV. Match the following terms with their meanings below:

phosphorus	sinus	temporomandibular joint
pubic symphysis	styloid process	trabeculae
red bone marrow	tubercle	trochanter
sella turcica		

1. Soft bone tissue found in cancellous bone; contains hematopoietic
   stem cells and blood cells _____

2. Supporting bundles of bony fibers in cancellous bone_____

3. Depression in the sphenoid bone; location of the pituitary gland _____

4. Rounded, small process on a bone; attachment site for
   muscles and tendons _____

5. Pole-like process extending downward from the temporal bone on each side of the skull _____

6. Area where the two pubic bones come together in the pelvis _____

7. Connection on either side of the head between the temporal bone of the skull and the mandibular bone of the jaw _____

8. Large process at the neck of the femur _____

9. Mineral substance found in bones in combination with calcium _____

10. Hollow air cavity with a bone_____

V. Match the following terms with their meanings below:

epiphyseal plate	tuberosity	xiphoid process
ribs	vertebra	yellow bone marrow

1. Lower, narrow portion of the sternum _____

2. Rounded process on bone; attachment for muscles and tendons _____

3. Twelve pairs of elongated, curved bones that form the chest wall _____

4. Fatty tissue found in the medullary cavity of most adult long bones _____

5. Individual backbone _____

6. Cartilaginous area at the ends of long bones _____

B. JOINTS AND MUSCLES

I. Match the following terms with their meanings below:

articulation	suture joint	synovial joint
bursa	synovial cavity	synovial membrane
ligament	synovial fluid	tendon

1. Sticky material within the synovial cavity; lubricates the joint space _____

2. Joint in which apposed surfaces are closely united; motion is minimal _____

3. Any joint _____

4. Connective tissue that binds muscles to bones_____

5. Space between bones at a freely movable joint _____

6. Lining of the synovial cavity; produces fluid in the joint space _____

7. Connective tissue binding bones to other bones_____

8. Sac of fluid near a joint _____

9. A freely movable joint_____

II. Match the following terms with their meanings below:

adduction	flexion	rotation
adduction	insertion of a muscle	skeletal muscle
dorsiflexion	origin of a muscle	supination
extension	plantar flexion	visceral muscle
fascia	pronation	

1. Bending at a joint _____

2. Fibrous membrane separating and enveloping muscles _____

3. Movement away from the midline of the body _____

4. Bending the sole of the foot downward toward the ground _____

5. Straightening of a flexed limb _____

6. Backward bending of the foot _____

7. Connection of a muscle to a bone that moves_____

8. Turning the palm backward _____

9. Connection of a muscle to a stationary bone _____

10. Movement toward the midline of the body _____

11. Smooth muscle connected to internal organs _____

12. Circular movement around a central point _____

13. Turning the palm forward _____

14. Striated muscle connected to bones _____

Chapter Fifteen
REVIEW SHEET QUIZ

Name: _____

A. *Give meanings for the following combining forms:*

1. acetabul/o _____
2. ankyl/o _____
3. arthr/o _____
4. articul/o _____
5. burs/o _____

6. calc/o _____
7. calcane/o _____
8. carp/o _____
9. cervic/o _____
10. chondr/o _____

B. *Give combining forms for the following meanings:*

1. collar bone _____
2. tailbone _____
3. ribs _____
4. skull _____
5. fascia _____

6. thigh bone _____
7. smooth muscle _____
8. upper arm bone _____
9. ilium _____
10. ischium _____

C. *Give meanings for the following combining forms:*

1. kyph/o _____
2. lamin/o _____
3. lord/o _____
4. lumb/o _____
5. malleol/o _____

6. maxill/o _____
7. metacarp/o _____
8. metatars/o _____
9. my/o _____
10. myel/o _____

D. *Give meanings for the following combining forms:*

1. myos/o _____
2. olecran/o _____
3. orth/o _____
4. oste/o _____
5. patell/o _____

6. perone/o _____
7. phalang/o _____
8. vertebr/o _____
9. rhabdomy/o _____
10. spondyl/o _____

E. *Give combining forms for the following meanings:*

1. sacrum _____

2. flesh _____

3. shoulder blade _____

4. crooked, bent (lateral _____ curvature of spine)

5. breast bone _____

6. chest _____

7. larger lower leg bone _____

8. lower arm bone (little finger side) _____

9. lower arm bone (thumb side) _____

10. lower jaw bone _____

F. *Give meanings for the following suffixes:*

1. -algia _____

2. -asthenia _____

3. -blast _____

4. -clast _____

5. -desis _____

6. -emia _____

7. -listhesis _____

8. -malacia _____

9. -penia _____

10. -porosis _____

11. -tome _____

12. -trophy _____

G. *Give meanings for the following prefixes:*

1. a-, an- _____

2. ab- _____

3. ad- _____

4. dia- _____

5. dorsi- _____

6. epi- _____

7. exo- _____

8. meta- _____

9. peri- _____

10. poly- _____

11. sub- _____

12. supra- _____

Chapter Fifteen
CROSSWORD PUZZLE

Name: _____

Fill in the crossword puzzle below using the clues listed underneath it.

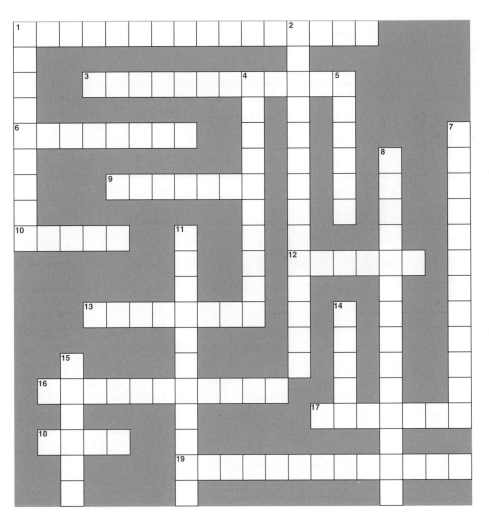

Across Clues

1. The process of recording the strength of muscle contraction.
3. Chronic inflammatory myopathy of uncertain etiology (inflammation of many muscles).
6. Rounded process on a bone; attachment for muscles and tendons
9. Decreasing the angle between two bones; bending a limb.
10. Cavity within a bone (cranial and facial bones).
12. Connective tissue that binds muscles to bones.
13. A cystic mass arising from a tendon in the wrist.
16. A partial or incomplete dislocation.
17. Clubfoot.
18. Flat, round, plate-like cartilaginous structure between vertebrae.
19. Inflammation of the bone and bone marrow.

Down Clues

1. Bony growth arising from the surface of bone.
2. Surgical puncture of the joint space with a needle.
4. As applied to the hand, the act of turning the palm forward.
5. Trauma to a joint with pain, swelling, and injury to ligaments.
7. Decrease in bone density; thinning and weakening of the bone.
8. Progressive, degenerative joint disease characterized by loss of articular cartilage; literally, inflammation of bone and joint.
11. Displacement of a bone from its joint. For example, a shoulder _____.
14. Shallow cavity in a bone.
15. Abnormal swelling of the joint between the big toe and the first metatarsal bone.

Chapter Fifteen

PRACTICAL APPLICATIONS

Name: _____

A. Chart Note

The patient is having pain around the medial aspect of his left knee. About 12 years ago he had a tear of his medial meniscus (crescent-shaped fibrocartilage), which was removed. On exam, he has a well-healed medial scar to his left knee; there was no effusion; full range of motion; and it is stable. X-rays show very slight scarring of the medial femoral condyle and a small accessory bone medially, but nothing in the interior of the joint. The great toe shows a healed fracture. There was no obvious exostosis impinging on the base of the nail.

1. **Effusion in a joint means:** ....
   A. The bones at the joint are broken
   B. The meniscus is torn
   C. The patella is fractured
   D. There is fluid in the joint space

2. **Where is the femoral condyle?** ....
   A. At the ankle joint
   B. At the knee joint
   C. At the distal end of the tibia
   D. At the distal end of the fibula

3. **An exostosis is:** ....
   A. A bony growth
   B. A fluid-filled cyst
   C. A healed fracture
   D. Type of tendon

4. **Where is the medial meniscus?** ....
   A. Near the big toe
   B. At the hip socket
   C. In the middle of the knee
   D. At the base of the nail of the big toe

B. Chart Note

Follow-up for the complications of osteoporosis as they affect the spine. Mrs. Smith had a 6-month history of progressive disabling back pain visibly associated with progressive kyphotic deformity of the thoracolumbar spine, with an attendant cervical lordosis. X-rays of the thoracic spine reveal a compression fracture of T11 and L1. I advised the patient that such fractures even without trauma may be complications of underlying osteoporosis as severe as hers.

1. **Which term best describes Mrs. Smith's condition?** ....
   A. Osteoarthritis
   B. Gouty arthritis
   C. Osteomalacia
   D. Osteopenia

2. **What type of spinal deformity is present?** ....
   A. Posterior curvature of the chest and anterior curvature of the neck
   B. Lateral curvature of the chest
   C. Cervical fracture
   D. Anterior curvature of the thorax

Chapter Fifteen
ANSWERS TO THE QUIZZES

Multiple Choice Quiz

1. E	4. D	7. B	10. D	13. A	16. C	19. A	22. D	25. D
2. C	5. E	8. E	11. D	14. A	17. C	20. A	23. C	
3. D	6. A	9. B	12. B	15. C	18. D	21. E	24. B	

Exercise Quiz

Part I:

A

1. calcium and phosphorus
2. diaphysis
3. epiphyses
4. cartilage
5. osteoblasts
6. cancellous
7. periosteum
8. compact bone
9. orthopedist
10. haversian canals

B

11. knuckle-like projection
12. shallow cavity in bone
13. rounded process on bone
14. large process on femur for attachment of muscles
15. opening for blood vessels and nerves
16. narrow, deep slit-like opening

C

17. frontal bone
18. zygomatic bone
19. maxilla
20. occipital bone
21. mandible
22. parietal bone
23. lacrimal bone
24. temporal bone

D

25. scapula
26. humerus
27. sternum
28. femur
29. phalanges
30. clavicle
31. carpals
32. patella
33. metatarsals
34. vertebra

E

35. heel bone
36. socket for femur in hip
37. projection of scapula
38. rounded process at the ankle
39. part of the vertebral arch
40. elbow bone
41. anterior part of the hip bone
42. decrease in bone density; thinning and weakening of bone
43. malignant tumor of bone

F

44. scoliosis
45. myelopoiesis
46. lordosis
47. exostoses
48. kyphosis
49. talipes
50. spondylolisthesis

Part II:

A

1. ligament
2. tendon
3. synovial fluid
4. bursa
5. articular cartilage
6. arthroplasty

B

7. tendinitis
8. rheumatologist
9. chondroma
10. arthrotomy
11. ankylosis
12. tenorrhaphy
13. chondromalacia
14. chondrosarcoma
15. bursitis

C

16. partial or incomplete dislocation
17. binding of a joint

18. sharp pain of big toe; associated with gouty arthritis
19. fever
20. pain radiating down the leg

D

21. fascia
22. abduction
23. myocardial
24. polymyalgia
25. supination
26. visceral
27. insertion
28. origin

E

29. achondroplasia
30. ganglion
31. gouty arthritis
32. osteoarthritis
33. ankylosing spondylitis
34. carpal tunnel syndrome
35. bunion
36. Lyme disease
37. rheumatoid arthritis
38. systemic lupus erythematosus
39. dislocation

F

40. pain of fibrous tissue and muscle
41. tumor (malignant) of smooth muscle
42. poor development of muscle; group of inherited diseases with progressive muscle weakness and degeneration
43. chronic inflammation of many muscles
44. inflammation of fascia

G

45. E
46. D
47. A
48. C
49. F
50. B

Dictation and Comprehension Quiz: Bones

A

1. acetabulum
2. calcaneus
3. cartilage
4. Colles fracture
5. comminuted fracture
6. epiphysis
7. ethmoid bone
8. osteogenic sarcoma
9. ischium
10. malleolus
11. myelopoiesis
12. occipital bone
13. olecranon
14. osteodystrophy
15. peroneal
16. scoliosis
17. sphenoid bone
18. spondylolisthesis
19. talipes
20. trochanter

B

16 Lateral curvature of the spinal column
17 Bat-shaped cranial bone behind the eyes
20 Large process below the neck of the femur
6 End of a long bone
3 Flexible connective tissue at joints
4 Bone break at the wrist
10 Round process on both sides of ankle
12 Forms the back and base of the skull
14 Poor development of bone
15 Pertaining to the smaller lower leg bone
1 Hip socket
7 Thin, delicate cranial bone; supports the nasal cavity
11 Formation of bone marrow
8 Malignant bone tumor
9 Upper part of the hip bone
18 Forward vertebral subluxation
5 Bone is splintered or crushed
2 Heel bone
13 Elbow bone
19 Club foot

Dictation and Comprehension Quiz: Joints and Muscles

A

1. abduction
2. achondroplasia
3. ankylosing spondylitis
4. arthrodesis
5. bunion
6. bursa
7. dorsiflexion
8. electromyography
9. hyperuricemia
10. leiomyosarcoma
11. podagra
12. polymyositis
13. pyrexia
14. rhabdomyosarcoma
15. rheumatoid arthritis
16. sprain
17. strain
18. supination
19. synovitis
20. tendinitis

B

8 Process of recording the electrical activity of muscles
3 Chronic, progressive arthritis with stiffening of joints (primarily the spine)
4 Bones are fused across the joint space
20 Inflammation of the tissue connecting bones and muscles
2 Bones of the arms and legs fail to grow to normal size (defect in cartilage formation)
7 Bending of the foot backward (upward)
18 Act of turning the palm forward
1 Movement away from the midline of the body
19 Inflammation of the membrane lining the joint
10 Malignant tumor of smooth muscle
17 Trauma to a muscle from violent contraction or excessive stretching
12 Inflammation of many muscles
16 Trauma to a joint due to injury to ligaments
13 Fever
9 Blood condition found in gouty arthritis
14 Malignant tumor of skeletal muscle

15 Chronic disease of joint inflammation (primarily the small joints of the hands and feet); an autoimmune reaction
5 Abnormal swelling of the metatarsophalangeal joint
6 Sac of fluid near a joint
11 Extreme pain of the big toe associated with gouty arthritis

Spelling Quiz

A

1. arthrocentesis—surgical puncture to remove fluid from a joint
2. osteoporosis—decrease in bone density and weakening of bone
3. cartilage—connective tissue at joints
4. atrophy—lack of development; shrinkage of muscle
5. chondrocostal—pertaining to rib cartilage
6. scoliosis—lateral curvature of the spine
7. Ewing sarcoma—malignant bone tumor
8. osteomyelitis—inflammation of bone and bone marrow
9. acetabulum—socket in the hip bone
10. osteodystrophy—poor development of bone

B

11. humerus
12. femur
13. epiphysis
14. kyphosis
15. calcaneus
16. phalanges
17. clavicle
18. patella
19. tibia
20. phosphorus

Pronunciation Quiz

A

1. ace<u>ta</u>bulum
2. osteo<u>dys</u>trophy
3. e<u>piph</u>ysis
4. <u>scap</u>ular
5. ky<u>pho</u>sis
6. mal<u>le</u>olus
7. fibromy<u>al</u>gia
8. pha<u>lan</u>ges
9. po<u>dag</u>ra
10. rheuma<u>tol</u>ogist

B

1. D
2. C
3. H
4. A
5. G
6. E
7. J
8. B
9. F
10. I

C

1. tenorrhaphy
2. patellapexy
3. calcaneal
4. leiomyoma
5. hypercalcemia
6. osteomyelitis
7. scoliosis
8. osteogenic sarcoma
9. ankylosing spondylitis

Abbreviations Quiz

1. anterior cruciate ligament J
2. rheumatoid arthritis H
3. systemic lupus erythematosus E
4. temporomandibular joint A
5. dual-energy x-ray absorptiometry C
6. electromyography G
7. intramuscular I
8. thoracic vertebrae 1–12 F
9. nonsteroidal anti-inflammatory drug D
10. carpal tunnel syndrome B

Diagram Quiz

1. Diaphysis
2. Epiphysis
3. Epiphyseal plate (line)
4. Metaphysis
5. Periosteum
6. Articular cartilage
7. Compact cortical bone
8. Haversian canals
9. Medullary cavity
10. Cancellous bone

Vocabulary Quiz

A

BONES

I. 1. cartilage
   2. cranial bones
   3. calcium
   4. acromion

5. cancellous bone
6. acetabulum
7. collagen
8. condyle
9. articular cartilage
10. compact bone

II. 1. fossa
   2. diaphysis
   3. disk (disc)
   4. fontanelle
   5. fissure
   6. facial bones
   7. haversian canals
   8. epiphysis
   9. foramen
   10. malleolus

III. 1. ossification
   2. osteoclast
   3. mastoid process
   4. medullary cavity
   5. manubrium
   6. osteoblast
   7. periosteum
   8. osseous tissue
   9. metaphysis
   10. olecranon

IV. 1. red bone marrow
   2. trabeculae
   3. sella turcica
   4. tubercle
   5. styloid process
   6. pubic symphysis
   7. temporomandibular joint
   8. trochanter
   9. phosphorus
   10. sinus

V. 1. xiphoid process
   2. tuberosity
   3. ribs
   4. yellow bone marrow
   5. vertebra
   6. epiphyseal plate

B

JOINTS AND MUSCLES

I. 1. synovial fluid
   2. suture joint
   3. articulation
   4. tendon
   5. synovial cavity
   6. synovial membrane
   7. ligament
   8. bursa
   9. synovial joint

II. 1. flexion
   2. fascia
   3. abduction
   4. plantar flexion

5. extension
6. dorsiflexion
7. insertion of a muscle
8. pronation
9. origin of a muscle
10. adduction
11. visceral muscle
12. rotation
13. supination
14. skeletal muscle

Review Sheet Quiz

A

1. acetabulum
2. stiff
3. joint
4. joint
5. bursa (sac of fluid near a joint)
6. calcium
7. calcaneus
8. wrist
9. neck
10. cartilage

B

1. clavicul/o
2. coccyg/o
3. cost/o
4. crani/o
5. fasci/o
6. femor/o
7. leiomy/o
8. humer/o
9. ili/o
10. ischi/o

C

1. humpback
2. lamina (part of the vertebral arch)
3. curve, swayback
4. loins, lower back
5. malleolus (rounded portion of ankle bone)
6. maxilla (upper jaw bone)
7. hand bones
8. foot bones
9. muscle
10. bone marrow

D

1. muscle
2. olecranon (elbow)
3. straight
4. bone
5. patella (knee cap)
6. fibula (smaller lower leg bone)
7. finger and toe bones
8. vertebra, backbone

9. skeletal, striated muscle
10. vertebra, backbone

E

1. sacr/o
2. sarc/o
3. scapul/o
4. scoli/o
5. stern/o
6. thorac/o
7. fibul/o
8. uln/o
9. radi/o
10. mandibul/o

F

1. pain
2. lack of strength
3. immature cell, embryonic
4. to break
5. to bind, tie together
6. blood condition
7. slipping
8. softening
9. deficiency
10. pore, passage
11. instrument to cut
12. nourishment, development

G

1. no, not, without
2. away from

3. toward
4. complete, through
5. back
6. above, upon
7. out, outside
8. between, beyond
9. surrounding
10. many, much
11. under, below
12. above

Crossword Puzzle

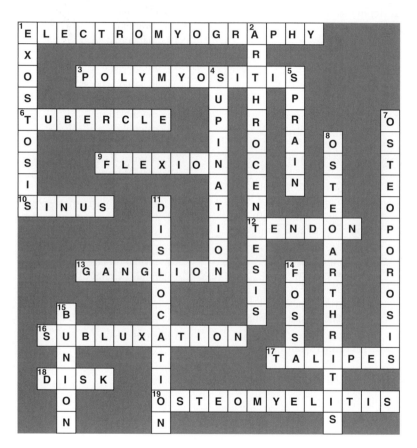

Practical Applications

A

1. D
2. B
3. A
4. C

B

1. D
2. A

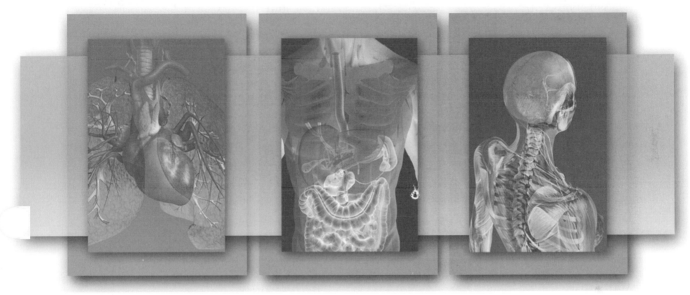

chapter 16

Chapter Sixteen

MULTIPLE CHOICE QUIZ

Name: _____

In the box write the letter of the choice that is the definition of the term or best answers the question. There is only one correct answer for each question.

1. **A type of epithelial cell in the epidermis is a:** .... ☐
   A. Lipocyte
   B. Neuron
   C. Chondrocyte
   D. Histiocyte
   E. Squamous cell

2. **Dermis:** .... ☐
   A. Basal layer of skin
   B. Middle layer of skin
   C. Epithelial layer
   D. Above the epidermis
   E. Subcutaneous tissue

3. **A hard protein material found in the epidermis:** .... ☐
   A. Melanin
   B. Sebum
   C. Keratin
   D. Collagen
   E. Cerumen

4. **Structural protein found in skin and connective tissue:** .... ☐
   A. Cartilage
   B. Collagen
   C. Cerumen
   D. Melanin
   E. Sebum

5. **Xer/o means:** .... ☐
   A. Dry
   B. Scaly
   C. Thick
   D. Yellow
   E. White

6. **Pertaining to under a nail:** .... ☐
   A. Hypodermic
   B. Hypoglossal
   C. Epidermis
   D. Subcutaneous
   E. Subungual

7. **What is a combining form meaning skin?** .... ☐
   A. Ichthy/o
   B. Adip/o
   C. Cutane/o
   D. Pachy/o
   E. Xanth/o

8. **Absence of pigment in skin:** .... ☐
   A. Erythroderma
   B. Melanism
   C. Xanthoderma
   D. Dermatitis
   E. Albinism

9. **Inflammation of the soft tissue around a nail:** .... ☐
   A. Onychomycosis
   B. Erythema
   C. Epidermolysis
   D. Paronychia
   E. Dermatitis

10. **Profuse sweating:** .... ☐
    A. Anhidrosis
    B. Diaphoresis
    C. Hidradenitis
    D. Seborrhea
    E. Keratosis

11. **Fungal infection:** .... ☐
    A. Leukoderma
    B. Keratosis
    C. Erythema
    D. Trichomycosis
    E. Seborrhea

12. **Fatty mass within a sebaceous gland:** .... ☐
    A. Steatoma
    B. Lipoma
    C. Pilosebaceous
    D. Onychophagia
    E. Verrucae

13. **A wheal is a/an:** .... ☐
    A. Macule
    B. Wart
    C. Polyp
    D. Ulcer
    E. Hive

14. **Bullae:** .... ☐
    A. Papules
    B. Macules
    C. Fissures
    D. Large blisters
    E. Nodules

15. **Pustule:** .... ☐
    A. Cyst
    B. Pruritus
    C. Urticaria
    D. Small abscess
    E. Ecchymoses

16. **Itching:** .... ☐
    A. Pruritis
    B. Petechiae
    C. Alopecia
    D. Purpura
    E. Pruritus

17. **Keloid:** .... ☐
    A. Thickened scar
    B. Leukoplakia
    C. Comedo
    D. Callus
    E. Wart

18. **Inflammatory disease of the joints and collagen of the skin; can affect other organs of the body:** .... ☐
    A. Impetigo
    B. Systemic lupus erythematosus
    C. Mycosis fungoides
    D. Actinic keratosis
    E. Eczema

19. **Moles that can develop into malignant melanoma:** .... ☐
    A. Basal cell carcinomas
    B. Squamous cell carcinomas
    C. Verrucae
    D. Dysplastic nevi
    E. Polyps

20. **Bed sore; break in continuity of skin:** .... ☐
    A. Leukoplakia
    B. Psoriasis
    C. Tinea
    D. Decubitus ulcer
    E. Scleroderma

21. **Chronic recurrent dermatosis with silvery gray scales covering red patches in skin:** .... ☐
    A. Leukoplakia
    B. Psoriasis
    C. Tinea
    D. Decubitus ulcer
    E. Scleroderma

22. **A dermatomycosis:** .... ☐
    A. Leukoplakia
    B. Psoriasis
    C. Tinea
    D. Decubitus ulcer
    E. Scleroderma

23. **White patches on a mucous membrane of tongue or cheek:** .... ☐
    A. Leukoplakia
    B. Psoriasis
    C. Tinea
    D. Decubitus ulcer
    E. Scleroderma

24. **Connective tissue in the skin hardens:** .... ☐
    A. Leukoplakia
    B. Psoriasis
    C. Tinea
    D. Decubitus ulcer
    E. Scleroderma

25. **Layers of growth are removed and examined microscopically:** .... ☐
    A. Fungal test
    B. Scratch test
    C. Mohs surgery
    D. Cryosurgery
    E. Punch biopsy

Chapter Sixteen
EXERCISE QUIZ

Name: _____

A. *Select from the following to complete the sentences below:*

basal layer   dermis   lunula   stratum corneum
collagen   keratin   melanin
cuticle   lipocyte   sebum

1. A fat cell is a _____

2. The half-moon shaped white area at the base of a nail is called the _____

3. A structural protein found in skin and connective tissue is _____

4. A black pigment found in the epidermis is _____

5. The deepest region of the epidermis is the _____

6. The outermost layer of the epidermis, consisting of flattened keratinized
   cells is the _____

7. An oily substance secreted by sebaceous glands is _____

8. The middle layer of the skin is the corium or _____

9. A hard, protein material found in epidermis, hair, and nails is _____

10. A band of epidermis at the base and side of the nail plate is the _____

B. *Complete the following terms from their meanings given below:*

11. The outermost layer of skin: **epi** _____

12. Profuse sweating: **dia** _____

13. Excessive secretion from sebaceous glands: **sebo** _____

14. Inflammation and swelling of soft tissue around a nail: **par** _____

15. Fungal infection of the skin: **dermato** _____

16. Burning sensation (pain) in the skin: **caus** _____

C. *Build medical terms from the definitions and word parts given:*

17. surgical repair of the skin: **dermato** _____

18. pertaining to under the skin: **sub** _____

19. abnormal condition of lack of sweat: **an** _____

20. abnormal condition of proliferation of keratinized cells: **kerat** _____

21. abnormal condition of dry, scaly skin: _____ **osis**

22. loosening of the epidermis: **epidermo** _____

23. yellow tumor (nodule under the skin): _____ oma

24. under the nail: **sub** _____

25. abnormal condition of nail fungus: **onycho** _____

D. Match the cutaneous lesion with its meaning below:

cyst	macule	papule	pustule	vesicle
fissure	nodule	polyp	ulcer	wheal

26. circumscribed collection of clear fluid (blister) _____

27. smooth, slightly elevated edematous area (hive) _____

28. discolored, flat lesion (freckle) _____

29. groove or crack-like sore _____

30. mushroom-like growth extending from the surface of a mucous membrane _____

31. circumscribed collection of pus _____

32. closed sac containing fluid or semi-solid material _____

33. open sore or erosion of skin _____

34. solid elevation of the skin (pimple) _____

35. larger than 1 cm solid elevation of the skin _____

E. Give medical terms for the following:

36. baldness _____   39. purplish, macular patch _____

37. itching _____   40. loss of pigment in skin _____

38. blackhead _____   41. small, pinpoint hemorrhages _____

F. Give the term that fits the definition (some letters or word parts are given):

42. contagious parasitic infection with intense pruritus: **sc** _____

43. white patches on mucous membrane of tongue or cheek: **leuko** _____

44. characterized by a rash: **ex** _____

45. colored pigmentation of the skin (mole): **n** _____

46. acute, allergic reaction in which hives develop: **u** _____

47. large blisters: b _____

48. raised, thickened scar: k _____

49. sac of fluid and hair over the sacral region of the back: p _____ cyst

50. chickenpox: v _____

G. Match the pathological skin condition with its description below:

acne	gangrene	psoriasis	tinea
decubitus ulcer	impetigo	scleroderma	
eczema	malignant melanoma	systemic lupus erythematosus	

51. build-up of sebum and keratin in pores of the skin
    leading to papular and pustular eruptions   _____

52. fungal skin infection _____

53. chronic hardening and shrinking of connective tissue _____

54. bedsore _____

55. necrosis of skin tissue resulting from ischemia _____

56. contagious, infectious pyoderma _____

57. chronic, recurrent dermatosis marked by silvery gray scales
    covering red patches on the skin   _____

58. cancerous tumor composed of melanocytes _____

59. widespread inflammatory disease of joints and collagen
    of the skin with "butterfly" rash on the face   _____

60. chronic or acute inflammatory skin disease with
    erythematous, pustular, or papular lesions   _____

H. Give short answers for the following:

61. Two skin tests for allergy are _____ and

    _____

62. A surgical procedure to core out a disk of skin for microscopic analysis is a _____

63. The procedure in which thin layers of malignant growth are removed
    and each is microscopically analyzed is   _____

64. Moles that do not form properly and may progress to form
    melanomas are called   _____

65. Destruction of tissue by intensely cold temperatures is called _____

Chapter Sixteen
DICTATION AND COMPREHENSION QUIZ: VOCABULARY, COMBINING FORMS, AND SUFFIXES

Name: _____

A. Dictation of Terms

1. _____   11. _____

2. _____   12. _____

3. _____   13. _____

4. _____   14. _____

5. _____   15. _____

6. _____   16. _____

7. _____   17. _____

8. _____   18. _____

9. _____   19. _____

10. _____   20. _____

B. Comprehension of Terms: Match the number of the above term with its meaning below:

_____ Tumor of fatty tissue

_____ Half-moon shaped, white area at the base of a nail

_____ Condition of absence of pigment in the skin

_____ Pigment that gives the skin color

_____ Band of epidermis at the base and sides of the nail plate

_____ Intensely unpleasant burning sensation in skin

_____ Scraping away of skin (to remove tattoos or fine wrinkles)

_____ Pertaining to redness of the skin

_____ Condition of absence of sweating

_____ Baldness

_____ Condition of white plaques (spots or patches) on the tongue or cheek

_____ Separation of the nail plate from the nail bed

_____ Inflammation of skin with yellow or brown-gray greasy scales (dandruff)

_____ Pertaining to under a nail

_____ Inflammation and swelling of the soft tissue around the nail

_____ Dry skin

_____ Pertaining to hair and glands that secrete sebum

_____ Abnormal condition of thickened area of the epidermis

_____ Abnormal condition of a fungal infection of the skin

_____ Structural protein found in the skin and connective tissue

Chapter Sixteen
DICTATION AND COMPREHENSION QUIZ: LESIONS, SYMPTOMS, ABNORMAL CONDITIONS, AND NEOPLASMS

Name: _____

A. Dictation of Terms

1. _____   11. _____

2. _____   12. _____

3. _____   13. _____

4. _____   14. _____

5. _____   15. _____

6. _____   16. _____

7. _____   17. _____

8. _____   18. _____

9. _____   19. _____

10. _____   20. _____

B. Comprehension of Terms: Match the number of the above term with its meaning below:

_____ Infection of the skin caused by a fungus

_____ Increased growth of cells in the horny (keratinized) layer of the epidermis

_____ Hypertrophied, thickened scar that occurs after trauma or surgical incision

_____ Normal scar left by a healed wound

_____ Bacterial inflammatory skin disease; a contagious pyoderma

_____ Papular and pustular eruption of the skin; comedones occur

_____ Chronic, recurrent dermatosis marked by itchy, scaly, red patches covered by silvery, gray scales

_____ Inflammatory skin disease with erythematous, papulovesicular lesions; common allergic reaction in children and adults

_____ Loss of pigment in areas of the skin

_____ Itching

_____ Bluish-black marks on the skin caused by hemorrhages into the skin

_____ Large areas of bleeding under the skin

_____ Death of tissue associated with loss of blood supply

_____ A small solid elevation of the skin (pimple)

_____ A smooth, slightly elevated, edematous area that is redder or paler than the surrounding skin

_____ An acute allergic reaction of the skin with hives and itching

_____ Bedsore

_____ Malignant tumor of cells in the epidermal layer of the skin

_____ An exanthematous viral disease; German measles

_____ Large vesicles

Chapter Sixteen
SPELLING QUIZ

Name: _____

A. *Circle the term that is spelled correctly and write its meaning in the space provided:*

1. paroncyhia   paronychia _____

2. pilosebaceous   pillosebaecous _____

3. subungwnal   subungual _____

4. xanthoma   xanantoma _____

5. dermatophytosis   dermatophitosis _____

6. wheel   wheal _____

7. verruca   veruca _____

8. callis   callus _____

9. keratosis   carrotosis _____

10. tinnea   tinea _____

B. *Circle the term that is spelled correctly. The meaning of each term is given.*

11. inflammatory skin disease .... ezcema   eksema   eczema

12. itching .... pruritis   purtritis   pruritus

13. red, round wheals (hives) .... urticaria   urtakaria   urtikaria

14. malignant tumor of pigmented
    skin cells .... melenoma   melonoma   melanoma

15. mole .... nevus   nevas   nevis

16. blackhead .... komedo   comedo   comeddo

17. absence of skin pigment .... albinism   allbinism   albenism

18. chronic recurrent dermatosis with itchy,
    scaly patches .... psoriesis   psoraisis   psoriasis

19. structural protein found in skin and
    connective tissue .... collegen   kollagen   collagen

20. profuse sweating .... diaphoresis   diaforesis   diaphoriesis

Chapter Sixteen
PRONUNCIATION QUIZ

Name: _____

A. *Underline the accented syllable in the following terms:*

1. impetigo
2. erythema
3. eczema
4. pilonidal cyst
5. dermatomycosis
6. steatoma
7. vitiligo
8. sebaceous gland
9. epithelium
10. albinism

B. *Match the term in Column I with its meaning in Column II:*

Column I

1. adipose _____
2. dermis _____
3. epithelium _____
4. urticaria _____
5. paronychia _____
6. tinea _____
7. melanin _____
8. nevus _____
9. keratin _____
10. collagen _____

Column II

A. A collection of pigmented cells on the skin surface.
B. Layer of skin cells on outer and inner surfaces on the body.
C. Pertaining to fat.
D. Hard protein material found in the skin, hair, and nails.
E. Structural protein found in the skin and connective tissue.
F. Hives.
G. A black pigment formed by cells in the skin.
H. Fungal infection of the skin.
I. The middle layer of the skin; corium.
J. Inflammation of soft tissue around the skin.

C. *Complete the following terms using the definitions given:*

1. epidermo_____ Loosening of the epidermis.
2. _____itis Inflammation of sweat glands.
3. _____ocyte Fat cell.
4. _____esis Excessive or profuse sweating.
5. _____ous Pertaining to under the skin.
6. _____o A blackhead.
7. _____osis A purplish patch on the skin caused by hemorrhage.
8. _____ous Pertaining to hair and oil glands.
9. _____oid Hypertrophied, thickened scar.
10. _____a Fungal infection of the skin.

Chapter Sixteen
DIAGRAM QUIZ

Name: _____

Label the diagram below using the terms listed below:

Fissure	Nodule
Crust	Papule
Cyst	Wheal
Erosion	Ulcer
Polyp	Vesicle
Macule	Pustule

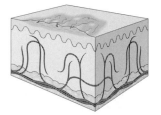

1. _____
(dried serum and cellular debris)

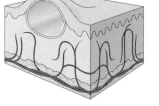

2. _____
(fluid or semisolid filled sac)

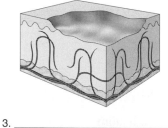

3. _____
(wearing away, loss of epidermis)

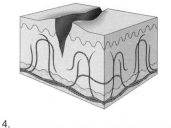

4. _____
(slit, groove)

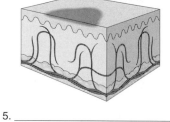

5. _____
(discolored, flat)

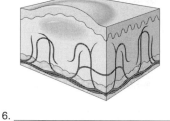

6. _____
(solid, elevated mass, more than 1 cm)

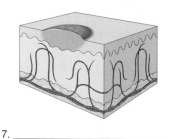

7. _____
(small, solid elevation)

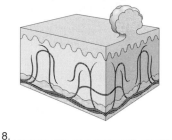

8. _____
(growth)

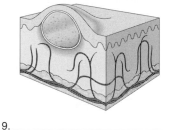

9. _____
(pus-filled)

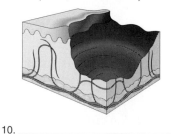

10. _____
(open sore, erosion)

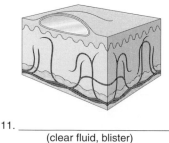

11. _____
(clear fluid, blister)

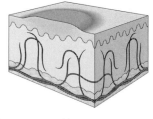

12. _____
(smooth, slightly elevated, edema)

Chapter Sixteen
VOCABULARY QUIZ

Name: _____

A. *Match the following terms with their meanings below:*

albino	cuticle	epidermis
apocrine sweat gland	dermis	epithelium
basal layer	eccrine sweat gland	hair follicle
collagen		

1. Structural protein found in the skin and connective tissue _____

2. Middle layer of the skin _____

3. Layer of skin cells forming the outer and inner surfaces of the body _____

4. Sac within which each hair grows _____

5. Person with skin deficient in pigment (melanin) _____

6. Band of epidermis at the base and sides of the nail plate _____

7. Most numerous of sweat-producing glands in the skin _____

8. Deepest region of the epidermis; it gives rise to all the epidermal cells _____

9. Large dermal exocrine gland; located in axilla and genitals _____

10. Outermost layer of the skin _____

B. Match the following terms with their meanings below:

integumentary system	paronychium	squamous epithelium
keratin	pore	stratified
lipocyte	sebaceous gland	stratum corneum
lunula	sebum	subcutaneous layer
melanin		

1. Fat cell _____

2. Tiny opening on the surface of the skin _____

3. Oily substance secreted by sebaceous glands _____

4. Half-moon shaped, white area at the base of a nail _____

5. Soft tissue surrounding the nail border _____

6. Arranged in layers _____

7. Flat, scale-like cells composing the epidermis _____

8. Major skin pigment _____

9. Hard protein material found in the epidermis, hair, and nails _____

10. Innermost layer of the skin, containing fatty tissue _____

11. The skin and its accessory structures, such as hair and nails _____

12. Outermost layer of the epidermis; consisting of flattened keratinized cells _____

13. Oil secreting gland in the dermis; associated with hair follicles _____

Chapter Sixteen
REVIEW SHEET QUIZ

Name: _____

A. *Give meanings for the following combining forms:*

1. adip/o _____

2. albin/o _____

3. caus/o _____

4. cutane/o _____

5. dermat/o _____

6. diaphor/o _____

7. erythem/o _____

8. hidr/o _____

9. hydr/o _____

10. trich/o _____

11. onych/o _____

12. myc/o _____

13. ungu/o _____

14. lip/o _____

15. pil/o _____

B. *Give combining forms for the following meanings:*

1. pus _____

2. black _____

3. dry _____

4. yellow _____

5. wrinkle_____

6. scaly, fish-like _____

C. *Give meanings for the following suffixes:*

1. -algia _____

2. -derma _____

3. -lysis _____

4. -osis _____

5. -ous _____

6. -plakia _____

7. -plasty _____

8. -rrhea _____

Chapter Sixteen
CROSSWORD PUZZLE

Name: _____

Fill in the crossword puzzle below using the clues listed underneath it.

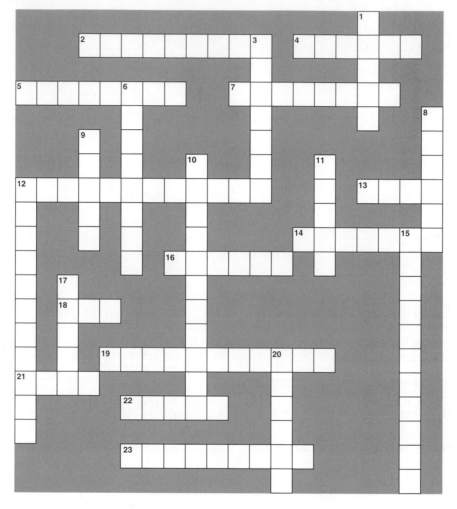

Across Clues

2. Chronic recurrent dermatosis marked by itchy, scaly, red patches covered by silvery scales.
4. Small, solid elevation of the skin.
5. Depigmentation in areas of the skin.
7. Death of tissue from loss of blood supply.
12. Innermost layer of the skin (under the skin).
13. Papular and pustular eruption of the skin.
14. Wart.
16. Increased growth of cells in the horny layer of the epidermis due to pressure or friction.
18. Outer layer of the skin:_____dermis.
19. White, thickened patches on mucous membrane tissue of the tongue or cheek.
21. A "butterfly_____"; as in SLE.
22. A mushroom-like growth extending on a stalk from the surface of a mucous membrane.
23. Thickened area of the epidermis; actinic and seborrheic are types.

Down Clues

1. Injuries to tissue caused by heat contact.
3. A contagious, parasitic infection of the skin with intense pruritus.
6. Bacterial, inflammatory, contagious skin disease characterized by vesicles and pustules.
8. Inflammatory skin disease with erythematous, papulovesicular lesions.
9. An open sore or erosion of the skin.
10. Study of the skin.
11. Infection of the skin caused by a fungus.
12. A chronic disease of the skin with hardening and shrinking of connective tissue.
15. Tissue is destroyed by the application of intensely cold liquid nitrogen.
17. Colored (pigmented) lesion of the skin; a mole.
20. An enlarged, thickened scar after trauma or surgery.

Chapter Sixteen

PRACTICAL APPLICATIONS

Name: _____

The following questions can be used with the Disease Descriptions on page 649 of the text:

1. **Which condition is caused by a fungal infection?** .... ☐
   A. Mycosis fungoides
   B. Candidiasis
   C. Cellulitis
   D. Both A and B

2. **Which condition is a cancerous condition?** .... ☐
   A. Mycosis fungoides
   B. Candidiasis
   C. Cellulitis
   D. Both B and C

3. **Which condition is caused by a bacterial infection?** .... ☐
   A. Mycosis fungoides
   B. Candidiasis
   C. Cellulitis
   D. Both A and C

4. **What is a common location for candidiasis?** .... ☐
   A. Soles of the feet
   B. Lumbar area of the spine
   C. Mouth and genital area
   D. Underarm

5. **Paronychial lesions occur around the:** .... ☐
   A. Nails
   B. Hair follicles
   C. Groin
   D. Armpit

6. **Thrush can occur:** .... ☐
   A. In the mouth
   B. In the vagina
   C. Between the fingers
   D. A and B

7. **Cellulitis is a nonsuppurative infection. This means:** .... ☐
   A. It is not contagious
   B. It is caused by a virus
   C. It affects the epidermis
   D. It is not purulent

8. **Edematous skin means:** .... ☐
   A. Swollen tissue
   B. Reddish-brown color
   C. White plaques
   D. Skin ulcer

9. **Streptococci are:** .... ☐
   A. Berry-shaped bacteria in clusters
   B. Berry-shaped bacteria in twisted chains
   C. A type of fungus
   D. A type of bacillus

10. **Mycosis fungoides involves malignant:** .... ☐
    A. Erythrocytes
    B. Leukocytes
    C. Thrombocytes
    D. Neutrophils

11. **Generalized erythroderma means:** ...... ☐
    A. Lymph nodes are involved
    B. Tumor has invaded the spleen
    C. Widespread red skin
    D. Ulcerations are present

12. **Treatment for mycosis fungoides includes:** .... ☐
    A. Surgery
    B. Dermatologic chemotherapy
    C. Radiotherapy
    D. Both B and C

Chapter Sixteen
ANSWERS TO THE QUIZZES

Multiple Choice Quiz

1. E	4. B	7. C	10. B	13. E	16. E	19. D	22. C	25. C
2. B	5. A	8. E	11. D	14. D	17. A	20. D	23. A	
3. C	6. E	9. D	12. A	15. D	18. B	21. B	24. E	

Exercise Quiz

A

1. lipocyte
2. lunula
3. collagen
4. melanin
5. basal layer
6. stratum corneum
7. sebum
8. dermis
9. keratin
10. cuticle

B

11. epidermis
12. diaphoresis
13. seborrhea
14. paronychia
15. dermatomycosis
16. causalgia

C

17. dermatoplasty
18. subcutaneous
19. anhidrosis
20. keratosis
21. ichthyosis
22. epidermolysis
23. xanthoma
24. subungual
25. onychomycosis

D

26. vesicle
27. wheal
28. macule
29. fissure
30. polyp
31. pustule
32. cyst
33. ulcer
34. papule
35. nodule

E

36. alopecia
37. pruritus
38. comedo

39. purpura
40. albinism
41. petechiae

F

42. scabies
43. leukoplakia
44. exanthematous
45. nevus
46. urticaria
47. bullae
48. keloid
49. pilonidal cyst
50. varicella

G

51. acne
52. tinea
53. scleroderma
54. decubitus ulcer
55. gangrene
56. impetigo
57. psoriasis
58. malignant melanoma
59. systemic lupus erythematosus
60. eczema

H

61. patch and scratch
62. punch biopsy
63. Mohs surgery
64. dysplastic nevi
65. cryosurgery

Dictation and Comprehension: Vocabulary, Combining Forms, and Suffixes

A

1. albinism
2. alopecia
3. anhidrosis
4. causalgia
5. collagen
6. cuticle
7. dermabrasion
8. dermatomycosis
9. erythematous

10. keratosis
11. leukoplakia
12. lipoma
13. lunula
14. melanin
15. onycholysis
16. paronychia
17. pilosebaceous
18. seborrheic dermatitis
19. subungual
20. xeroderma

B

12 Tumor of fatty tissue
13 Half-moon shaped, white area at the base of a nail
1 Condition of absence of pigment in the skin
14 Pigment that gives the skin color
6 Band of epidermis at the base and sides of the nail plate
4 Intensely unpleasant burning sensation in skin
7 Scraping away of skin (to remove tattoos or fine wrinkles)
9 Pertaining to redness of the skin
3 Condition of absence of sweating
2 Baldness
11 Condition of white plaques (spots or patches) on the tongue or cheek
15 Separation of the nail plate from the nail bed
18 Inflammation of skin with yellow or brown-gray greasy scales (dandruff)
19 Pertaining to under a nail
16 Inflammation and swelling of the soft tissue around the nail
20 Dry skin
17 Pertaining to hair and glands that secrete sebum
10 Abnormal condition of thickened area of the epidermis
8 Abnormal condition of a fungal infection of the skin
5 structural protein found in the skin and connective tissue

Dictation and Comprehension: Lesions, Symptoms, Abnormal Conditions, and Neoplasms

A

1. acne
2. basal cell carcinoma
3. bullae
4. callus
5. cicatrix
6. decubitus ulcer
7. ecchymoses
8. eczema
9. gangrene
10. impetigo
11. keloid
12. papule
13. pruritus
14. psoriasis
15. purpura
16. rubella
17. tinea
18. urticaria
19. vitiligo
20. wheal

B

17 Infection of the skin caused by a fungus
4 Increased growth of cells in the horny (keratinized) layer of the epidermis
11 Hypertrophied, thickened scar that occurs after trauma or surgical incision
5 Normal scar left by a healed wound
10 Bacterial inflammatory skin disease; a contagious pyoderma
1 Papular and pustular eruption of the skin; comedones occur
14 Chronic, recurrent dermatosis marked by itchy, scaly, red patches covered by silvery, gray scales
8 Inflammatory skin disease with erythematous, papulovesicular lesions; common allergic reaction in children and adults
19 Loss of pigment in areas of the skin
13 Itching
7 Bluish-black marks on the skin caused by hemorrhages into the skin
15 Large areas of bleeding under the skin
9 Death of tissue associated with loss of blood supply

12 A small solid elevation of the skin (pimple)
20 A smooth, slightly elevated, edematous area that is redder or paler than the surrounding skin
18 An acute allergic reaction of the skin with hives and itching
6 Bedsore
2 Malignant tumor of cells in the epidermal layer of the skin
16 An exanthematous viral disease; German measles
3 Large vesicles

Spelling Quiz

A

1. paronychia—infection of the nail bed
2. pilosebaceous—pertaining to hair and sebaceous gland
3. subungual—pertaining to under a nail
4. xanthoma—lipid collection under the skin
5. dermatophytosis—abnormal condition of fungal infection of the skin
6. wheal—smooth, slightly elevated swollen area
7. verruca—wart
8. callus—increased growth in epidermis due to pressure
9. keratosis—thickened area of the epidermis
10. tinea—fungal infection of the skin

B

11. eczema
12. pruritus
13. urticaria
14. melanoma
15. nevus
16. comedo
17. albinism
18. psoriasis
19. collagen
20. diaphoresis

Pronunciation Quiz

A

1. impe<u>ti</u>go
2. ery<u>the</u>ma
3. ec<u>ze</u>ma
4. pilo<u>ni</u>dal cyst
5. dermatomy<u>co</u>sis
6. stea<u>to</u>ma
7. viti<u>li</u>go

8. se<u>ba</u>ceous gland
9. epi<u>the</u>lium
10. <u>al</u>binism

B

1. C
2. I
3. B
4. F
5. J
6. H
7. G
8. A
9. D
10. E

C

1. epidermolysis
2. hidradenitis
3. lipocyte
4. diaphoresis
5. subcutaneous
6. comedo
7. ecchymosis
8. pilosebaceous
9. keloid
10. tinea

Diagram Quiz

1. Crust
2. Cyst
3. Erosion
4. Fissure
5. Macule
6. Nodule
7. Papule
8. Polyp
9. Pustule
10. Ulcer
11. Vesicle
12. Wheal

Vocabulary Quiz

A

1. collagen
2. dermis
3. epithelium
4. hair follicle
5. albino
6. cuticle
7. eccrine sweat gland
8. basal layer
9. apocrine sweat gland
10. epidermis

B

1. lipocyte
2. pore
3. sebum

4. lunula
5. paronychium
6. stratified
7. squamous epithelium
8. melanin
9. keratin
10. subcutaneous layer
11. integumentary system
12. stratum corneum
13. sebaceous gland

Review Sheet Quiz

A

1. fat
2. white
3. burn, burning
4. skin
5. skin
6. profuse sweating
7. redness
8. sweat
9. water
10. hair
11. nail
12. fungus
13. nail
14. fat
15. hair

B

1. py/o
2. melan/o
3. xer/o
4. xanth/o
5. rhytid/o
6. ichyth/o

C

1. pain
2. skin
3. separation, breakdown
4. condition, abnormal condition
5. pertaining to
6. plaque
7. surgical repair
8. flow, discharge

Practical Applications

1. B
2. A
3. C
4. C
5. A
6. D
7. D
8. A
9. B
10. B
11. C
12. D

Crossword Puzzle

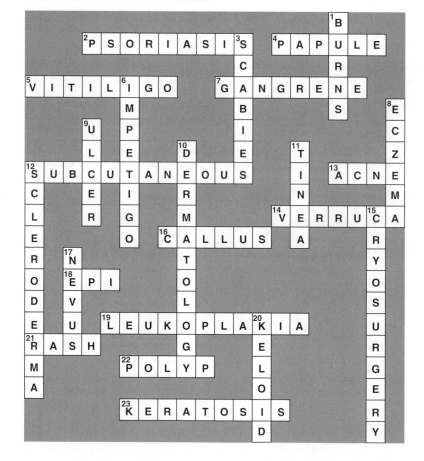

Chapter Sixteen

Answers to Combining Forms and Terminology Sections

(textbook pages 632–636)

Terminology	Meaning

Combining Forms

adipose	Pertaining to fat.
albinism	Condition of no pigment in skin, hair, and eyes (white skin).
causalgia	Intense burning sensation in the skin (due to nerve damage).
electrocautery	Wires used during surgery to burn through tissue.
subcutaneous	Pertaining to beneath the skin.
epidermis	Outermost layer of skin.
dermatitis	Inflammation of skin.
dermatoplasty	Surgical repair of the skin.
dermatologist	Specialist in diseases of the skin.
dermabrasion	A surgical procedure to remove acne scars, tattoos, and fine wrinkles. Skin is scraped away; sandpaper or mechanical methods are used on frozen skin.
epidermolysis	Loosening of the skin.
diaphoresis	Condition of profuse sweating.
erythema	Condition of redness of the skin (flushing).
anhidrosis	Condition of lack of sweat.
ichthyosis	Abnormal condition of dry, scaly skin (fish-like skin).
keratosis	Abnormal condition of thickened areas of the skin (horny cells accumulate).
leukoplakia	Condition of white plaques on the skin.
lipoma	Tumor (benign) of fat tissue.
liposuction	Removal of subcutaneous fat tissue with a blunt-tipped cannula (tube) through which suction (aspiration) is applied.
melanocyte	Cell that forms melanin and is found in the epidermis of the skin.
melanoma	Tumor (malignant) of melanocytes.
mycosis	Any disease caused by fungus.
onycholysis	Separation of nail plate from the nail bed in fungal infections or after trauma.
onychomycosis	Abnormal condition of fungal infection of nails.
paronychia	Condition of inflammation and swelling (infection) of the tissue around the nail.
dermatophytosis	Abnormal condition of fungus (plant) infection in the skin.
pilosebaceous	Pertaining to a sebaceous gland and hair.
pyoderma	Condition of pus infection within the skin.
rhytidectomy	Removal of wrinkles.
seborrhea	"Flow of sebum"; disturbance of sebaceous glands marked by increase in the flow of sebum.
squamous epithelium	Pertaining to scale-like cells that cover the outside of the body (epidermis) and line the inner tubes of the body.
steatoma	Mass, tumor arising from sebaceous glands; sebaceous cyst.
trichomycosis	Disease of the hair due to a fungal infection.
subungual	Pertaining to under a nail.
xanthoma	Flat, slightly elevated, rounded plaque or nodule usually found on the eyelids.
xeroderma	Abnormal condition of dry, rough skin.

chapter 17

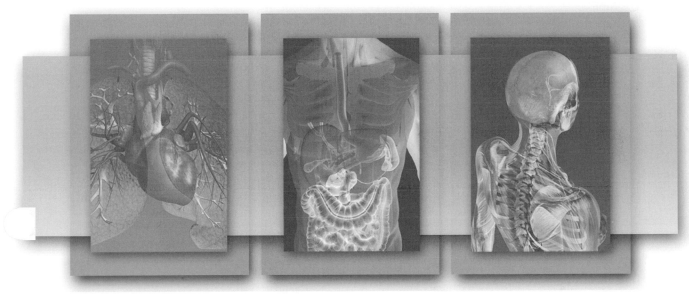

Chapter Seventeen

MULTIPLE CHOICE QUIZ

Name: _____

In the box write the letter of the choice that is the definition of the term or best answers the question. There is only one correct answer for each question.

1. **Fibrous layer of clear tissue that extends over the anterior portion of the eye and is continuous with the white of the eye:** .... ☐
   A. Fundus
   B. Ciliary body
   C. Pupil
   D. Cornea
   E. Iris

2. **Yellowish region in the retina; contains the fovea centralis:** .... ☐
   A. Optic disc
   B. Posterior chamber
   C. Macula lutea
   D. Sclera
   E. Choroid

3. **What eye structure is transparent, biconvex, and focuses light on the retina?** .... ☐
   A. Conjunctiva
   B. Lens
   C. Vitreous body
   D. Aqueous humor
   E. Sclera

4. **Place where optic nerve fibers cross in the brain:** .... ☐
   A. Optic disc
   B. Optic chiasma
   C. Retina
   D. Olfactory lobe
   E. Cerebral cortex

5. **Adjustment of the lens by the ciliary body:** .... ☐
   A. Accommodation
   B. Refraction
   C. Binocular vision
   D. Photophobia
   E. Amblyopia

6. **Photosensitive receptor cells of the retina; make the perception of color possible:** .... ☐
   A. Rods
   B. Cones
   C. Megakaryocyte
   D. Optic disc
   E. Optic chiasm

7. **The combining form for cornea is:** ...... ☐
   A. Ocul/o
   B. Opt/o
   C. Scler/o
   D. Choroid/o
   E. Kerat/o

8. **The combining form for the ciliary body is:** .... ☐
   A. Phak/o
   B. Lacrim/o
   C. Irid/o
   D. Cycl/o
   E. Dacry/o

9. **The meaning of palpebr/o is:** .... ☐
   A. Eyelid
   B. Cornea
   C. Tear gland
   D. Lens of the eye
   E. Optic disc

10. **An eye inflammation commonly called "pinkeye" is:** .... ☐
    A. Iritis
    B. Conjunctivitis
    C. Dacryoadenitis
    D. Scleritis
    E. Uveitis

11. **Impairment of vision due to old age:** .... ☐
    A. Emmetropia
    B. Diplopia
    C. Esotropia
    D. Presbyopia
    E. Anisocoria

12. **Myopia:** ....
    A. Nearsightedness
    B. Farsightedness
    C. Astigmatism
    D. Strabismus
    E. Glaucoma

13. **Astigmatism:**.............................
    A. Localized purulent infection of the eye
    B. Atrophy of the retina
    C. Esotropia
    D. Exotropia
    E. Defective curvature of the cornea or lens

14. **Glaucoma is primarily diagnosed by:**...............................
    A. Tonometry
    B. Ophthalmoscopy
    C. Slit lamp biomicroscopy
    D. Fluorescein angiography
    E. Visual field exam

15. **A blind spot; area of depressed vision surrounded by an area of normal vision:** ....
    A. Nyctalopia
    B. Exotropia
    C. Scotoma
    D. Esotropia
    E. Strabismus

16. **Macular degeneration produces:**...........
    A. Loss of central vision
    B. Hemianopia
    C. Retinal detachment
    D. Nystagmus
    E. Cataracts

17. **Small hard mass on the eyelid; formed from a sebaceous gland enlargement:**..
    A. Scleral buckle
    B. Blepharochalasis
    C. Chalazion
    D. Cataract
    E. Steatoma

18. **Snail-shaped, spirally wound tube in the inner ear is the:** ....
    A. Auricle
    B. Cochlea
    C. Auditory meatus
    D. Utricle
    E. Pinna

19. **Channel between the middle ear and the nasopharynx:**..............................
    A. Organ of Corti
    B. Semicircular canal
    C. Labyrinth
    D. Eustachian tube
    E. Oval window

20. **Myring/o means:**..............................
    A. Cerumen
    B. Tympanic membrane
    C. Stapes
    D. Auditory canal
    E. Semicircular canals

21. **Bacterial infection of the middle ear:** ....
    A. Serous otitis media
    B. Cholesteatoma
    C. Mastoiditis
    D. Barotitis
    E. Suppurative otitis media

22. **Tinnitus:** ....
    A. Hearing loss occurring with old age
    B. Dizziness associated with nausea and sensations of whirling motion
    C. Ringing sound in ears
    D. Dysphonia
    E. Aural discharge

23. **Visual examination of the ear:** ....
    A. Audiometry
    B. Otoscopy
    C. Tympanometry
    D. Tuning fork test
    E. Ophthalmoscopy

24. **Nerve deafness occurring with aging:** ....
    A. Vertigo
    B. Ménière disease
    C. Acoustic neuroma
    D. Presbycusis
    E. Otopyorrhea

25. **Fungal infection of the ear:**................
    A. Macrotia
    B. Salpingitis
    C. Otomycosis
    D. Cholesteatoma
    E. Labyrinthitis

Chapter Seventeen
EXERCISE QUIZ

Name: _____

EYE

A. *Match the structure of the eye with its description below:*

choroid	conjunctiva	iris	pupil	sclera
ciliary body	cornea	lens	retina	vitreous humor

1. Contains sensitive cells (rods and cones) that transmit light energy to nervous impulses _____

2. Contains muscles that control the shape of the lens and secrete aqueous humor _____

3. Transparent body behind the iris and in front of the vitreous humor; refracts light rays to bring them into focus on the retina _____

4. Jelly-like material behind the lens; helps to maintain the shape of the eyeball _____

5. Dark center of the eye through which light rays enter_____

6. Vascular layer of the eyeball that is continuous with the iris_____

7. Delicate membrane lining the eyelids and covering the anterior eyeball _____

8. Fibrous layer of clear tissue that extends over the anterior portion of the eyeball _____

9. Colored portion of the eye; surrounds the pupil _____

10. Tough, white outer coat of the eyeball _____

B. *Supply the term to complete the following:*

11. Region at the back of the eye where the retina meets the optic nerve is _____

12. The normal adjustment of the lens to bring an object into focus is _____

13. A yellowish region on the retina lateral to the optic disc is _____

14. Bending of light rays by the cornea, lens, and fluids of the eye is _____

15. Photosensitive receptor cells in the retina that make color perception possible are _____

16. Photosensitive receptor cells that make vision in dim light possible are _____

C. *Give meanings for the following terms:*

17. anisocoria _____

18. papilledema _____

19. photophobia _____

20. scotoma _____

D. *Complete the medical term from its definition and word parts given:*

21. inflammation of an eyelid: _____ itis

22. inflammation of the cornea: _____ itis

23. inflammation of the iris: _____ itis

24. inflammation of the conjunctiva: _____ itis

25. pertaining to within the eye: intra _____

E. *Match the following terms with their meanings below:*

aphakia   esotropia   hemianopsia
exotropia   xerophthalmia   uveitis

26. Inflammation of the vascular layer of the eye _____

27. Condition of dry eyes _____

28. Outward deviation of the eye _____

29. Inward deviation of the eye _____

30. Absence of the lens of the eye _____

31. Absence of vision in half of the visual field _____

F. *Describe the following visual conditions:*

32. presbyopia _____

33. myopia _____

34. diplopia _____

35. amblopia _____

36. hyperopia _____

37. emmetropia _____

G. Match the following abnormal conditions of the eye with their meanings below:

cataract   glaucoma   macular degeneration
diabetic retinopathy   hordeolum (stye)   strabismus

38. Abnormal deviations of the eye _____

39. Increased intraocular pressure results in retinal and optic nerve damage _____

40. Localized purulent infection of a sebaceous gland in the eyelid _____

41. Clouding of the lens causes decreased vision _____

42. Retinal microaneurysms, hemorrhages occur secondary to an endocrine condition _____

43. Deterioration of the macula lutea of the retina _____

H. Give the meanings for the following abbreviations:

44. OU _____

45. OD _____

46. OS _____

47. PERRLA _____

48. c. gl. _____

49. VF _____

50. s. gl. _____

Chapter Seventeen
EXERCISE QUIZ

Name: _____

EAR

A. *Arrange the following in the correct order to indicate their sequence in the transmission of sound waves to the brain from the outer ear:*

auditory liquids and receptors	external auditory canal	pinna
auditory nerve fibers	incus	stapes
cerebral cortex	malleus	tympanic membrane
cochlea	oval window	

1. _____   7. _____

2. _____   8. _____

3. _____   9. _____

4. _____   10. _____

5. _____   11. _____

6. _____

B. *Give meanings for the following medical terms:*

12. semicircular canals _____

13. cerumen _____

14. perilymph and endolymph _____

15. tympanic membrane _____

C. *Complete the following medical terms from their definitions given:*

16. removal of the third bone of the middle ear: _____ ectomy

17. instrument to measure hearing: _____ meter

18. deafness due to old age: _____ cusis

19. inflammation of the middle ear: ot _____

20. surgical repair of the eardrum: _____ plasty

D. Give the meanings for the following medical terms:

21. vertigo _____

22. otosclerosis _____

23. tinnitus _____

24. labyrinthitis _____

25. myringitis _____

26. suppurative otitis media _____

27. mastoiditis _____

28. Ménière disease _____

29. acoustic neuroma _____

30. cholesteatoma _____

E. Give meanings for the following abbreviations:

31. AS _____

32. ENG _____

33. EENT _____

34. AD _____

35. ENT _____

Chapter Seventeen
DICTATION AND
COMPREHENSION QUIZ: EYE

Name: _____

A. *Dictation of Terms*

1. _____   11. _____

2. _____   12. _____

3. _____   13. _____

4. _____   14. _____

5. _____   15. _____

6. _____   16. _____

7. _____   17. _____

8. _____   18. _____

9. _____   19. _____

10. _____   20. _____

B. *Comprehension of Terms: Match the number of the above term with its meaning below.*

_____ Visual examination of the eye

_____ White portion of the eye

_____ Fluid produced by the ciliary body; circulates through the anterior chamber of the eye

_____ Pupils are of unequal size

_____ Delicate membrane lining the eyelids and covering the anterior eyeball

_____ Inflammation of the cornea

_____ Paralysis of the ciliary muscles of the eye

_____ Double vision

_____ Clouding of the lens, causing decreased vision

_____ Abnormal deviation of the eye (esotropia and exotropia)

_____ Defective curvature of the cornea or lens of the eye

_____ Small, hard cystic mass on the eyelid

_____ Impairment of vision due to old age

_____ Nearsightedness

_____ Inflammation of the iris

_____ Loss of vision in one half of the visual field

_____ Swelling in the region of the optic disc

_____ Process of recording blood vessels in the back of the eye after IV injection of a dye

_____ Progressive damage to the yellowish region on the retina (lateral to and slightly below the optic disc)

_____ Absence of the lens of the eye

Chapter Seventeen

DICTATION AND
COMPREHENSION QUIZ: EAR

Name: _____

A. *Dictation of Terms*

1. _____   11. _____
2. _____   12. _____
3. _____   13. _____
4. _____   14. _____
5. _____   15. _____
6. _____   16. _____
7. _____   17. _____
8. _____   18. _____
9. _____   19. _____
10. _____   20. _____

B. *Comprehension of Terms: Match the number of the above term with its meaning below.*

_____ Fluid contained in the inner part of the ear

_____ Maze-like series of canals of the inner ear

_____ The outer flap of the ear; auricle

_____ Channel between the middle ear and the nasopharynx

_____ Waxy substance secreted by the external ear

_____ Collection of skin cells and cholesterol in a sac within the middle ear

_____ Incision of the eardrum

_____ Hardening of bony tissue in the inner ear; ankylosis of the stapes may occur

_____ Passages in the inner ear that are associated with maintaining equilibrium

_____ Specialist in the study of the ear and voice box

_____ Sensation of noises (ringing, buzzing, whistling) in the ears

_____ Sensation of irregular or whirling motion either of oneself or of external objects

_____ Surgical repair of a small bone in the middle ear

_____ Instrument to measure hearing

_____ Fungal infection of the ear

_____ Channel leading from the outer ear flap to the eardrum

_____ Benign tumor arising from the 8th cranial nerve in the brain

_____ A snail-shaped, spirally wound tube in the inner ear; contains hearing-sensitive cells

_____ Surgical repair of the eardrum

_____ Inflammation of the middle ear with pus formation

Chapter Seventeen
SPELLING QUIZ

Name: _____

A. *Circle the term that is spelled correctly and write its meaning in the space provided:*

1. anisocoria   anisocorea _____

2. acqueous humer   aqueous humor _____

3. blepharitis   blepheritis _____

4. cateract   cataract _____

5. conjuntivia   conjunctiva _____

6. cornea   kornea _____

7. cilliary body   ciliary body _____

8. dacryorhea   dacryorrhea _____

9. glaucoma   glaukoma _____

10. opthalmologist   ophthalmologist _____

B. *Circle the term that is spelled correctly. The meaning of each term is given.*

11. pertaining to sound	acoustic	acustic	akustic
12. outer flap of the ear	pina	penna	pinna
13. fungal ear condition	otomicosis	automycosis	otomycosis
14. ringing in the ears	tinnitis	tinitus	tinnitus
15. surgical repair of the eardrum	tympanoplasty	tinpanoplasty	timpanoplasty
16. incision of the eardrum...........................	myringotomy	myringetomy	miringotomy
17. waxy discharge from the ear	ceremen	serumen	cerumen
18. dizziness...	virtigo	vertigo	vertego
19. hearing impairment due to old age	presbycussis	presbicusis	presbycusis
20. removal of a middle ear bone...................	stapedectomy	stapidectomy	stapidectomy

Chapter Seventeen
PRONUNCIATION QUIZ

Name: _____

A. *Underline the accented syllable in the following words:*

1. prosthesis   4. malleus   7. mydriatic   10. macrotia
2. corneoscleral   5. palpebral   8. blepharitis
3. audiometer   6. presbycusis   9. retinopathy

B. *Match the term in Column I with its meaning in Column II:*

Column I   ### Column II

1. cerumen   _____   A. Clouding of the lens.

2. cochlea   _____   B. Small bone in the middle ear.

3. cornea   _____   C. Abnormal deviation of the eye caused by muscle weakness.

4. chalazion   _____   D. Wax found in the outer ear.

5. cataract   _____   E. Clear tissue that covers the front portion of the eyeball.

6. pinna   _____   F. Ringing sound in the ears.

7. eustachian tube _____   G. The flap, or outside part, of the ear.

8. stapes   _____   H. A snail-shaped, spirally wound tube in the inner ear.

9. tinnitus   _____   I. Small hard mass on the eyelid.

10. strabismus   _____   J. Tube connecting the middle ear to the throat.

C. *Complete the following medical terms from their definitions:*

1. _____ opia   Impairment of vision due to old age.

2. _____oplasty   Surgical repair of the eardrum.

3. _____o_____   Paralysis of the eye.

4. _____ eal   Pertaining to the eustachian tube and the throat.

5. hemi _____   Loss of one half of the visual field.

6. _____itis   Inflammation of the vascular layer of the eye.

7. a _____   Condition of the absence of the lens.

8. oto _____   Hardening of the bony tissue in the inner ear.

B. *Match the following terms with their meanings below:*

fundus of the eye	optic chiasm	refraction
iris	optic disc	retina
lens	optic nerve	pupil
macula	thalamus	sclera

1. Colored, pigmented membrane surrounding the pupil of the eye _____

2. Light-sensitive nerve cell layer containing photoreceptor
   cells (rods and cones) _____

3. Dark opening of the eye _____

4. Yellowish region on the retina, slightly below the optic disc;
   contains the fovea centralis _____

5. Point at which optic nerve fibers cross in the brain. _____

6. Bending of light rays by the cornea, lens, and fluids of the eye to bring them
   into focus on the retina _____

7. Region at the back of the eye where the optic nerve meets the retina _____

8. Cranial nerve carrying impulses from the retina to
   the brain (cerebral cortex) _____

9. Transparent, biconvex body behind the pupil; it bends light rays
   to focus them on the retina _____

10. Posterior, inner portion of the eye _____

11. Tough, white outer coat of the eyeball. _____

12. Relay center of the brain; optic nerve fibers pass through the thalamus
    on their way to the cerebral cortex _____

EAR

A. *Match the following terms with their meanings below:*

auditory canal   cochlea   incus
auditory nerve fibers   endolymph   labyrinth
auricle   eustachian tube   malleus
cerumen

1. Snail-shaped, spirally wound tube in the inner ear; contains hearing-sensitive receptor cells _____

2. Carry impulses from the inner ear to the brain (cerebral cortex) _____

3. Waxy substance secreted by the external ear; ear wax _____

4. Second little bone of the middle ear; shaped like an anvil _____

5. Channel between the middle ear and the nasopharynx; auditory tube _____

6. Flap of the ear _____

7. First little bone of the middle ear; shaped like a hammer _____

8. Fluid within the labyrinth of the ear _____

9. Maze-like series of canals within the inner ear _____

10. Channel that leads from the auricle to the eardrum; auditory meatus _____

B. *Match the following terms with their meanings below:*

organ of Corti   perilymph   stapes
ossicle   pinna   tympanic membrane
oval window   semicircular canals vestibule

1. Third small bone of the middle ear; shaped like a stirrup _____

2. Flap of the ear; auricle _____

3. Central cavity of the labyrinth, connecting the semicircular canals and the cochlea _____

4. Eardrum _____

5. Membrane between the middle and inner ear _____

6. Sensitive auditory receptive area in the cochlea of the inner ear _____

7. Passages in the inner ear associated with maintenance of equilibrium _____

8. Small bone _____

9. Fluid contained in the labyrinth of the inner ear _____

Chapter Seventeen
REVIEW SHEET QUIZ

Name: _____

A. *Give meanings for the following combining forms:*

1. acous/o _____

2. ambyl/o _____

3. anis/o _____

4. aque/o _____

5. audit/o _____

6. aur/o _____

7. blephar/o _____

8. cochle/o _____

9. conjunctiv/o _____

10. cor/o _____

B. *Give meanings for the following combining forms:*

1. corne/o _____

2. cycl/o _____

3. dacry/o _____

4. dipl/o _____

5. glauc/o _____

6. ir/o _____

7. kerat/o _____

8. lacrim/o _____

9. mi/o _____

10. mydr/o _____

C. *Give meanings for the following combining forms:*

1. myring/o _____

2. nyct/o _____

3. ocul/o _____

4. ophthalm/o _____

5. opt/o _____

6. ossicul/o _____

7. ot/o _____

8. palpebr/o _____

9. papill/o _____

10. phac/o _____

11. phot/o _____

12. presby/o _____

D. Give meanings for the following combining forms:

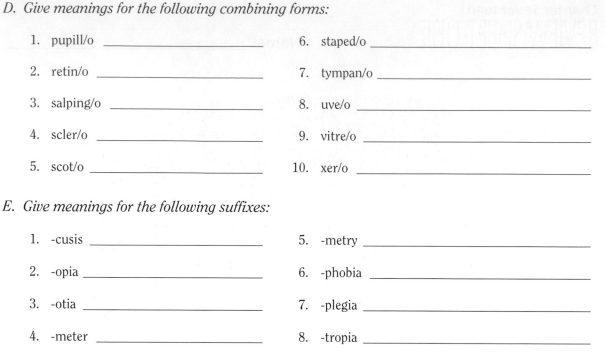

1. pupill/o _____
2. retin/o _____
3. salping/o _____
4. scler/o _____
5. scot/o _____

6. staped/o _____
7. tympan/o _____
8. uve/o _____
9. vitre/o _____
10. xer/o _____

E. Give meanings for the following suffixes:

1. -cusis _____
2. -opia _____
3. -otia _____
4. -meter _____

5. -metry _____
6. -phobia _____
7. -plegia _____
8. -tropia _____

Chapter Seventeen
CROSSWORD PUZZLE

Name: _____

Fill in the crossword puzzle below using the clues listed underneath it.

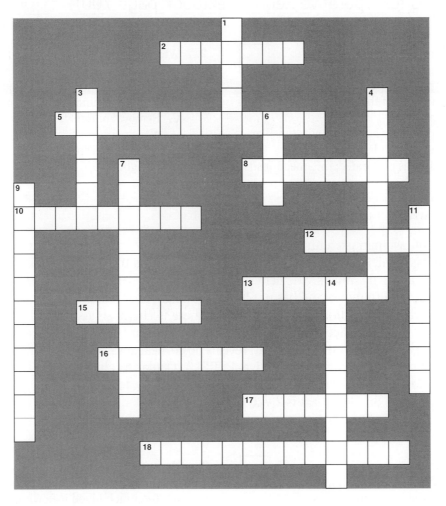

Across Clues

2. Small bone.
5. Normal adjustment of the lens by the ciliary muscle.
8. Having two sides that are rounded, elevated, and curved evenly.
10. Pertaining to the sense of smell. From the Latin, *olfacere*, meaning "to smell."
12. Nearsightedness.
13. A snail-shaped, spirally wound tube in the inner ear.
15. One of the tiny bones in the middle ear; stirrups.
16. Ringing sound in the ear; means "tinkling" in Latin.
17. Sensation of irregular or whirling motion either of oneself or of external objects.
18. Collection of skin cells and cholesterol in a sac within the middle ear.

Down Clues

1. Auricle; ear flap.
3. Tough, white, outer coat of the eyeball.
4. Farsightedness.
6. Colored portion of the eye.
7. Defective curvature of the cornea or lens of the eye.
9. Delicate membrane lining the eyelids and covering the exposed surfaces of the sclera.
11. Clouding of the lens, causing decreased vision.
14. Maze-like series of canals in the inner ear.

Chapter Seventeen
PRACTICAL APPLICATIONS

Name: _____

A. Questions for Operative Report (textbook page 700)

1. **What was the patient's diagnosis before surgery?** .... ☐
   A. Inflammation of the right eye and ear
   B. Inflammation of the left ear, adenoids, and tonsils
   C. Inflammation of both ears with tonsillar and adenoidal inflammation
   D. Eardrum was perforated; inflamed tonsils and adenoids

2. **What operation was performed?** .... ☐
   A. Removal of adenoids and tonsils
   B. Incision of the eardrums and placement of PE tubes; removal of adenoids and tonsils
   C. Removal of tonsils and adenoids and tube placement in left ear
   D. Removal of tonsils and placement of tubes in right ear

B. Chart Note

This 36-year-old woman presents with the complaint of dacryorrhea and irritation OS for about 48 hours. She has a thick mucous discharge that sticks the lids together overnight. Vision seems fine except for blurring by mucus. She denies trauma or ocular pathology. No symptoms of URI or allergy. She has no photophobia and has not been around anyone with pinkeye.

The conjunctiva (OS) is diffusely hyperemic, and there is chemosis (edema of the conjunctiva) and moderate lid edema. Traces of mucopurulent discharge are evident on the lid. Exam with Pontocaine (local anesthetic) and fluorescein reveals no corneal abrasions or ulceration. No foreign bodies are noted on the palpebral conjunctiva. PERRLA. Ocular fundus is normal. Slit-lamp exam shows no pathology in the cornea, anterior chamber, or lens. Tonometry is deferred. Far point vision testing with the Snellen chart is 20/20 in each eye.

Diagnosis is acute bacterial conjunctivitis OS.

1. **What are the patient's main symptoms?** .... ☐
   A. Blurred vision and itchy eyes
   B. Right eye irritation and excessive tearing
   C. Left eye irritation and excessive tearing
   D. Both eyes are tearing and irritated

2. **Where is the eye problem?** .... ☐
   A. In the cornea of the right eye
   B. Under the eyelids of both eyes
   C. In the cornea of the left eye
   D. The conjunctiva and lid of the left eye

3. **Hyperemic means:** .... ☐
   A. Not enough blood is flowing to the area
   B. Too much blood is flowing to an area
   C. There is blood and pus in the area
   D. The conjunctiva is purulent

4. **What is the condition of the patient's pupils?** .... ☐
   A. Pupils were not tested
   B. No foreign bodies were found in the pupils
   C. No abrasions or ulcerations noticed
   D. Pupils equal, round, reactive to light and accommodation

Chapter Seventeen
ANSWERS TO THE QUIZZES

Multiple Choice Quiz

1. D	4. B	7. E	10. B	13. E	16. A	19. D	22. C	25. C
2. C	5. A	8. D	11. D	14. A	17. C	20. B	23. B	
3. B	6. B	9. A	12. A	15. C	18. B	21. E	24. D	

Exercise Quiz

EYE

A
1. retina
2. ciliary body
3. lens
4. vitreous humor
5. pupil
6. choroid
7. conjunctiva
8. cornea
9. iris
10. sclera

B
11. optic disc (disk)
12. accommodation
13. macula lutea
14. refraction
15. cones
16. rods

C
17. pupils are unequal in size
18. swelling; fluid accumulation in the back of the eye
19. sensitivity to light
20. blind spot

D
21. blepharitis
22. keratitis
23. iritis
24. conjunctivitis
25. intraocular

E
26. uveitis
27. xerophthalmia
28. exotropia
29. esotropia
30. aphakia
31. hemianopsia

F
32. decreased vision in old age
33. nearsightedness
34. double vision
35. dim vision; lazy eye
36. farsightedness
37. normal vision

G
38. strabismus
39. glaucoma
40. hordeolum (stye)
41. cataract
42. diabetic retinopathy
43. macular degeneration

H
44. both eyes
45. right eye
46. left eye
47. pupils equal, round, reactive to light and accommodation
48. with glasses
49. visual field
50. without glasses

EAR

A
1. pinna
2. external auditory canal
3. tympanic membrane
4. malleus
5. incus
6. stapes
7. oval window
8. cochlea
9. auditory liquids and receptors
10. auditory nerve fibers
11. cerebral cortex

B
12. passages in the inner ear associated with equilibrium
13. waxy substance secreted by the external ear
14. auditory fluids in the labyrinth of the inner ear
15. eardrum

C
16. stapedectomy
17. audiometer
18. presbycusis
19. otitis media
20. tympanoplasty

D
21. sensation of irregular or whirling motion; dizziness
22. hardening of bony tissue in the labyrinth of the ear
23. noise sound (ringing) in the ears
24. inflammation of the inner ear (labyrinth)
25. inflammation of the eardrum
26. inflammation of middle ear with pus formation
27. inflammation of the mastoid bone near the ear
28. labyrinth disorder with elevated endolymph pressure in the cochlea
29. benign tumor of the acoustic nerve in the brain
30. collection of skin cells and cholesterol in a sac within the middle ear

E
31. left ear
32. electronystagmography
33. eyes, ears, nose, and throat
34. right ear
35. ear, nose, and throat

Dictation and Comprehension Quiz: Eye

A
1. anisocoria
2. aphakia
3. aqueous humor
4. astigmatism
5. cataract
6. chalazion
7. conjunctiva
8. cycloplegia
9. diplopia
10. fluorescein angiography
11. hemianopsia
12. iritis

13. keratitis
14. macular degeneration
15. myopia
16. ophthalmoscopy
17. papilledema
18. presbyopia
19. sclera
20. strabismus

B

16 Visual examination of the eye
19 White portion of the eye
3   Fluid produced by the ciliary body; circulates through the anterior chamber of the eye
1   Pupils are of unequal size
7   Delicate membrane lining the eyelids and covering the anterior eyeball
13 Inflammation of the cornea
8   Paralysis of the ciliary muscles of the eye
9   Double vision
5   Clouding of the lens, causing decreased vision
20 Abnormal deviation of the eye (esotropia and exotropia)
4   Defective curvature of the cornea or lens of the eye
6   Small, hard cystic mass on the eyelid
18 Impairment of vision due to old age
15 Nearsightedness
12 Inflammation of the iris
11 Loss of vision in one half of the visual field
17 Swelling in the region of the optic disc
10 Process of recording blood vessels in the back of the eye after IV injection of a dye
14 Progressive damage to the yellowish region on the retina (lateral to and slightly below the optic disc)
2   Absence of the lens of the eye

Dictation and Comprehension Quiz: Ear

A

1. acoustic neuroma
2. audiometer
3. auditory meatus
4. cerumen
5. cholesteatoma
6. cochlea
7. eustachian tube
8. labyrinth

9. myringotomy
10. ossiculoplasty
11. otolaryngologist
12. otomycosis
13. otosclerosis
14. perilymph
15. pinna
16. semicircular canals
17. suppurative otitis media
18. tinnitus
19. tympanoplasty
20. vertigo

B

14 Fluid contained in the inner part of the ear
8   Maze-like series of canals of the inner ear
15 The outer flap of the ear; auricle
7   Channel between the middle ear and the nasopharynx
4   Waxy substance secreted by the external ear
5   Collection of skin cells and cholesterol in a sac within the middle ear
9   Incision of the eardrum
13 Hardening of bony tissue in the inner ear; ankylosis of the stapes may occur
16 Passages in the inner ear that are associated with maintaining equilibrium
11 Specialist in the study of the ear and voice box
18 Sensation of noises (ringing, buzzing, whistling) in the ears
20 Sensation of irregular or whirling motion either of oneself or of external objects
10 Surgical repair of a small bone in the middle ear
2   Instrument to measure hearing
12 Fungal infection of the ear
3   Channel leading from the outer ear flap to the eardrum
1   Benign tumor arising from the 8th cranial nerve in the brain
6   A snail-shaped, spirally wound tube in the inner ear; contains hearing-sensitive cells
19 Surgical repair of the eardrum
17 Inflammation of the middle ear with pus formation

Spelling Quiz

A

1. anisocoria—pupils are unequal size

2. aqueous humor—fluid in the anterior and posterior chambers of the eye
3. blepharitis—inflammation of the eyelid
4. cataract—clouding of the lens, causing decreased vision
5. conjunctiva—delicate membrane lining the eyelids and covering the anterior eyeball
6. cornea—fibrous, transparent layer of clear tissue over the anterior of the eyeball
7. ciliary body—on each side of the lens to control the shape of lens
8. dacryorrhea—excessive flow of tears
9. glaucoma—increased intraocular pressure
10. ophthalmologist—doctor who examines the eye and treats eye disorders

B

11. acoustic
12. pinna
13. otomycosis
14. tinnitus
15. tympanoplasty
16. myringotomy
17. cerumen
18. vertigo
19. presbycusis
20. stapedectomy

Pronunciation Quiz

A

1. prosthesis
2. corneoscleral
3. audiometer
4. malleus
5. palpebral
6. presbycusis
7. mydriatic
8. blepharitis
9. retinopathy
10. macrotia

B

1. D
2. H
3. E
4. I
5. A
6. G
7. J
8. B
9. F
10. C

C

1. presbyopia
2. tympanoplasty
3. ophthalmoplegia
4. salpingopharyngeal
5. hemianopsia
6. uveitis
7. aphakia
8. otosclerosis

Abbreviations Quiz

1. intraocular lens <u>H</u>
2. acute otitis media <u>E</u>
3. electronystagmography <u>J</u>
4. visual acuity <u>A</u>
5. intraocular pressure <u>D</u>
6. ear, nose and throat <u>I</u>
7. pupils equal, round, reactive to light and accommodation <u>G</u>
8. age-related macular degeneration <u>F</u>
9. visual field <u>C</u>
10. pressure equalizing tube <u>B</u>

Diagram Quiz

EYE

1. Pupil
2. Conjunctiva
3. Cornea
4. Sclera
5. Choroid
6. Iris
7. Ciliary body
8. Lens
9. Anterior chamber
10. Vitreous humor
11. Retina
12. Optic nerve
13. Optic disc
14. Macula
15. Fovea centralis

EAR

1. Pinna (auricle)
2. External auditory meatus (auditory canal)
3. Tympanic membrane (eardrum)
4. Malleus
5. Incus
6. Stapes
7. Oval window
8. Eustachian (auditory) tube
9. Cochlea
10. Auditory nerve fibers
11. Vestibule
12. Semicircular canals

Vocabulary Quiz

EYE

A

1. aqueous humor
2. cone
3. choroid
4. accommodation
5. fovea centralis
6. anterior chamber
7. biconvex
8. conjunctiva
9. cornea
10. ciliary body
11. vitreous humor
12. rod

B

1. iris
2. retina
3. pupil
4. macula
5. optic chiasm
6. refraction
7. optic disc
8. optic nerve
9. lens
10. fundus of the eye
11. sclera
12. thalamus

EAR

A

1. cochlea
2. auditory nerve fibers
3. cerumen
4. incus
5. eustachian tube
6. auricle
7. malleus
8. endolymph
9. labyrinth
10. auditory canal

B

1. stapes
2. pinna
3. vestibule
4. tympanic membrane
5. oval window
6. organ of Corti
7. semicircular canals
8. ossicle
9. perilymph

Review Sheet Quiz

A

1. hearing
2. dull, dim
3. unequal
4. water
5. hearing
6. ear
7. eyelid
8. cochlea
9. conjunctiva
10. pupil

B

1. cornea
2. ciliary body
3. tears; tear duct
4. double
5. gray
6. iris
7. cornea
8. tears
9. smaller, less
10. widen, enlarge

C

1. eardrum
2. night
3. eye
4. eye
5. eye, vision
6. ossicle (small bone)
7. ear
8. eyelid
9. optic disc
10. lens
11. light
12. old age

D

1. pupil
2. retina
3. eustachian tube, auditory tube
4. sclera
5. darkness
6. stapes
7. eardrum, tympanic membrane
8. uvea (vascular layer of the eye)
9. glassy
10. dry

E

1. hearing
2. vision
3. ear condition
4. instrument to measure
5. process of measurement
6. fear
7. paralysis
8. to turn

Crossword Puzzle

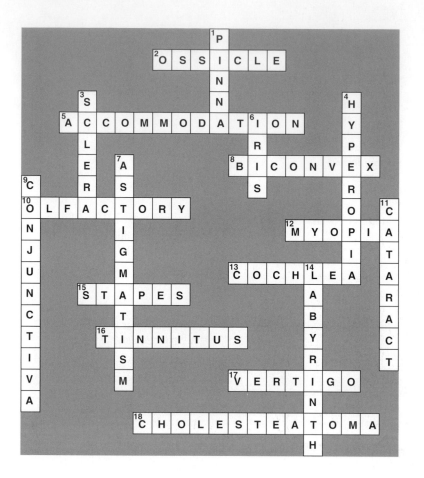

Practical Applications

A

1. C
2. B

B

1. C
2. D
3. B
4. D

chapter 18

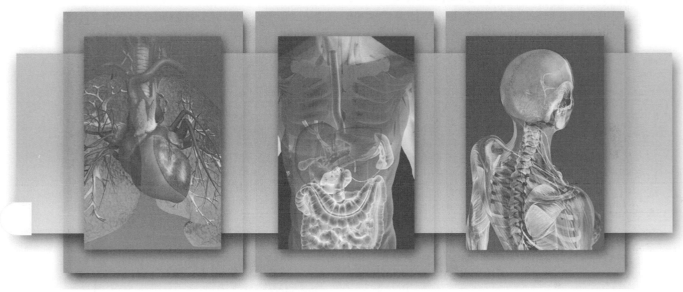

Chapter Eighteen
MULTIPLE CHOICE QUIZ

Name: _____

In the box write the letter of the choice that is the definition of the term or best answers the question. There is only one correct answer for each question.

1. **Which is a function of the thyroid gland?** ....☐
   A. Secretes immunologic substances
   B. Secretes thymosin
   C. Secretes corticosteroids
   D. Secretes thyroid-stimulating hormone
   E. Secretes thyroxine

2. **What is another name for the anterior lobe of the pituitary gland?** ....☐
   A. Hypophysis
   B. Hypothalamus
   C. Adenohypophysis
   D. Neurohypophysis
   E. Thalamus

3. **Which of the following secretes cortisol?** ....☐
   A. Testes
   B. Ovaries
   C. Adrenal medulla
   D. Adrenal cortex
   E. Pituitary gland

4. **Which is a hormone secreted by the pancreas?** ....☐
   A. Estrogen
   B. Insulin
   C. Vasopressin
   D. Epinephrine
   E. Glucose

5. **Which hormone regulates calcium in the blood and bones?** ....☐
   A. Parathyroid hormone
   B. Thyroxine
   C. Thyroid-stimulating hormone
   D. Prolactin
   E. Prostaglandins

6. **Which hormone stimulates the adrenal cortex to secrete hormones?** ....☐
   A. Growth hormone
   B. ADH
   C. ACTH
   D. Cortisone
   E. Secretin

7. **Which is an example of an electrolyte?** ....☐
   A. Insulin
   B. Sodium
   C. Renin
   D. Glucagon
   E. Steroid

8. **Which is an element that is present in thyroxine?** ....☐
   A. Iron
   B. Calcium
   C. Vitamin D
   D. Glucose
   E. Iodine

9. **Which is a hormone secreted by the ovary and adrenal cortex?** ....☐
   A. Follicle-stimulating hormone
   B. Luteinizing hormone
   C. Androgen
   D. Estrogen
   E. Oxytocin

10. **Which is a description of gonadotropins?** ....☐
    A. Secreted by the anterior lobe of the pituitary gland
    B. Stimulate the growth of long bones
    C. Stimulate glucose uptake in cells
    D. Secreted by the testes
    E. Stimulate the secretion of milk

11. **What is the term for excessive development of mammary tissue in a male?** ....☐
    A. Homeostasis
    B. Hypogonadism
    C. Galactorrhea
    D. Gynecomastia
    E. Hypernatremia

12. **Kal/i is a combining form for which substance?** ....☐
    A. Phosphorus
    B. Sodium
    C. Calcium
    D. Milk
    E. Potassium

13. **Insulin deficiency or resistance leads to hyperglycemia and ketoacidosis:**.....................
    A. Graves disease
    B. Diabetes mellitus
    C. Cushing syndrome
    D. Acromegaly
    E. Myxedema

14. **A group of symptoms produced by excess of cortisol from the adrenal cortex:**............................
    A. Graves disease
    B. Diabetes mellitus
    C. Cushing syndrome
    D. Acromegaly
    E. Myxedema

15. **Advanced hypothyroidism in adulthood:**..............................
    A. Graves disease
    B. Diabetes mellitus
    C. Cushing syndrome
    D. Acromegaly
    E. Myxedema

16. **Post-puberty hypersecretion of growth hormone from the anterior pituitary gland:**........................
    A. Graves disease
    B. Diabetes mellitus
    C. Cushing syndrome
    D. Acromegaly
    E. Myxedema

17. **Thyrotoxicosis; hypersecretion of the thyroid gland:**.....................
    A. Graves disease
    B. Diabetes mellitus
    C. Cushing syndrome
    D. Acromegaly
    E. Myxedema

18. **Which term means enlargement of the thyroid gland?**.........................
    A. Hypergonadism
    B. Euthyroid
    C. Goiter
    D. Hypophyseal enlargement
    E. Tetany

19. **Exophthalmos is a symptom of which endocrine disorder?**.........................
    A. Endemic goiter
    B. Thyroid carcinoma
    C. Graves disease
    D. Nodular goiter
    E. Pituitary gland hypertrophy

20. **Which is a description of tetany?**.........
    A. Constant muscle contraction
    B. Increased bone growth
    C. Hypercalcemia
    D. Hypokalemia
    E. Hypernatremia

21. **Natr/o is the combining form for which substance?**..............................
    A. Sugar
    B. Milk
    C. Sodium
    D. Iodine
    E. Potassium

22. **Characteristic of type 1 diabetes mellitus?**..............................
    A. Gradual onset; patient is asymptomatic
    B. Ketoacidosis seldom occurs
    C. Treatment is diet and oral hypoglycemic agents
    D. Little or no insulin produced
    E. Usually occurs after age 30

23. **Which of the following is associated with neuropathy, nephropathy, and retinopathy?**...................
    A. Hyperthyroidism
    B. Deficient ADH secretion
    C. Secondary complications of diabetes mellitus
    D. Hypergonadism
    E. Panhypopituitarism

24. **Which is a description of achondroplasia?**............................
    A. Enlargement of extremities
    B. Defective cartilage formation that affects bone growth
    C. Tumor of the sella turcica
    D. Abnormal formation of cartilage in an adult
    E. Hyperfunctioning of pituitary gland

25. **Which is a description of a thyroid scan?**............................
    A. CT image of thyroid gland
    B. Radioimmunoassay of thyroxine in the bloodstream
    C. Ultrasound image of the neck
    D. Skull x-ray of the brain
    E. Administration of radioactive compound and visualization with a scanner to detect tumors or nodules

Chapter Eighteen
EXERCISE QUIZ

Name: _____

A. *Name the endocrine organs that produce the following hormones:*

1. insulin _____

2. cortisol _____

3. epinephrine _____

4. follicle-stimulating hormone _____

5. thyroxine _____

6. aldosterone _____

7. vasopressin _____

8. estradiol _____

9. growth hormone _____

10. progesterone _____

B. *Give the meaning of the following abbreviations for hormones:*

11. ACTH _____

12. ADH _____

13. TSH _____

14. PTH _____

15. T_4 _____

16. T_3 _____

17. LH _____

18. GH _____

C. *Match the following hormones with their actions:*

ACTH	cortisol	insulin	thyroxine
ADH	epinephrine	parathyroid hormone	
aldosterone	estradiol	testosterone	

19. Sympathomimetic; elevates heart rate, blood pressure _____

20. Promotes growth and maintenance of male sex characteristics _____

21. Stimulates water reabsorption by kidney tubules; decreases urine _____

22. Increases metabolism in body cells _____

23. Raises blood calcium _____

24. Increases reabsorption of sodium by kidney tubules _____

25. Stimulates secretion of hormones from adrenal cortex _____

26. Increases blood sugar _____

27. Helps transport glucose to cells and decreases blood sugar _____

28. Develops and maintains female sex characteristics _____

D. *Build medical terms from their definitions and word parts given:*

29. abnormal condition (hypersecretion) of the thyroid gland: thyro _____

30. removal of the pancreas: _____ ectomy

31. condition of deficiency or underdevelopment of sex organs: hypo _____

32. pertaining to producing female characteristics: _____ genic

33. removal of the pituitary gland: _____ ectomy

34. deficiency of calcium in the blood: hypo _____

35. excessive sugar in the blood: _____ emia

E. *Indicate whether the following are related to hyposecretion or hypersecretion and name the endocrine gland involved:*

	Hypo- or Hyper-	Gland
36. acromegaly	_____	_____
37. tetany	_____	_____
38. diabetes mellitus	_____	_____
39. Graves disease	_____	_____
40. myxedema	_____	_____
41. Cushing syndrome	_____	_____
42. cretinism	_____	_____

F. *Give the meanings for the following conditions:*

43. hyponatremia _____

44. polydipsia _____

45. glycosuria _____

46. euthyroid _____

G. *Give the meanings for the following terms or abbreviations related to diabetes mellitus:*

47. type 1 _____

48. diabetic neuropathy _____

49. ketoacidosis _____

50. type 2 _____

Chapter Eighteen
DICTATION AND COMPREHENSION QUIZ: VOCABULARY AND TERMINOLOGY

Name: _____

A. *Dictation of Terms*

1. _____   11. _____

2. _____   12. _____

3. _____   13. _____

4. _____   14. _____

5. _____   15. _____

6. _____   16. _____

7. _____   17. _____

8. _____   18. _____

9. _____   19. _____

10. _____   20. _____

B. *Comprehension of Terms: Match the number of the above term with its meaning below.*

_____ Hormone secreted by the posterior part of the pituitary gland; increases reabsorption of water

_____ Hormone secreted by the adrenal cortex; increases salt (sodium) reabsorption by the kidney

_____ A mineral salt found in the blood and tissues; potassium is an example

_____ Excessive thirst

_____ Hormone secreted by the thyroid gland; lowers blood calcium

_____ Resection of a gland near and behind the stomach

_____ Hormone secreted by the posterior pituitary gland; stimulates contraction of the uterus during labor

_____ Sugar present in the urine

_____ Hormone secreted by the thyroid gland; thyroxine

_____ Tendency of an organism to maintain a constant internal environment

_____ Blood condition of deficient sodium

_____ Type of hormone secreted by the adrenal cortex; necessary for the use of sugars, fats, and proteins

_____ Anterior lobe of the pituitary gland

_____ Resection of four small glands in the neck region

_____ Hormone secreted by the ovaries

_____ Blood condition of deficient potassium

_____ Region of the brain that produces factors to stimulate the pituitary gland

_____ Hormone secreted by the anterior lobe of the pituitary gland; stimulates the adrenal cortex

_____ Condition of sugar in the blood

_____ Hormone derived from an amino acid and secreted by the adrenal medulla; epinephrine is an example

Chapter Eighteen
DICTATION AND COMPREHENSION QUIZ: ABNORMAL CONDITIONS, LABORATORY TESTS, PROCEDURES

Name: _____

A. *Dictation of Terms*

1. _____
2. _____
3. _____
4. _____
5. _____
6. _____
7. _____
8. _____
9. _____

10. _____
11. _____
12. _____
13. _____
14. _____
15. _____
16. _____
17. _____
18. _____

B. *Comprehension of Terms: Match the number of the above term with its meaning below.*

_____ Test that measures hormone levels in plasma

_____ Test that measures levels of sugar in the blood

_____ Radioactive compound is given and localizes in the thyroid gland

_____ Enlargement of extremities caused by excessive growth hormone after puberty

_____ Insufficient secretion of antidiuretic hormone produces this condition

_____ Malignant tumor of an endocrine gland in the neck

_____ Extreme hypothyroidism during infancy and childhood produces this condition

_____ Advanced hypothyroidism in adulthood produces this condition

_____ Enlargement and bulging of the eyeballs caused by hyperthyroidism

_____ Excessive hair on the face and body of adult women

_____ Group of symptoms produced by excess of cortisol from the adrenal cortex

_____ Enlargement of the thyroid gland

_____ Overactivity of the thyroid gland (Graves disease)

_____ Benign tumor of the adrenal medulla

_____ Lack of insulin secretion or resistance of insulin to promoting sugar, starch, and fat metabolism in cells

_____ Constant muscle contraction

_____ Fats are improperly burned, leading to accumulation of ketones in the body

_____ Hypofunctioning of the adrenal cortex

Chapter Eighteen
SPELLING QUIZ

Name: _____

A. Circle the term that is spelled correctly and write its meaning in the space provided.

1. courtisol   cortisol _____
2. goiter   goyter _____
3. estrogen   estrogin _____
4. pitiutary gland pituitary gland _____
5. gonadotrophan   gonadotropin _____
6. uthyroid   euthyroid _____
7. hypocalemia   hypokalemia _____
8. hypophysectomy   hypophisectomy _____
9. pancrease   pancreas _____
10. corticosteroid cortikosteroid _____

B. Circle the term that is spelled correctly. The meaning of each term is given.

11. hormone secreted by the
    thyroid gland .... thyroixine   thiroxine   thyroxine

12. condition of eyeballs that
    protrude outward...................... exopthalmos   exophthmalmos   exophthalmos

13. hormone secreted by the ovary .... progesterone   projesterone   progesteron

14. constant muscle contraction .... tetany   teteny   tettany

15. hormone secreted by the islet cells
    of Langerhans........................... insalin   insulin   insulen

16. state of equilibrium or constancy .... homeiostasis   homostasis   homeostasis

17. part of the brain that controls
    the secretions of the pituitary gland........ hypothalmus   hypothalmis   hypothalamus

18. excessive thirst .... polydipsea   pollydipsia   polydipsia

19. enlargement of extremities due to
    hypersecretion of growth hormone .... acromegaly   accromegaly   acromeagaly

20. hyposecretion of the thyroid gland
    in adulthood .... mixadema   myxedema   myxademae

Chapter Eighteen
PRONUNCIATION QUIZ

Name: _____

A. *Underline the accented syllable in the following terms:*

1. glucagon
2. parathormone
3. adenohypophysis

4. testosterone
5. sella turcica
6. goiter

7. exophthalmos
8. homeostasis
9. mineralocorticoid

10. gonadotropin

B. *Match the term in Column I with its meaning in Column II:*

Column I

1. aldosterone _____
2. diabetes insipidus _____
3. diabetes mellitus _____
4. progesterone _____
5. glycogen _____
6. cretinism _____
7. epinephrine _____
8. thyroxine _____
9. electrolyte _____
10. prolactin _____

Column II

A. Starch; storage form of sugar.

B. A mineral salt found in the blood and in tissues.

C. Hormone secreted by the adrenal cortex.

D. Hormone secreted by the adrenal medulla.

E. Hormone secreted by the ovary.

F. Disease condition due to malfunction of the posterior lobe of the pituitary gland.

G. Extreme hypothyroidism in childhood.

H. Disease condition due to malfunction of cells in pancreas.

I. Hormone secreted by anterior lobe of pituitary gland.

J. Hormone secreted by thyroid gland.

C. *Complete the following terms from their definitions below:*

1. hyper _____ Excessive amount of calcium in the blood.

2. hypo _____ Deficient amount of potassium in the blood.

3. hypo _____ Deficient sodium in the blood.

4. _____ ectomy Removal of the pancreas.

5. adreno _____ Disease condition of adrenal gland.

6. poly _____ Excessive thirst.

7. _____ thyroid Normal thyroid function.

8. tri _____ Hormone secreted by the thyroid gland.

Chapter Eighteen

ABBREVIATIONS QUIZ

Name: _____

Give meanings for the following abbreviations in Column I and match each with an associated explanation in Column II:

Column I	Column II
1. TSH _____ _____	A. Type 1 and type 2 are forms of this condition
2. RAI _____ _____	B. This is an electrolyte
3. Na+ _____ _____	C. This test assesses the function of an endocrine gland in the neck
4. GH _____ _____	
5. T$_4$ _____ _____	D. Secretion of this hormone stimulates an endocrine gland above the kidney
6. GTT _____ _____	E. Secretion of this hormone from the anterior pituitary gland stimulates an endocrine gland in the neck
7. ACTH _____ _____	
8. TFT _____ _____	F. Hormone secreted from the thyroid gland
9. DM _____ _____	G. Treatment for Graves disease to destroy an overactive thyroid gland
10. DI _____ _____	H. Posterior pituitary gland fails to release vasopressin
	I. Somatotropin
	J. Test to assess the sugar levels in the blood

Chapter Eighteen

DIAGRAM QUIZ

Name: _____

Label the diagram below using the terms listed below:

Adrenal glands
Ovaries
Pancreas
Parathyroid glands
Pineal gland
Pituitary gland
Testes
Thymus gland
Thyroid gland

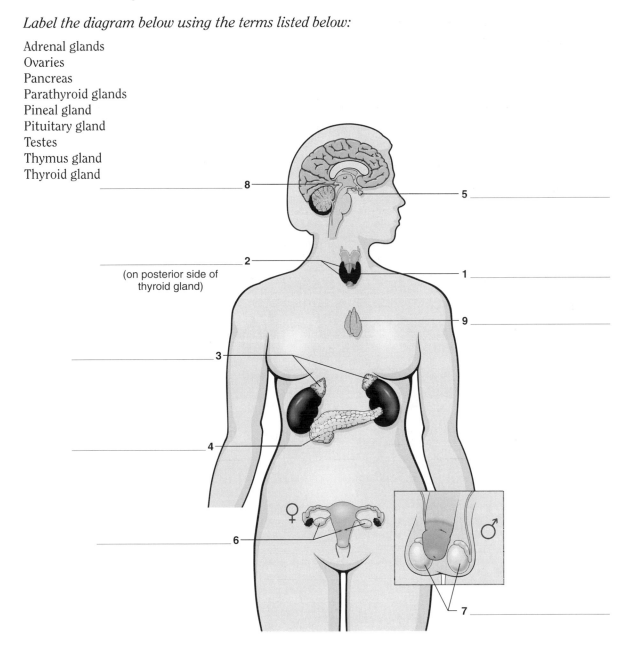

8 _____

(on posterior side of
thyroid gland)

2 _____

5 _____

1 _____

9 _____

3 _____

4 _____

6 _____

7 _____

Chapter Eighteen
VOCABULARY QUIZ

Name: _____

A. *Match the following glands with their descriptions below:*

adrenal cortex   pancreas   testes
adrenal medulla   parathyroid glands   thyroid gland
ovaries   pituitary gland

1. Two glands enclosed in the scrotal sac of a male _____

2. Located behind the stomach; alpha and beta islet cells secrete hormones _____

3. Located in the neck on either side of the trachea; secretes thyroxine _____

4. Inner section of a gland above each kidney; secretes epinephrine _____

5. Located at the base of the brain in the sella turcica; hypophysis _____

6. Outer section of a gland above each kidney: secretes cortisol, aldosterone, and sex hormones _____

7. Located in the lower abdomen of a female; responsible for egg cell production and estrogen secretion _____

8. Four small glands on the posterior side of the thyroid gland _____

B. *Match the following hormones with their descriptions below:*

adrenaline (epinephrine)   antidiuretic hormone (ADH)   estradiol
adrenocorticotropic hormone (ACTH)   calcitonin   follicle-stimulating hormone
aldosterone   cortisol   glucagon
androgen

1. Male hormone secreted by the testes _____

2. Female hormone secreted by the ovaries _____

3. Secreted by the posterior lobe of the pituitary gland; vasopressin _____

4. Secreted by the adrenal medulla; increases heart rate and blood pressure _____

5. Secreted by the thyroid gland; decreases blood calcium levels _____

6. Secreted by the adrenal cortex; increases salt reabsorption _____

7. Secreted by the anterior lobe of the pituitary gland; stimulates hormone secretion and egg production by the ovaries _____

8. Secreted by the pancreas; increases blood sugar by conversion of glycogen to glucose _____

9. Secreted by the anterior lobe of the pituitary gland; stimulates secretions of the adrenal cortex _____

10. Secreted by the adrenal cortex; increases blood sugar _____

C. *Match the following hormones with their descriptions below:*

growth hormone (somatotropin)   parathormone   testosterone
insulin   progesterone   thyroid-stimulating hormone
luteinizing hormone   prolactin   thyronine
oxytocin

1. Secreted by the ovaries; prepares the uterus for pregnancy _____

2. Secreted by beta islet cells of the pancreas; lowers blood sugar _____

3. Secreted by the anterior lobe of the pituitary gland; promotes milk secretion _____

4. Secreted by the anterior lobe of the pituitary gland; stimulates
    secretion by the thyroid gland _____

5. Male hormone secreted by the testes _____

6. Secreted by the posterior lobe of the pituitary gland; stimulates
    contraction of the uterus during childbirth _____

7. Secreted by the thyroid gland; increases metabolism in cells; T4 _____

8. Secreted by the anterior lobe of the pituitary gland; stimulates ovulation _____

9. Secreted by the anterior lobe of the pituitary gland; stimulates
    growth of bones and soft tissues _____

10. Secreted by the parathyroid glands; increases blood calcium _____

D. Match the following terms with their descriptions below:

catecholamines   homeostasis   sella turcica
corticosteroids   hypothalamus   sympathomimetic
electrolyte   mineralocorticoid   target tissue
glucocorticoid

1. Region of the brain lying below the thalamus; secretes factors and hormones that affect the pituitary gland _____

2. Cavity in the skull that contains the pituitary gland _____

3. Tendency of an organism to maintain a constant internal environment _____

4. Mimicking or copying the effect of the sympathetic nervous system; adrenaline is an example _____

5. Mineral salt found in the blood and tissues and necessary for proper functioning of cells; potassium is an example _____

6. Hormones derived from an amino acid and secreted by the adrenal medulla _____

7. Cells of an organ that are affected or stimulated by specific hormones _____

8. Steroid hormone secreted by the adrenal cortex; regulates mineral salts and water balance _____

9. Steroid hormones secreted by the adrenal cortex; cortisol, aldosterone, and sex hormones are examples _____

10. Steroid hormone secreted by the adrenal cortex; regulates glucose, fat, and protein metabolism _____

Chapter Eighteen
REVIEW SHEET QUIZ

Name: _____

A. *Give meanings for the following combining forms:*

1. aden/o _____
2. adren/o _____
3. andr/o _____
4. calc/o _____
5. cortic/o _____

6. dips/o _____
7. estr/o _____
8. gluc/o _____
9. glyc/o _____
10. gonad/o _____

B. *Give meanings for the following combining forms:*

1. kal/i _____
2. lact/o _____
3. myx/o _____
4. natr/o _____
5. pancreat/o _____

6. somat/o _____
7. thyr/o _____
8. toxic/o _____
9. ur/o _____
10. home/o _____

C. *Give meanings for the following suffixes and prefixes:*

1. -agon _____
2. -ectomy _____
3. -emia _____
4. -genic _____
5. -tropin _____
6. -uria _____
7. -megaly _____

8. hyper- _____
9. hypo- _____
10. pan- _____
11. tetra- _____
12. poly- _____
13. tri- _____
14. eu- _____

Chapter Eighteen
CROSSWORD PUZZLE

Name: _____

Fill in the crossword puzzle below using the clues listed underneath it.

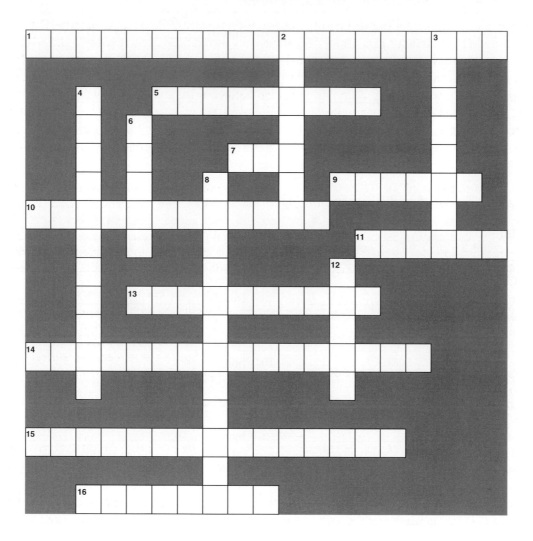

Across Clues

1. ACTH.
5. Kal/i means _____ .
7. Pan- means _____ .
9. Two endocrine glands in the scrotal sac of a male.
10. A hormone produced by the ovaries.
11. Toxic/o means _____.
13. Enlargement of the extremities; pituitary gland hypersecretion after puberty.
14. T_3
15. Pertaining to mimicking or copying the effect of the sympathetic nervous system.
16. Home/o means _____ .

Down Clues

2. Produced by the islet cells of the pancreas.
3. Endocrine gland behind the stomach.
4. Tendency in an organism to return to an equilibrium or constant, stable state.
6. Tri- means _____.
8. A male hormone produced by the testes.
12. Aden/o means _____.

Chapter Eighteen
PRACTICAL APPLICATIONS

Name: _____

A. Cushing Syndrome

Hypertension, both systolic and diastolic, is a common feature of Cushing syndrome. Other clinical features are likely to attract more attention than the hypertension: obesity with "buffalo hump" and "moon face," muscular weakness, scattered bruises, and osteoporosis. The excessive secretion of adrenocortical steroids that is responsible for the syndrome is frequently due to primary disease of the adrenals, either hyperplasia or discrete tumors. However, the hyperactivity of the adrenal cortex may be secondary to a tumor or malfunction of the pituitary or a neoplasm secreting an ACTH-like substance elsewhere in the body. Appropriate x-ray studies, including arteriograms or retrograde venograms of the adrenals, may disclose a tumor in the adrenals, hypophysis, or elsewhere.

1. **Which is a common clinical feature of Cushing syndrome?** .... ☐
   A. Decreased blood flow to the heart
   B. Abnormal sounds in the heart
   C. Peripheral edema
   D. High blood pressure when the heart is contracting and relaxing

2. **Cushing syndrome is associated with which of the following?** .... ☐
   A. Tendency to accumulate fat in tissues
   B. Tetany
   C. Bone tumors
   D. Low blood pressure

3. **What is a probable etiology of Cushing syndrome?** .... ☐
   A. Excessive porosity of bones
   B. Decreased secretion of adrenal hormones
   C. Decreased secretion of pituitary hormones
   D. Tumor or disease of the adrenal cortex

4. **What is a likely secondary cause of Cushing syndrome?** .... ☐
   A. Decreased secretion of ACTH
   B. Blocked artery in the kidney
   C. Tumor of the adenohypophysis
   D. Muscular weakness

B. Chart Note

A 26-year-old woman is referred for Graves disease. The patient was first found to be hyperthyroid shortly after she became pregnant. She has a tremor in her hands, a sensation of being hot, insomnia, weakness in her legs, and exophthalmos.

Physical examination reveals thyromegaly; the gland is rather mushy and soft. No nodules were noted. T_3 and T_4 levels were ordered and an appointment was made to have an uptake scan.

1. **What is the cause of Graves disease?** ... ☐
   A. The thyroid gland is slow to function
   B. The pancreas is hyperfunctioning
   C. The thyroid gland is oversecreting
   D. Hyperactive ovarian function

2. **Why were T_3 and T_4 levels ordered?** ..... ☐
   A. To measure the extent of eyelid prolapse
   B. To assess the function of the thyroid gland
   C. To measure the size of the thyroid gland
   D. To assess heart function

Chapter Eighteen

ANSWERS TO THE QUIZZES

Multiple Choice Quiz

1. E	4. B	7. B	10. A	13. B	16. D	19. C	22. D	25. E
2. C	5. A	8. E	11. D	14. C	17. A	20. A	23. C	
3. D	6. C	9. D	12. E	15. E	18. C	21. C	24. B	

Exercise Quiz

A

1. pancreas
2. adrenal cortex
3. adrenal medulla
4. ovary
5. thyroid gland
6. adrenal cortex
7. posterior pituitary gland
8. ovary; adrenal cortex
9. anterior pituitary gland
10. ovary

B

11. adrenocorticotropic hormone
12. antidiuretic hormone
13. thyroid-stimulating hormone
14. parathyroid hormone; parathormone
15. tetraiodothyronine (thyroxine)
16. triiodothyronine
17. luteinizing hormone
18. growth hormone

C

19. epinephrine
20. testosterone
21. ADH
22. thyroxine
23. parathyroid hormone
24. aldosterone
25. ACTH
26. cortisol
27. insulin
28. estradiol

D

29. thyrotoxicosis
30. pancreatectomy
31. hypogonadism
32. estrogenic
33. hypophysectomy
34. hypocalcemia
35. hyperglycemia

E

36. hyper/adenohypophysis
37. hypo/parathyroid
38. hypo/pancreas
39. hyper/thyroid
40. hypo/thyroid
41. hyper/adrenal cortex
42. hypo/thyroid

F

43. low levels of sodium in the blood
44. excessive thirst
45. sugar in the urine
46. normal thyroid function

G

47. insulin-dependent diabetes mellitus
48. disease of nerves secondary to diabetes mellitus
49. abnormal condition of ketones in the blood (acid-forming); complication of diabetes mellitus
50. non-insulin dependent diabetes mellitus

Dictation and Comprehension Quiz: Vocabulary and Terminology

A

1. adenohypophysis
2. adrenocorticotropin
3. aldosterone
4. calcitonin
5. catecholamine
6. electrolyte
7. glucocorticoid
8. glycemia
9. glycosuria
10. homeostasis
11. hypokalemia
12. hyponatremia
13. hypothalamus
14. oxytocin
15. pancreatectomy
16. parathyroidectomy
17. polydipsia
18. progesterone
19. tetraiodothyronine
20. vasopressin

B

20 Hormone secreted by the posterior part of the pituitary gland; increases reabsorption of water
 3 Hormone secreted by the adrenal cortex; increases salt (sodium) reabsorption by the kidney
 6 A mineral salt found in the blood and tissues; potassium is an example
17 Excessive thirst
 4 Hormone secreted by the thyroid gland; lowers blood calcium
15 Resection of a gland near and behind the stomach
14 Hormone secreted by the posterior pituitary gland; stimulates contraction of the uterus during labor
 9 Sugar present in the urine
19 Hormone secreted by the thyroid gland; thyroxine
10 Tendency of an organism to maintain a constant internal environment
12 Blood condition of deficient sodium
 7 Type of hormone secreted by the adrenal cortex; necessary for the use of sugars, fats, and proteins
 1 Anterior lobe of the pituitary gland
16 Resection of four small glands in the neck region
18 Hormone secreted by the ovaries
11 Blood condition of deficient potassium
13 Region of the brain that produces factors to stimulate the pituitary gland
 2 Hormone secreted by the anterior lobe of the pituitary gland; stimulates the adrenal cortex

8 Condition of sugar in the blood
5 Hormone derived from an amino acid and secreted by the adrenal medulla; epinephrine is an example

Dictation and Comprehension Quiz: Abnormal Conditions, Laboratory Tests, Procedures

A

1. acromegaly
2. Addison disease
3. cretinism
4. Cushing syndrome
5. diabetes insipidus
6. diabetes mellitus
7. exophthalmos
8. glucose tolerance test
9. goiter
10. hirsutism
11. ketoacidosis
12. myxedema
13. pheochromocytoma
14. radioimmunoassay
15. tetany
16. thyroid carcinoma
17. thyroid scan
18. thyrotoxicosis

B

14 Test that measures hormone levels in plasma
8 Test that measures levels of sugar in the blood
17 Radioactive compound is given and localizes in the thyroid gland
1 Enlargement of extremities caused by excessive growth hormone after puberty
5 Insufficient secretion of antidiuretic hormone produces this condition
16 Malignant tumor of an endocrine gland in the neck
3 Extreme hypothyroidism during infancy and childhood produces this condition
12 Advanced hypothyroidism in adulthood produces this condition
7 Enlargement and bulging of the eyeballs caused by hyperthyroidism

10 Excessive hair on the face and body of adult women
4 Group of symptoms produced by excess of cortisol from the adrenal cortex
9 Enlargement of the thyroid gland
18 Overactivity of the thyroid gland (Graves disease)
13 Benign tumor of the adrenal medulla
6 Lack of insulin secretion or resistance of insulin to promoting sugar, starch, and fat metabolism in cells
15 Constant muscle contraction
11 Fats are improperly burned, leading to accumulation of ketones in the body
2 Hypofunctioning of the adrenal cortex

Spelling Quiz

A

1. cortisol—hormone secreted by the adrenal cortex
2. goiter—enlargement of the thyroid gland
3. estrogen—hormone secreted by the ovaries
4. pituitary gland—located at the base of the brain
5. gonadotropin—hormone secreted by the pituitary gland
6. euthyroid—normal thyroid function
7. hypokalemia—low potassium in the blood
8. hypophysectomy—removal of the pituitary gland
9. pancreas—endocrine gland behind the stomach
10. corticosteroid—type of hormone secreted by the adrenal cortex

B

11. thyroxine
12. exophthalmos
13. progesterone
14. tetany
15. insulin
16. homeostasis
17. hypothalamus
18. polydipsia
19. acromegaly
20. myxedema

Pronunciation Quiz

A

1. glucagon
2. para<u>thor</u>mone
3. adenohy<u>pophy</u>sis
4. test<u>oste</u>rone
5. <u>sella</u> <u>tur</u>cica
6. goiter
7. exoph<u>thal</u>mos
8. homeo<u>sta</u>sis
9. mineralo<u>cortic</u>oid
10. gonado<u>tropin</u>

B

1. C
2. F
3. H
4. E
5. A
6. G
7. D
8. J
9. B
10. I

C

1. hypercalcemia
2. hypokalemia
3. hyponatremia
4. pancreatectomy
5. adrenopathy
6. polydipsia
7. euthyroid
8. triiodothyronine

Abbreviations Quiz

1. thyroid-stimulating hormone <u>E</u>
2. radioactive iodine <u>G</u>
3. sodium <u>B</u>
4. growth hormone <u>I</u>
5. thyroxine <u>F</u>
6. glucose tolerance test <u>J</u>
7. adrenocorticotropic hormone <u>D</u>
8. thyroid function test <u>C</u>
9. diabetes mellitus <u>A</u>
10. diabetes insipidus <u>H</u>

Diagram Quiz

1. Thyroid gland
2. Parathyroid glands
3. Adrenal glands
4. Pancreas
5. Pituitary gland
6. Ovaries
7. Testes
8. Pineal gland
9. Thymus gland

Vocabulary Quiz

A
1. testes
2. pancreas
3. thyroid gland
4. adrenal medulla
5. pituitary gland
6. adrenal cortex
7. ovaries
8. parathyroid glands

B
1. androgen
2. estradiol
3. antidiuretic hormone (ADH)
4. adrenaline (epinephrine)
5. calcitonin
6. aldosterone
7. follicle-stimulating hormone
8. glucagon
9. adrenocorticotropic hormone (ACTH)
10. cortisol

C
1. progesterone
2. insulin
3. prolactin
4. thyroid-stimulating hormone
5. testosterone
6. oxytocin
7. thyroxine
8. luteinizing hormone
9. growth hormone (somatotropin)
10. parathormone

D
1. hypothalamus
2. sella turcica
3. homeostasis
4. sympathomimetic
5. electrolyte
6. catecholamines
7. target tissue
8. mineralocorticoid
9. corticosteroids
10. glucocorticoid

Review Sheet Quiz

A
1. gland
2. adrenal gland
3. male
4. calcium
5. cortex; outer area
6. thirst
7. female
8. sugar
9. sugar
10. sex glands; gonads (organs that produce sex cells or gametes)

B
1. potassium
2. milk
3. mucus
4. sodium
5. pancreas
6. body
7. thyroid gland
8. poison
9. urine
10. sameness

C
1. assemble, gather together
2. removal, excision, resection
3. blood condition
4. pertaining to producing
5. stimulating the function of
6. urine condition
7. enlargement
8. excessive, above
9. deficient, below
10. all
11. four
12. many, much
13. three
14. good, normal

Crossword Puzzle

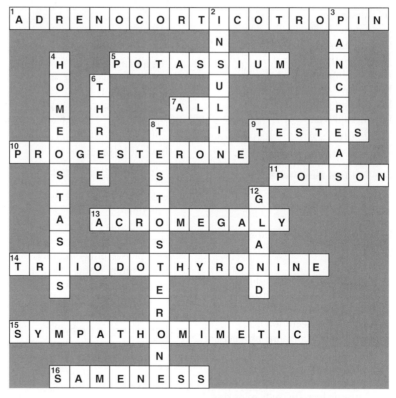

Practical Applications

A
1. D
2. A
3. D
4. C

B
1. C
2. B

Chapter Eighteen
Answers to Combining Forms and Terminology Sections

(textbook pages 736–739)

Terminology	Meaning
adenectomy	Removal of a gland.
adrenopathy	Disease of adrenal glands.
adrenalectomy	Removal of an adrenal gland.
gonadotropin	Hormone that is secreted from the pituitary gland and acts on the gonads (ovaries and testes).
hypogonadism	Condition of decreased function of the gonads, with decreased growth and sexual development.
pancreatectomy	Removal of the pancreas.
parathyroidectomy	Removal of the parathyroid glands.
hypopituitarism	Condition resulting from decreased secretion by the pituitary gland.
thyroidtropic hormone	Hormone secreted by the anterior pituitary gland that acts on the thyroid gland (TSH or thyroid-stimulating hormone).
thyroiditis	Inflammation of the thyroid gland.
androgen	Hormone producing or stimulating male characteristics (e.g., testosterone).
hypercalcemia	Increased calcium in the blood.
hypercalciuria	High levels of calcium in urine.
hypocalcemia	Decreased calcium in the blood.
corticosteroid	Any of the hormones produced by the adrenal cortex.
endocrinologist	Specialist in diagnosis and treatment of endocrine gland disorders.
polydipsia	Condition of excessive thirst.
estrogenic	Pertaining to having properties similar to estrogen (producing estrogen-like effects).
glucagon	Hormone from the pancreas that causes sugar to be released into the bloodstream when blood sugar levels are low.
hyperglycemia	Blood condition of increased sugar.
glycemic	Pertains to sugar in the blood.
glycogen	An animal starch; produced from sugar by the liver.
homeostasis	State of equilibrium (constancy) of the body's internal environment.
hormonal	Pertaining to hormones.
hypokalemia	Low levels of potassium in the blood.
prolactin	Hormone secreted by the anterior pituitary that promotes the growth of breast tissue and stimulates milk production.
myxedema	Condition of mucous-like swelling of the face and soft tissues; due to hyposecretion of the thyroid gland in adults.
hyponatremia	Blood condition of deficiency of sodium.
hypophysectomy	Removal of the pituitary gland.
somatotropin	Hormone secreted by the anterior pituitary gland; stimulates growth of bones and tissues (growth hormone).
steroid	An organic (containing carbon) compound with a ring structure; bile acids, vitamin D, certain hormones.
oxytocin	Hormone secreted by the posterior lobe of the pituitary gland; stimulates childbirth.
thyrotoxicosis	Condition of increased secretion from the thyroid gland with symptoms such as sweating, rapid pulse, tremors, and exophthalmos.
antidiuretic hormone	Secreted by the posterior lobe of the pituitary gland; causes water to be retained in the body.

Suffixes

glucagon	Hormone from the pancreas that "assembles" sugar from starch and increases blood sugar when it is low.
hypoglycemia	Low levels of sugar in blood.
epinephrine	Hormone secreted by the adrenal medulla; raises blood pressure.
adrenocorticotropin	Hormone secreted by the anterior lobe of the pituitary gland; stimulates the adrenal cortex to release its hormones.
glycosuria	Condition of sugar in the urine.

Prefixes

euthyroid	Normal thyroid function.
hyperkalemia	High levels of potassium in blood.
hypoinsulinism	Low levels of insulin.
oxytocin	Hormone from the neurohypophysis that stimulates childbirth.
panhypopituitarism	Condition of deficient secretion of all hormones from the pituitary gland.
tetraiodothyronine	Thyroid gland hormone containing 4 atoms of iodine; thyroxine.
triiodothyronine	Thyroid gland hormone containing 3 atoms of iodine.

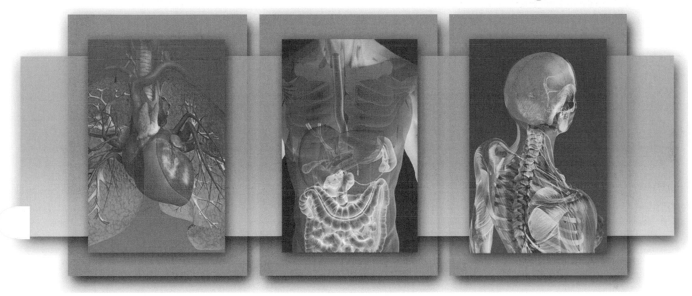

chapter 19

Chapter Nineteen

MULTIPLE CHOICE QUIZ

Name: _____

In the box write the letter of the choice that is the definition of the term or best answers the question. There is only one correct answer for each question.

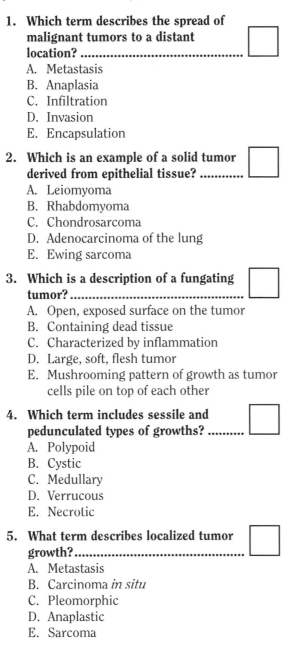

1. **Which term describes the spread of malignant tumors to a distant location?** .... ☐
    A. Metastasis
    B. Anaplasia
    C. Infiltration
    D. Invasion
    E. Encapsulation

2. **Which is an example of a solid tumor derived from epithelial tissue?** .... ☐
    A. Leiomyoma
    B. Rhabdomyoma
    C. Chondrosarcoma
    D. Adenocarcinoma of the lung
    E. Ewing sarcoma

3. **Which is a description of a fungating tumor?** .... ☐
    A. Open, exposed surface on the tumor
    B. Containing dead tissue
    C. Characterized by inflammation
    D. Large, soft, flesh tumor
    E. Mushrooming pattern of growth as tumor cells pile on top of each other

4. **Which term includes sessile and pedunculated types of growths?** .... ☐
    A. Polypoid
    B. Cystic
    C. Medullary
    D. Verrucous
    E. Necrotic

5. **What term describes localized tumor growth?** .... ☐
    A. Metastasis
    B. Carcinoma *in situ*
    C. Pleomorphic
    D. Anaplastic
    E. Sarcoma

6. **Which is a description of scirrhous type tumors?** .... ☐
    A. Form small nipple-like projections
    B. Form small, microscopic glandular-type sacs
    C. Hard, densely packed tumor cells
    D. Resemble squamous epithelial cells
    E. Contain a variety of tumor cells

7. **What does staging a tumor mean?** .... ☐
    A. Assessing the degree of differentiation
    B. Analyzing the microscopic appearance of tumor cells
    C. The tumor has spread
    D. Assessing the extent of tumor spread
    E. Treatment involves radiotherapy

8. **What does mutagenic mean?** .... ☐
    A. Producing a change in the DNA of a cell
    B. Increased cell growth
    C. New growth in numbers of cells
    D. Tumors are large and fleshy
    E. Cells are very differentiated

9. **What does the notation T1N2M0 mean?** .... ☐
    A. Tumor is localized and no lymph nodes are involved
    B. Tumor cannot be assessed
    C. Lymph nodes are not demonstrably abnormal
    D. Tumor is present with palpable regional lymph nodes and no metastases
    E. Metastasis to distant lymph nodes is detectable

10. **What is the definition of a mutation?** .... ☐
    A. Inheritable change in a cell
    B. Specialization of cells
    C. Plan for treatment of an illness
    D. Cell division
    E. Giving radiation in small doses

11. **Which is an example of genetic material that causes cancer?** .... ☐
    A. Vinyl chloride
    B. Hydrocarbons
    C. Diethylstilbestrol
    D. Alkylating agents
    E. Oncogenes

12. **Which is a description of exenteration?** .... ☐
    A. Malignant tissue is frozen
    B. Cells are scraped from region
    C. Tumors are burned
    D. Wide resection of tumor and removal of surrounding tissue
    E. Material is taken from the vagina or cervix and analyzed microscopically

13. **What is the meaning of fulguration? ...** ☐
    A. Destruction of tissue by electric sparks
    B. Treatment with drugs
    C. Treatment with radiation
    D. Tumor is removed by surgical excision
    E. Aspiration biopsy technique

14. **Which is an example of a known type of inherited cancer?** .... ☐
    A. Bone cancer
    B. Lung cancer
    C. Retinoblastoma
    D. Basal cell carcinoma
    E. Adenocarcinoma of the cervix

15. **What is a definition of modality?** .... ☐
    A. Method of treatment
    B. Damage to normal tissue
    C. Change in genetic material
    D. Description of the diagnosis
    E. Death of cells

16. **Which is a definition of a radio-resistant tumor?** .... ☐
    A. Tumor is completely eradicated by chemical therapy
    B. Tumor requires large doses of radiation to produce death of cells
    C. Tumor in which irradiation causes death of cancer cells without damage to surrounding tissue
    D. Tumor is not significantly affected by drug treatment
    E. Tumor is resistant to surgical intervention

17. **Which is a description of cauterization?** .... ☐
    A. Treating a tumor with freezing temperatures
    B. Treating tissue with heat
    C. Drying tissue electrically
    D. Surgical puncture to remove fluid
    E. Removing cells by scraping the walls of an organ

18. **Which is a description of pharmacokinetics?** .... ☐
    A. Type of ionizing radiation
    B. Study of the distribution and removal of drugs in the body
    C. Method of giving x-ray treatment
    D. Use of drugs to increase the sensitivity of tumors to x-rays
    E. Abnormal growth of cells

19. **What term means assisting or aiding?** .... ☐
    A. Lethal
    B. Fractionation
    C. Aspiration
    D. Adjuvant
    E. Grading

20. **Which term is used in treatment of tumors with radiation?** .... ☐
    A. Steroid
    B. Antibiotic
    C. Antimetabolite
    D. Linear accelerator
    E. Plant alkaloid

21. **Which is a description of an estrogen receptor assay?** .... ☐
    A. Tests for the presence of carcinoembryonic antigen in the blood
    B. Tests for a portion of human chorionic gonadotropin in serum of patients
    C. Tests the presence of a protein antigen in serum of liver and testicular cancer patients
    D. Tests the concentration of hormone receptor sites in cells of breast cancer patients
    E. Tests for the amount of carcinogenic hormones in the bloodstream of cancer patients

22. **Which best describes a wide surgical incision of the abdomen to detect disease?**.....................
    A. Staging laparotomy
    B. Liver and spleen scan
    C. Peritoneoscopy
    D. Bone marrow biopsy
    E. Laparoscopy

23. **What best describes interferon?** ....
    A. Carcinogen
    B. Molecularly targeted drug
    C. Alkylating agent used for chemotherapy
    D. Type of electron beam
    E. Biological response modifier

24. **What term means return of symptoms of disease?**.................................
    A. Remission
    B. Mutation
    C. Metastasis
    D. Relapse
    E. Differentiation

25. **Which term means cancerous tumor derived from bone?** ....
    A. Adenocarcinoma
    B. Osteogenic sarcoma
    C. Osteoma
    D. Chondrosarcoma
    E. Wilms tumor

26. **A side effect of radiation therapy (redness of skin):** ....
    A. Alopecia
    B. Myelosuppression
    C. Mucositis
    D. Fibrosis
    E. Erythema

27. **A side effect of chemotherapy or radiotherapy (hair loss):** ....
    A. Alopecia
    B. Myelosuppression
    C. Mucositis
    D. Fibrosis
    E. Erythema

28. **A side effect of radiation therapy to the lungs (abnormal growth of connective tissue):**...............................
    A. Alopecia
    B. Myelosuppression
    C. Mucositis
    D. Fibrosis
    E. Erythema

29. **Hypoplasia of bone marrow:**................
    A. Alopecia
    B. Myelosuppression
    C. Mucositis
    D. Fibrosis
    E. Erythema

30. **Inflammation of the inner lining of an organ:**..
    A. Alopecia
    B. Myelosuppression
    C. Mucositis
    D. Fibrosis
    E. Erythema

Chapter Nineteen
EXERCISE QUIZ

Name: _____

A. *Identify the following characteristics of malignant tumors from their definitions below. Word parts are given as clues.*

1. Loss of differentiation of cells and reversion to a more primitive cell type: ana _____

2. Extending beyond the normal tissue boundaries: in _____

3. Having the ability to enter and destroy surrounding tissue: in _____

4. Spreading to a secondary site: meta _____

B. *Match the following terms or abbreviations with their meanings below:*

| chemical carcinogen | mitosis | oncogene | RNA | virus |
| DNA | mutation | radiation | ultraviolet radiation | |

5. replication of cells; two identical cells are produced from a parent cell _____

6. cellular substance (ribonucleic acid) that is important in protein synthesis _____

7. infectious agent that reproduces by entering a host cell and using the host's genetic material to

   make copies of itself _____

8. rays given off by the sun _____

9. an agent (hydrocarbon, insecticide, hormone) that causes cancer _____

10. genetic material within the nucleus that controls replication and protein synthesis _____

11. region of genetic material that causes cancer; found in tumor cells or viruses _____

12. change in the genetic material of a cell _____

13. energy carried by a stream of particles _____

C. *Give meanings for the following terms:*

14. adenocarcinoma _____

15. osteosarcoma _____

16. benign _____

17. differentiation _____

18. neoplasm _____

D. Name the terms that describe microscopic tumor growth. Definitions and word parts are given.

19. forming small nipple-like projections: papill _____

20. abnormal formation of cells: dys _____

21. localized growth of cells: carcin _____

22. densely packed; containing fibrous connective tissue: _____ ous

23. patterns resembling small, microscopic sacs: alveol _____

24. small gland-type sacs: foll _____

25. lacking structures typical of mature cells: un _____

E. Match the following gross descriptions of tumors with their meanings:

cystic	inflammatory	necrotic	ulcerating
fungating	medullary	polypoid	verrucous

26. characterized by redness, swelling, and heat _____

27. tumors are large, soft, fleshy _____

28. containing dead tissue _____

29. mushrooming pattern of growth _____

30. characterized by large, open, exposed surfaces _____

31. tumors form large, open spaces filled with fluid _____

32. tumors resemble wart-like growths _____

33. growths are projections from a base (sessile and pedunculated) _____

F. Match the surgical procedure in Column I with its meaning in Column II.

Column I

34. fulguration _____

35. en bloc resection _____

36. incisional biopsy _____

37. excisional biopsy _____

38. cryosurgery _____

39. cauterization _____

40. pelvic exenteration _____

Column II

A. Removal of tumor and a margin of abnormal tissue for diagnosis and possible cure for small tumors.

B. Removal of entire tumor with large area of surrounding tissue and lymph nodes.

C. Burning a lesion.

D. Destruction of tissue using heat.

E. Cutting into tumor and removing a piece to establish diagnosis.

F. Freezing a lesion.

G. Wide resection involving tumor, organ of origin, and surrounding tissue in the area of the hip.

G. *Give meanings for the following terms:*

41. relapse _____

42. morbidity _____

43. protocol _____

44. modality _____

45. remission _____

46. adjuvant therapy _____

H. *Match the test or procedure with its description below:*

beta-HCG test	CEA test	laparoscopy	staging laparotomy
bone marrow biopsy	estrogen receptor assay	needle biopsy	
CA-125	exfoliative cytology	PSA test	

47. Test for the presence of a portion of human chorionic gonadotropin hormone (a marker for testicular cancer) _____

48. Incision of the abdomen to determine extent of disease _____

49. Protein marker test to detect ovarian cancer cells in blood _____

50. Visual examination of the abdominal cavity; peritoneoscopy _____

51. Test for the presence of a hormone receptor on breast cancer cells _____

52. Removal and microscopic examination of bone marrow tissue _____

53. Aspiration of tissue for microscopic examination _____

54. Blood test for the presence of an antigen related to prostate cancer _____

55. Blood test for carcinoembryonic antigen (marker for GI cancer) _____

56. Cells are scraped off tissue and microscopically examined _____

Chapter Nineteen

DICTATION AND COMPREHENSION QUIZ

Name: _____

A. Dictation of Terms

1. _____   11. _____

2. _____   12. _____

3. _____   13. _____

4. _____   14. _____

5. _____   15. _____

6. _____   16. _____

7. _____   17. _____

8. _____   18. _____

9. _____   19. _____

10. _____   20. _____

B. Comprehension of Terms: Match the number of the above term with its meaning below.

_____ Programmed cell death

_____ Specialization of cells

_____ Giving radiation therapy in small, repeated doses

_____ Spread of a malignant tumor to a secondary site

_____ Condition of being diseased

_____ Drug that increases the sensitivity of tumors to radiation therapy

_____ Loss of specialization of cells; reversion to a more primitive type

_____ Malignant tumor of connective tissue

_____ Possessing a stem or stalk; characteristic of some polypoid tumors

_____ Formation of blood vessels

_____ Region of DNA found in tumor cells; examples are *abl, ras, src*

_____ Synthetic chemicals containing groups that interfere with DNA synthesis

_____ Visual examination of the abdomen using small incisions and an endoscope

_____ Removal of tumor along with a large area of surrounding tissue and lymph nodes

_____ Microscopic description of tumors possessing a variety of cells

_____ Localized cancer; confined to the site of origin

_____ Malnutrition associated with chronic disease (such as malignancy) and ill health

_____ Malignant tumor of epithelial tissue (glandular cells)

_____ Cells are scraped from an area of suspected disease and examined microscopically

_____ Pertaining to producing change in cells

Chapter Nineteen
SPELLING QUIZ

Name: _____

A. *Circle the term that is spelled correctly and write its meaning in the space provided.*

1. retinoblastoma   retinoblasoma _____

2. metastasis   matestasis _____

3. bengine   benign _____

4. chemotherapy   chemotheraphy _____

5. oncology   onkocology _____

6. malignent   malignant _____

7. carsinoma in situ   carcinoma *in situ* _____

8. hyperplasia   hyperplayzea _____

9. displastic   dysplastic _____

10. polypoid   polipoid _____

B. *Circle the term that is spelled correctly. The meaning of each term is given.*

11. malignant tumor of fibrous ....fibrosacroma   fibrosarcoma   fibrosarkoma
    tissue

12. additional treatment..........................adjuvant therapy   adjivent theraphy   adjuvent therapy

13. replication of cells ....miteosis   mitosis   meiosis

14. specialization of cells.........................differentiation   differantiation   differentsheation

15. return of disease symptoms ....relaspe   relapse   relapze

16. plan for treatment ....protocal   protokol   protocol

17. densely packed tumors.......................scirrhous   skirrus   scirrhus

18. complex, naturally occurring ....steroids   stairoids   steriods
    chemicals

19. pertaining to tumors filled ....mucinous   mucanous   musinous
    with mucus

20. condition of being diseased...............morbitity   morbidity   morbitidy

Chapter Nineteen

PRONUNCIATION QUIZ

Name: _____

A. *Underline the accented syllable in the following terms:*

1. papillary tumor	4. laparoscopy	7. adjuvant	10. mucinous
2. exenteration	5. anaplasia	8. pharmacokinetics	
3. cauterization	6. alkylating	9. antimetabolites	

B. *Match the term in Column I with its meaning in Column II:*

Column I

Column II

1. benign _____   A. In glass; an experiment performed in a laboratory with chemicals.

2. neoplasm _____   B. Harmless; not cancerous.

3. morbidity _____   C. Production of two identical cells from a parent cell.

4. protocol _____   D. Plan for treatment.

5. *in vitro* _____   E. To remove substances from a cavity using suction.

6. *in vivo* _____   F. In life; an experiment performed in a living animal.

7. lethal _____   G. The condition of being diseased.

8. mitosis _____   H. A new growth; tumor.

9. carcinogen _____   I. A substance that produces cancer.

10. aspiration _____   J. Pertaining to producing death.

C. *Complete the following medical terms from their definitions:*

1. cach _____   Malnutrition associated with cancer.

2. _____oma   Cancerous tumor of a gland.

3. _____oma   Tumor of embryonic retinal cells.

4. meta _____   Beyond control; spreading of a cancer tumor to secondary origin.

5. angio _____   Formation of blood vessels.

6. in _____   Extending beyond normal boundaries; local invasion of tissue.

7. chemo _____   Treatment using drugs.

8. ped_____   Possessing a stem or stalk.

9. dif _____   Specialization of cells.

Chapter Nineteen
ABBREVIATIONS QUIZ

Name: _____

Give the meaning of the abbreviation related to oncology in Column I and then match it with an associated explanation in Column II.

Column I

1. MOAB _____ _____

2. Gy _____ _____

3. VEGF _____ _____

4. PSCT _____ _____

5. TNM _____ _____

6. EPO _____ _____

7. CSF _____ _____

8. XRT _____ _____

9. bx _____ _____

10. mets _____ _____

Column II

A. Promotes the growth of red blood cells

B. Microscopic examination of living tissue for diagnosis of disease

C. Unit of radiation equal to one hundredth of a rad

D. Secreted by tumors to stimulate formation of new blood vessels

E. Type of biological response modifier used in cancer treatment

F. Spread of malignant cells to a distant site

G. Infusion of undifferentiated blood cells into a patient to repopulate the bone marrow

H. Protein factor that promotes growth of white blood cells

I. Brachytherapy and teletherapy are examples

J. Staging system for evaluating malignancies

Chapter Nineteen
VOCABULARY QUIZ

Name: _____

A. *Match the following terms with their meanings below:*

adjuvant therapy   antibiotics   apoptosis
alkylating agents   antimetabolites   benign tumor
anaplasia   antimitotics   biologic response modifiers
angiogenesis

1. Substances produced by normal cells that either directly block tumor
   growth or stimulate the immune system to fight cancer _____

2. Synthetic chemicals containing alkyl groups that interfere with DNA synthesis _____

3. Loss of differentiation of cells _____

4. Programmed cell death _____

5. Chemicals that prevent cell division by inhibiting formation of
   substances necessary to make DNA _____

6. Process of forming new blood vessels _____

7. Noncancerous growth _____

8. Chemical substances, produced by bacteria or primitive plants; inhibit
   the growth of cells in cancer chemotherapy _____

9. Drugs that block mitosis (cell division) _____

10. Assisting primary treatment _____

B. *Match the following terms with their meanings below:*

biological therapy   chemotherapy   differentiating agents
carcinogens   dedifferentiation   differentiation
carcinoma   deoxyribonucleic acid (DNA)   electron beams
cellular oncogenes

1. Treatment with drugs _____

2. Genetic material within the nucleus of a cell _____

3. Cancerous tumor _____

4. Drugs that promote tumor cells to differentiate, stop growing, and die _____

5. Pieces of DNA that can cause a normal cell to become malignant _____

6. Loss of differentiation of cells; reversion to a more primitive type; anaplasia _____

7. Agents that cause cancer; chemicals, drugs, radiation, viruses _____

8. Use of the body's own defenses to destroy tumor cells _____

9. Low-energy beams of radiation for treatment of skin or surface tumors _____

10. Specialization of cells _____

C. Match the following terms with their meanings below:

external beam radiation	gray (Gy)	mitosis
fractionation	irradiation	modality
genetic screening	metastasis	morbidity
grading of tumors		

1. Unit of absorbed radiation dose _____

2. Exposure to any form of radiant energy such as light, heat or x-rays _____

3. Evaluation of the degree of maturity of tumor cells _____

4. Giving radiation in small, repeated doses _____

5. Replication of cells; two identical cells from a parent cell _____

6. Spread of a malignant tumor to a secondary site _____

7. Condition of being diseased _____

8. Family members are tested to determine whether they have inherited a cancer-causing gene _____

9. Radiation applied to a tumor from a distant source _____

10. Method of treatment, such as surgery, chemotherapy, or radiation _____

D. Match the following terms with their meanings listed below:

mutation	palliative	protocol
neoplasm	pedunculated	proton therapy
nucleotide	pharmacokinetics	radiation
oncogene		

1. Study of the distribution in and removal of drugs from the body over a period of time _____

2. Unit of DNA composed of a sugar, phosphate, and base _____

3. Possessing a stem or stalk (peduncle) _____

4. Subatomic particles produced by a cyclotron deposit an absorbed dose of radiation at a focused point in the body _____

5. New growth (tumor) _____

6. Detailed plan for treatment _____

7. Region of DNA in tumor cells or in viruses that cause cancer _____

8. Change in genetic material (DNA) of a cell _____

9. Relieving, but not curing, symptoms _____

10. Energy carried by a stream of particles _____

E. Match the following terms with their meanings listed below:

radiocurable tumor	radiotherapy	sarcoma
radioresistant tumor	relapse	simulation
radiosensitive tumor	remission	steroids
radiosensitizers	ribonucleic acid (RNA)	stereotactic radiosurgery

1. Study using CT scan or MRI to map treatment prior to radiation treatment _____

2. Return of symptoms of disease _____

3. Treatment of tumors using radiation; radiation oncology _____

4. Dose of radiation delivered under highly precise guidance

   (gamma knife surgery) _____

5. Tumor cells that are destroyed by radiation therapy _____

6. Partial or complete disappearance of symptoms of disease _____

7. Tumor cells that require large doses of radiation to be destroyed _____

8. Cellular substance that along with DNA plays an important role in

   protein synthesis _____

9. Drugs that increase the sensitivity of tumors to x-rays _____

10. Complex, naturally occurring chemicals (such as hormones) that are

    used in cancer chemotherapy _____

11. Cancerous tumor derived from connective or flesh tissue _____

12. Tumor in which radiation can cause the death of cells without serious

    damage to surrounding tissue _____

Chapter Nineteen
REVIEW SHEET QUIZ

Name: _____

A. *Give meanings for the following combining forms:*

1. aden/o _____
2. cac/o _____
3. carcin/o _____
4. cauter/o _____
5. chem./o _____

6. cry/o _____
7. cyst/o _____
8. fibr/o _____
9. follicul/o _____
10. fung/i _____

B. *Give meanings for the following combining forms:*

1. medull/o _____
2. mucos/o _____
3. mut/a _____
4. necr/o _____
5. onc/o _____
6. papill/o _____
7. pharmac/o _____

8. plas/o _____
9. ple/o _____
10. polyp/o _____
11. radi/o _____
12. sarc/o _____
13. scirrh/o _____
14. xer/o _____

C. *Give meanings for the following suffixes and prefixes:*

1. -blastoma _____
2. -oid _____
3. -oma _____
4. -plasia _____
5. -plasm _____
6. -ptosis _____
7. -stasis _____
8. -genesis _____
9. -suppression _____

10. -therapy _____
11. ana- _____
12. anti- _____
13. apo- _____
14. brachy- _____
15. dys- _____
16. meta- _____
17. tele- _____
18. epi- _____

Chapter Nineteen
CROSSWORD PUZZLE

Name: _____

Fill in the crossword puzzle below using the clues listed underneath it.

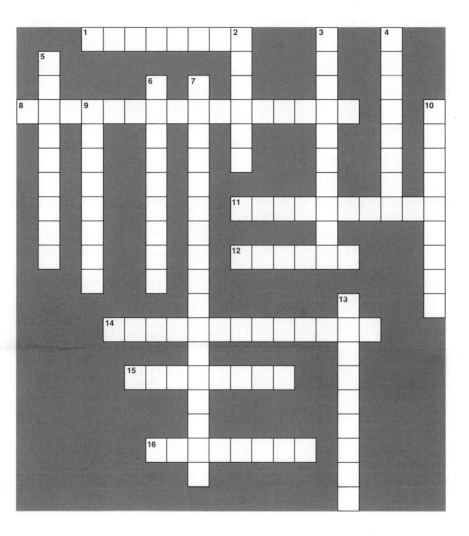

Across Clues

1. Containing dead tissue.
8. Lacking microscopic structures typical of normal, fully matured cells.
11. Forming small, microscopic gland-type sacs.
12. Noncancerous, not harmful.
14. Giving radiation in small, repeated doses.
15. Method of treatment, such as surgery, chemotherapy, or radiation.
16. New growth.

Down Clues

2. Forming large open sacs filled with fluid.
3. Characterizing an open, exposed surface resulting from death of overlying tissue.
4. An explicit detailed plan for treatment.
5. Mushrooming pattern of growth.
6. Resembling a wart-like growth.
7. Loss of differentiation cells.
9. Having the ability to enter and destroy surrounding tissue.
10. Hard, densely packed tumors, overgrown with fibrous tissue.
13. Damage to normal tissue; state of being diseased.

Chapter Nineteen
PRACTICAL APPLICATIONS

Name: _____

A. Case Study

The patient is a 63-year-old woman with a history (10 years ago) of squamous cell carcinoma *in situ* of the cervix, which was treated with a total abdominal hysterectomy. Three years ago, a pelvic mass was palpated, and exploratory laparotomy revealed a multinodular solid cystic mass of 10 cm–12 cm. The mass arose from the right ovary and was adherent to the right pelvic wall. The patient underwent resection of the mass, and the pathology revealed squamous cell carcinoma of the ovary. She subsequently had combined modality treatment with chemotherapy (cisplatin and 5-fluorouracil) and radiation therapy to the pelvis. The latest CT scan of the abdomen revealed a new right retroperitoneal lymph node. CT-guided fine needle aspiration was consistent with metastatic ovarian squamous cell carcinoma.

1. **What best describes the patient's original diagnosis?** .... ☐
   A. Endometrial and cervical carcinoma
   B. Localized cancer of the lower portion of the uterus
   C. Cervical cancer that spread to the abdomen
   D. Ovarian cancer

2. **What was the initial primary treatment?** .... ☐
   A. Drug treatment
   B. Radiation treatment
   C. Drug and radiation treatment
   D. Surgical removal of the entire uterus

3. **What procedure identified the new pelvic mass?** .... ☐
   A. Incision of the abdomen
   B. Radiation therapy
   C. Total abdominal hysterectomy
   D. CT scan of the abdomen

4. **Which treatment modalities were used for the patient's ovarian carcinoma?** .... ☐
   A. Computed tomography of the abdomen
   B. Fine needle aspiration of the ovary
   C. Drug and radiation therapy in addition to surgical removal
   D. Surgical resection of the mass

5. **How would you characterize the disease in the patient's retroperitoneal lymph node?** .... ☐
   A. Cancer of the lymphatic system
   B. Cervical cancer that had spread
   C. Primary ovarian cancer
   D. Ovarian cancer that had spread

B. Research Report

In a recent trial comparing the antiemetics ondansetron (Zofran) and metoclopramide (Reglan), ondansetron was more effective and produced less severe side effects. The trial involved 24 medical centers and 307 cancer patients receiving high doses of cisplatin.

1. **What type of drug is ondansetron?** ..... ☐
   A. Chemotherapeutic
   B. Antipsychotic
   C. Antibiotic
   D. Antinauseant

2. **When is ondansetron prescribed?** ☐
   A. After cancer surgery
   B. In conjunction with metoclopramide
   C. When patients are receiving high-dose chemotherapy for cancer
   D. Before cancer surgery

C. Chart Note

Pt with metastatic squamous cell carcinoma of the tongue. Toward the end of XRT, the pt complained of some intermittent costal and low vertebral pain. The pt presented to the ER when pain control was no longer achieved using Percocet. CT scan and MRI were performed, revealing a number of vertebral bodies involved with tumor in the upper lumbar and lower thoracic region. Preliminary reading suggests no evidence of cord compression, yet there is evidence of disk protrusion at T6-T7. We are consulted for palliative XRT of the spine lesions for purpose of pain control.

1. **What was probably causing the patient's pain?** .... ☐
   A. Tuberculosis of the spine
   B. Pressure on the spinal cord
   C. Tumor of the oral cavity
   D. Metastatic tumor in the backbones ☐

2. **What does costal mean?** .... ☐
   A. Pertaining to ribs
   B. Pertaining to spinal cord
   C. Pertaining to the back
   D. Pertaining to the breast bone

3. **What is palliative XRT?** ☐
   A. Diagnostic workup for malignancy
   B. Chemotherapy for painful cancer treatment
   C. Radiotherapy to relieve symptoms but not to cure
   D. Surgery to relieve pain

4. **What type of doctor wrote this report?** ☐
   A. Radiologist
   B. Radiation oncologist
   C. Nuclear medicine specialist
   D. Orthopedist

Chapter Nineteen

ANSWERS TO THE QUIZZES

Multiple Choice Quiz

1. A	5. B	9. D	13. A	17. B	21. D	25. B	29. B
2. D	6. C	10. A	14. C	18. B	22. A	26. E	30. C
3. E	7. D	11. E	15. A	19. D	23. E	27. A	
4. A	8. A	12. D	16. B	20. D	24. D	28. D	

Exercise Quiz

A

1. anaplasia
2. infiltrative
3. invasive
4. metastasis

B

5. mitosis
6. RNA
7. virus
8. ultraviolet radiation
9. chemical carcinogen
10. DNA
11. oncogene
12. mutation
13. radiation

C

14. cancerous tumor of glandular tissue
15. cancerous tumor of bone
16. harmless; not cancerous
17. specialization of cells
18. new growth; tumor

D

19. papillary
20. dysplastic
21. carcinoma *in situ*
22. scirrhous
23. alveolar
24. follicular
25. undifferentiated

E

26. inflammatory
27. medullary
28. necrotic
29. fungating
30. ulcerating
31. cystic
32. verrucous
33. polypoid

F

34. D
35. B
36. E
37. A
38. F
39. C
40. G

G

41. return of symptoms of disease
42. the condition of being diseased
43. an explicit, detailed plan for treatment
44. method of treatment
45. absence of symptoms of disease
46. assisting primary treatment

H

47. beta-HCG test
48. staging laparotomy
49. CA-125
50. laparoscopy
51. estrogen receptor assay
52. bone marrow biopsy
53. needle biopsy
54. PSA test
55. CEA test
56. exfoliative cytology

Dictation and Comprehension Quiz

A

1. adenocarcinoma
2. alkylating agents
3. anaplasia
4. angiogenesis
5. apoptosis
6. cachexia
7. carcinoma in situ
8. differentiation
9. en bloc resection
10. exfoliative cytology
11. fibrosarcoma
12. fractionation
13. laparoscopy
14. metastasis
15. morbidity
16. mutagenic
17. oncogene
18. pedunculated
19. pleomorphic
20. radiosensitizer

B

5   Programmed cell death
8   Specialization of cells
12   Giving radiation therapy in small, repeated doses
14   Spread of a malignant tumor to a secondary site
15   Condition of being diseased
20   Drug that increases the sensitivity of tumors to radiation therapy
3   Loss of specialization of cells; reversion to a more primitive type
11   Malignant tumor of connective tissue
18   Possessing a stem or stalk; characteristic of some polypoid tumors
4   Formation of blood vessels
17   Region of DNA found in tumor cells; examples are *abl, ras, src*
2   Synthetic chemicals containing groups that interfere with DNA synthesis
13   Visual examination of the abdomen using small incisions and an endoscope
9   Removal of tumor along with a large area of surrounding tissue and lymph nodes
19   Microscopic description of tumors possessing a variety of cells

7 Localized cancer; confined to the site of origin

6 Malnutrition associated with chronic disease (such as malignancy) and ill health

1 Malignant tumor of epithelial tissue (glandular cells)

10 Cells are scraped from an area of suspected disease and examined microscopically

16 Pertaining to producing change in cells

Spelling Quiz

A

1. retinoblastoma—malignant tumor of the eye (inherited)
2. metastasis—spread of a malignant tumor
3. benign—harmless; not cancerous
4. chemotherapy—cancer treatment with drugs
5. oncology—the study of malignant tumors
6. malignant—harmful, cancerous
7. carcinoma *in situ*—localized cancer
8. hyperplasia—increased growth in numbers of cells
9. dysplastic—pertaining to abnormal formation of cells
10. polypoid—growths that are projections from a base

B

11. fibrosarcoma
12. adjuvant therapy
13. mitosis
14. differentiation
15. relapse
16. protocol
17. scirrhous
18. steroids
19. mucinous
20. morbidity

Pronunciation Quiz

A

1. papillary tumor
2. exenteration
3. cauterization
4. laparoscopy
5. anaplasia
6. alkylating
7. adjuvant

8. pharmacokinetics
9. antimetabolites
10. mucinous

B

1. B
2. H
3. G
4. D
5. A
6. F
7. J
8. C
9. I
10. E

C

1. cachexia
2. adenocarcinoma
3. retinoblastoma
4. metastasis
5. angiogenesis
6. infiltrative
7. chemotherapy
8. pedunculated
9. differentiation

Abbreviations Quiz

1. monoclonal antibody E
2. gray C
3. vascular endothelial growth factor D
4. peripheral stem cell transplant G
5. tumor, node, metastasis J
6. erythropoietin A
7. colony-stimulating factor H
8. radiation therapy I
9. biopsy B
10. metastases F

Vocabulary Quiz

A

1. biologic response modifiers
2. alkylating agents
3. anaplasia
4. apoptosis
5. antimetabolites
6. angiogenesis
7. benign tumor
8. antibiotics
9. antimitotics
10. adjuvant therapy

B

1. chemotherapy
2. deoxyribonucleic acid (DNA)
3. carcinoma

4. differentiating agents
5. cellular oncogenes
6. dedifferentiation
7. carcinogens
8. biological therapy
9. electron beams
10. differentiation

C

1. gray (Gy)
2. irradiation
3. grading of tumors
4. fractionation
5. mitosis
6. metastasis
7. morbidity
8. genetic screening
9. external beam radiation
10. modality

D

1. pharmacokinetics
2. nucleotide
3. pedunculated
4. proton therapy
5. neoplasm
6. protocol
7. oncogene
8. mutation
9. palliative
10. radiation

E

1. simulation
2. relapse
3. radiotherapy
4. stereotactic radiosurgery
5. radiocurable tumor
6. remission
7. radioresistant tumor
8. ribonucleic acid (RNA)
9. radiosensitizers
10. steroids
11. sarcoma
12. radiosensitive tumor

Review Sheet Quiz

A

1. gland
2. bad
3. cancer, cancerous
4. burn, heat
5. chemical, drug
6. cold
7. sac of fluid
8. fibers
9. small, glandular sacs
10. fungus, mushroom

B

1. soft, inner part
2. mucous membrane
3. genetic change
4. death
5. tumor
6. nipple-like
7. chemical, drug
8. formation
9. many, more
10. polyp
11. rays, x-rays
12. flesh, connective tissue
13. hard
14. dry

C

1. immature tumor
2. resembling, derived from
3. mass, tumor
4. formation, growth
5. formation, growth
6. falling, prolapse
7. stop, control
8. formation
9. to stop
10. treatment
11. backward
12. against
13. off, away
14. short (distance)
15. painful, difficult, abnormal
16. beyond, change
17. far
18. upon

Crossword Puzzle

Across / Down grid:

```
 N E C R O T I C        U        P
 F                Y      L        R
 F          V  D  S      C        O
 U N D I F F E R E N T I A T E D  T      S
 G          N  R  I      R        O  C
 A          V  R  I      A        C  I
 T          A  U  F      T        O  R
 I          S  C  F      F O L L I C U L A R
 N          I  O  E            N     H
 G          V  U  R      B E N I G N O
 E          E  S  E                  U
            N        M              S
 F R A C T I O N A T I O N
            I        R
 M O D A L I T Y     B
            T        I
            I        D
 N E O P L A S M     I
            N        T
                     Y
```

Practical Applications

A

1. B
2. D
3. A
4. C
5. D

B

1. D
2. C

C

1. D
2. A
3. C
4. B

Chapter Nineteen

Answers to Combining Forms and Terminology Sections

(textbook pages 795–797)

Terminology	Meaning
alveolar	Pertaining to tumor growth in small microscopic sacs (descriptive of connective tissue tumors—sarcomas).
cachexia	General ill health and malnutrition associated with chronic disease such as cancer.
carcinoma in situ	Localized tumor growth.
electrocauterization	Burning tissue to destroy it.
chemotherapy	Treatment using drugs.
cryosurgery	Destruction of tissue using cold temperatures.
cystic tumor	Tumor forms with large open spaces filled with fluid.
fibrosarcoma	Malignant tumor of fiber-producing cells (flesh or connective tissue origin).
follicular	Pertaining to microscopic description of tumor growth in small, gland-type sacs.
fungating tumor	Mushrooming pattern of growth in which tumor cells pile one on top of another and project from the tissue surface.
medullary tumor	Large, soft, fleshy tumor.
mucositis	Inflammation of mucous membranes.
mutation	Change in the genetic material of a cell.
mutagenic	Pertaining to producing mutation.
necrotic tumor	Tumor containing dead cells.
oncology	Study of tumors.
papillary	Pertaining to tumors that grow in small, nipple-like or finger-like pattern.
pharmacokinetics	Study of the distribution and removal of drugs in the body over a period of time.
dysplastic	Pertaining to abnormal growth of cells but not clearly cancerous.
pleomorphic	Pertaining to tumors that contain a variety of types of cells.
polypoid tumor	Tumors that grow as projections extending outward from a base.
radiotherapy	Treatment using radiation.
osteosarcoma	Malignant tumor (flesh tissue) of bone.
scirrhous	Pertaining to hard, densely packed tumors, overgrown with fibrous tissue.
xerostomia	Conditions of dry mouth.
retinoblastoma	Tumor of the retina of the eye (embryonic cells); congenital and hereditary tumor.
neuroblastoma	Cancerous tumor of embryonic nervous tissue; a sarcoma composed of neuroblasts and affecting infants and children up to 10 years of age. The tumor usually arises in the autonomic nervous system.
angiogenesis	Formation of blood vessels.
adenocarcinoma	Cancerous tumor of glandular tissue.
hyperplasia	Condition of increased growth of cells (in numbers).
neoplasm	New growth (tumor).
myelosuppression	Stopping or inhibiting the growth of bone marrow tissue. This means that blood cells (leukocytes, erythrocytes, and platelets), normally formed in bone marrow, are not produced.
biological therapy	Treatment using the body's own defense mechanisms to fight tumor cells.
anaplasia	Reversion of cells to a more embryonic type (as happens in malignancy).
apoptosis	Programmed cell death.
brachytherapy	Implantation of small, sealed containers or seeds of radioactive material directly or near tumors.
epidermoid	Resembling epidermal tissue (tumors that arise from aberrant epidermal cells).

metastasis	The spread of a malignant tumor from its original location to a distant site.
metaplasia	Abnormal transformation of adult differentiated cells to differentiated tissue of another kind.
protocol	Detailed plan for treatment of illness.
teletherapy	Radiation therapy using high-energy beams from a distant (tele-) source, such as a linear accelerator or cyclotron (proton therapy).

chapter 20

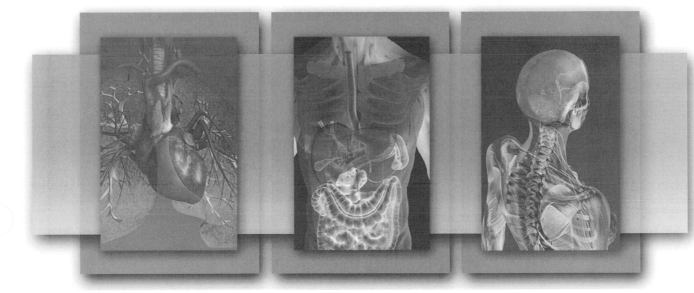

Chapter Twenty
MULTIPLE CHOICE QUIZ

Name: _____

In the box write the letter of the choice that is the definition of the term or best answers the question. There is only one correct answer for each question.

1. **What is the medical specialty that studies the characteristics and uses of radioactive substances in diagnosis of disease?** .... ☐
   A. Radiology
   B. Nuclear medicine
   C. Radiation oncology
   D. Roentgenology

2. **What does a radiologist do?** .... ☐
   A. Treats malignancy with radiation
   B. Aids a physician in administering x-ray procedures
   C. Specializes in the practice of administering diagnostic nuclear medicine procedures
   D. Specializes diagnostic techniques such as ultrasound, MRI, and CT scans.

3. **Which of the following is true of a radiopaque substance?** .... ☐
   A. Absorbs most of the x-rays it is exposed to
   B. Lung tissue is an example
   C. Is an air-containing structure
   D. Permits the passage of most x-rays

4. **Which best describes a barium enema?** .... ☐
   A. Iodine compound is given and x-rays are taken of the intestinal tract
   B. A fluorescent screen is used instead of a photographic plate to visualize images
   C. Metallic powder is introduced to the large intestine and x-rays are taken
   D. Radioactive substance is given and x-rays are taken

5. **X-ray of the renal pelvis and urinary tract after injecting dye into a vein:** .... ☐
   A. Venogram
   B. IVP
   C. RP
   D. Intravenous cholangiogram

6. **Myelogram:** .... ☐
   A. X-ray of lymphatic vessels
   B. X-ray of muscle
   C. X-ray of the bone marrow
   D. X-ray of the spinal cord

7. **Which is an x-ray of a joint?** .... ☐
   A. Pneumoencephalogram
   B. Ventriculogram
   C. Arthrogram
   D. Digital subtraction angiography

8. **Which term describes an x-ray test to show an organ in depth?** .... ☐
   A. Fluoroscopy
   B. Tomography
   C. Ultrasonography
   D. Arteriography

9. **What best characterizes a CT scan?** ..... ☐
   A. Uses radioactive substances to produce an x-ray image
   B. Gives a vertical front-to-back image of the body organs
   C. Magnetic and radio waves are used to create image
   D. Uses ionizing x-rays and a computer to produce a transverse image of the body organs

10. **What best characterizes an MRI?** .... ☐
    A. Sagittal, frontal, and cross-sectional images are produced using magnetic and radio waves
    B. Sound images are produced in addition to magnetic images
    C. X-rays and a contrast medium are used
    D. Radioactive matter enhances x-rays

11. **In which x-ray view is the patient upright with the back to the x-ray machine and the film to the chest?** .... ☐
    A. Oblique x-ray view
    B. Lateral x-ray view
    C. AP view
    D. PA view

12. **What is the meaning of adduction?** ..... ☐
    A. Bending a part of the body
    B. Moving the part of the body toward the midline of the body
    C. Moving the part away from the midline
    D. Turning inward

13. **What is a substance that gives off high-energy particles or rays?** ....
    A. Scanner
    B. Half-life
    C. Barium
    D. Radioisotope

14. **In which test is a radiopharmaceutical injected intravenously and traced within the vessels of the lung?** ....
    A. Chest x-ray of the lung
    B. CT scan of the thoracic cavity
    C. Perfusion study of the lung
    D. Ventilation scan of the lung

15. **What is an in vivo test?** ....
    A. Experiments are performed in a laboratory
    B. Radiopharmaceuticals are used
    C. Radionuclide is incorporated into a chemical substance
    D. Experiments are performed in a living organism

16. **What can liver and spleen scans detect?** ....
    A. Cirrhosis and splenomegaly due to abscess or tumor
    B. Blood flow through the heart and large vessels
    C. Areas of metabolic deficiency in the brain
    D. Thyroid carcinoma

17. **Interventional radiologists perform all of the following except** ....
    A. Administration of radiation therapy
    B. Placement of drainage catheters
    C. Occlusion of bleeding vessels
    D. Instillation of antibiotics or chemotherapy via catheters

18. **What is Thallium-201?** ....
    A. Gamma camera
    B. Contrast material
    C. Fluorescent material
    D. Radionuclide

19. **In which procedure is a transducer used?** ....
    A. MRI
    B. Ultrasound
    C. Bone scan
    D. CT Scan

20. **PACS is a** ....
    A. Radiopharmaceutical used in a PET scan
    B. Protocol for transmission between imaging devices
    C. Technique using a radioactive substance and a computer to create three-dimensional images
    D. System to replace traditional films with digital equivalents

21. **FDG is a** ....
    A. Radiopharmaceutical used in a PET scan
    B. Protocol for transmission between imaging devices
    C. Technique using a radioactive substance and a computer to create three-dimensional images
    D. System to replace traditional films with digital equivalents

22. **DICOM is a** ....
    A. Radiopharmaceutical used in a PET scan
    B. Protocol for transmission between imaging devices
    C. Technique using a radioactive substance and a computer to create three-dimensional images
    D. System to replace traditional films with digital equivalents

23. **SPECT is a:** ....
    A. Radiopharmaceutical used in a PET scan
    B. Protocol for transmission between imaging devices
    C. Technique using a radioactive substance and a computer to create three-dimensional images
    D. System to replace traditional films with digital equivalents

Chapter Twenty
EXERCISE QUIZ

Name: _____

A. *Name the medical term from its definition and word parts given:*

1. obstructing the passage of x-rays: radio _____

2. permitting the passage of x-rays: radio _____

3. aids physicians in performing ultrasound procedures:_____ grapher

4. radioactive element that gives off energy in the form of radiation: radio _____

5. radioactive drug administered for diagnostic purposes: radio _____

6. transformation of stable substances into changed particles: _____ ization

7. a physician who specializes in diagnostic radiology: radi _____

8. study of uses of radioactive substances in the diagnosis of disease: _____ medicine

B. *Match the special diagnostic technique below with its definition:*

cineradiography	fluoroscopy	positron emission tomography
computed tomography	interventional radiology	ultrasonography
contrast studies	magnetic resonance imaging	

9. Radiopaque substances are given and x-rays taken _____

10. Use of motion picture techniques to record x-ray images _____

11. Radioactive substance is given intravenously and a cross-sectional image is created of cellular metabolism based on local concentration of the radioactive substance _____

12. Echoes of high-frequency sound waves are used to diagnose disease _____

13. X-ray beams are focused from the body onto an image intensifier that glows as a result of the ionizing effect of x-rays _____

14. A magnetic field and radio waves are used to form images of the body _____

15. X-ray pictures are taken circularly around an area of the body and a computer synthesizes the information into a composite axial picture _____

16. Therapeutic procedures are performed by a radiologist under the guidance of fluoroscopy or ultrasound _____

C. *Give the meanings for the following medical terms:*

17. in vitro _____

18. in vivo _____

19. radiopharmaceutical _____

20. bone scan _____

D. *Match the diagnostic x-ray test in Column I with the part of the body that is imaged in Column II:*

Column I   Column II

21. myelography   _____   A. Joints

22. pyelography   _____   B. Spinal cord

23. angiography   _____   C. Uterus and fallopian tubes

24. arthrography   _____   D. Blood vessels

25. upper GI series   _____   E. Esophagus, stomach, and small intestine

26. cholangiography   _____   F. Lower gastrointestinal tract

27. barium enema   _____   G. Renal pelvis of kidney and the urinary tract

28. hysterosalpingography _____ H. Bile vessels (ducts)

E. *Give meanings for the following abbreviations:*

29. MRI _____   35. PACS _____

30. CT _____   36. DICOM _____

31. CXR _____   37. AP _____

32. U/S _____   38. KUB _____

33. PA _____   39. LAT _____

34. PET _____   40. ^{131}I _____

Chapter Twenty
DICTATION AND COMPREHENSION QUIZ

Name: _____

A. Dictation of Terms

1. _____   11. _____

2. _____   12. _____

3. _____   13. _____

4. _____   14. _____

5. _____   15. _____

6. _____   16. _____

7. _____   17. _____

8. _____   18. _____

9. _____   19. _____

10. _____   20. _____

B. Comprehension of Terms: Match number of the above term with its meaning below.

_____ Turning outward

_____ Use of motion picture techniques to record a series of x-ray images using fluoroscopy

_____ Measurement or observation within a living organism

_____ Permitting the passage of most x-rays

_____ Rate of absorption of a radionuclide into an organ or tissue

_____ A procedure in which something is measured or observed outside a living organism

_____ The emission of glowing light resulting from exposure to and absorption of radiation

_____ A radioactive form of a substance

_____ Process (two dimensional) used to detect radioactivity emitted in diagnostic imaging

_____ X-ray record of the uterus and fallopian tubes

_____ Movement toward the midline of the body

_____ Radioactive substances produce cross-sectional images of regions of the body

_____ Radioactive drug (radionuclide plus chemical) that is administered for diagnostic or therapeutic purposes

_____ Pertaining to treatment

_____ Obstructing the passage of x-rays

_____ Diagnostic x-ray procedure in which cross-sectional images are made of specific body segments

_____ X-ray record of the renal pelvis

_____ Process of recording x-ray images of bile vessels

_____ X-ray position; lying down and on one's side

_____ Process of recording sound waves in order to produce an image of the heart

Chapter Twenty
SPELLING QUIZ

Name: _____

A. *Circle the term that is spelled correctly and write its meaning in the space provided:*

1. floroscopy   fluoroscopy _____

2. therapeutic   therapreutic _____

3. colangiography   cholangiography _____

4. radionuclide   radioneuclide _____

5. radiolucent   radiolucant _____

6. anterioposterior   anteroposterior _____

7. transducer   transduser _____

8. radiopharmaceutical   radiopharmaseutical _____

9. traser studies   tracer studies _____

10. in vetro   in vitro _____

B. *Circle the term that is spelled correctly. The meaning of each term is given.*

11. X-ray record of the spinal cord .... myleogram	myelogram	mielogram
12. Moving toward the midline .... abduction	adduckshun	adduction
13. Lying down position .... rekumbent	recumbant	recumbent
14. Lying on the back .... supine	soupine	suppine
15. Obstructing the passage of x-rays .... radiopaquie	radiopaque	radioopaque
16. X-ray of the renal pelvis .... pyleogram	pyelogram	pyilogram
17. X-ray record of vessels .... anjiogram	angeiogram	angiogram
18. Radioactive form of a substance .... radioisotope	radioiceotope	radioisotop
19. Lying on the belly .... prone	proone	pron
20. Study of x-rays .... roentgenology	rentgenology	radology

Chapter Twenty
PRONUNCIATION QUIZ

Name: _____

A. *Underline the accented syllable in the following terms:*

1. radioisotope   4. supine   7. ionization   10. fluoroscopy
2. ultrasonography 5. recumbent   8. photopenic
3. angiography   6. echocardiography 9. lateral decubitus

B. *Match the term in Column I with its meaning in Column II:*

Column I

1. flexion _____
2. extension _____
3. prone _____
4. abduction _____
5. supine _____
6. eversion _____
7. oblique _____
8. cineradiography _____
9. tracer studies _____
10. ^{99m}Technetium _____
    sestamibi scan

Column II

A. Turning outward.
B. Lying on one's belly; face down.
C. Bending a part of the body.
D. Lying on one's back.
E. Radionuclides are used as tags attached to chemicals and followed throughout the body.
F. Test of blood flow to heart muscle.
G. Lengthening or straightening a flexed limb.
H. Carrying a limb away from the body.
I. Positioned at an angle.
J. Use of motion picture techniques to record a series of x-ray images.

C. *Complete the following medical terms from their definitions:*

1. _____ gram   X-ray record of the urinary tract.
2. _____ gram   X-ray record of the bile vessels.
3. radio _____   A radioactive drug used in diagnosis of disease.
4. _____ gram   X-ray record of the uterus and the fallopian tubes.
5. _____ ology   Study of x-rays.
6. radio _____   Permitting the passage of x-rays.
7. _____ scopy   The process of using x-rays to produce a fluorescent image on an image intensifier.

Chapter Twenty
VOCABULARY QUIZ

Name: _____

A. *Match the following terms with their meanings below:*

cineradiography	fluoroscopy	half-life
computed tomography (CT)	gamma camera	interventional radiology
contrast studies	gamma rays	ionization
fluorescence		

1. Time required for a radioactive substance to lose half its radioactivity by disintegration _____

2. Emission of glowing light resulting from exposure to and absorption of radiation from x-rays _____

3. High energy rays emitted by radioactive substances _____

4. Use of motion picture techniques to record a series of x-ray images during fluoroscopy _____

5. Therapeutic procedures performed by a radiologist _____

6. Transformation of electrically neutral substances into electrically charged particles _____

7. Diagnostic x-ray procedure whereby a cross-sectional and other images of a specific body segment are produced. _____

8. Materials are injected to obtain contrast with surrounding tissue when shown on x-ray film _____

9. Machine to detect gamma rays emitted from radiopharmaceuticals during scanning for diagnostic purposes _____

10. X-rays produce a fluorescent image on an image intensifier _____

B. Match the following terms with their meanings below:

in vitro   nuclear medicine   radioisotope
in vivo   positron emission tomography (PET)   radiology
labeled compound   radioimmunoassay   radiolucent
magnetic resonance (MR)

1. Permitting the passage of x-rays _____

2. Process, test, or procedure performed, measured, or observed in
   a living organism _____

3. Radioactive substance is given intravenously and a cross-sectional
   image is created of cellular metabolism based on local concentration
   of the radioactive substance _____

4. Process, test, or procedure performed, measured, or observed outside
   a living organism _____

5. Medical specialty that studies the uses of radioactive substances in
   diagnosis of disease _____

6. Magnetic field and radio waves produce images of the body in three
   planes (coronal, sagittal, and axial) _____

7. Radiopharmaceutical used in nuclear medicine studies _____

8. Test that combines radioactive chemicals and antibodies to detect
   minute quantities of substances in a patient's blood _____

9. Radioactive form of an element; radionuclide _____

10. Medical specialty concerned with the study of x-rays and their use in
    the diagnosis of disease _____

C. Match the following terms with their meanings below:

radiopaque   single-photon emission computed   ultrasound
radiopharmaceutical   tomography (SPECT)   uptake
roentgenology   tagging   ventilation/perfusion studies
scan   transducer

1. Rate of absorption of a radionuclide into an organ or tissue _____

2. Image of an area, organ, or tissue obtained from ultrasound, radioactive
   tracer studies, computed tomography, or magnetic resonance imaging _____

3. Handheld device that sends and receives ultrasound signals _____

4. Attaching a radionuclide to a chemical and following its path in the body _____

5. Radiopharmaceutical is inhaled and injected intravenously followed by
   imaging its passage through the respiratory tract _____

6. Obstructing the passage of x-rays _____

7. Diagnostic technique that projects and retrieves high-frequency sound
   waves as they echo off parts of the body _____

8. Radioactive tracer is injected intravenously and a computer reconstructs
   a three-dimensional image based on a composite of many views _____

9. Radioactive drug (radionuclide plus chemical) is administered for
   diagnostic and therapeutic purposes _____

10. Study of x-rays; radiology _____

Chapter Twenty
REVIEW SHEET QUIZ

Name: _____

A. *Give meanings for the following combining forms, suffixes, and prefixes:*

1. fluor/o _____

2. is/o _____

3. pharmaceut/o _____

4. radi/o _____

5. son/o _____

6. therapeut/o _____

7. vitr/o _____

8. viv/o _____

9. -gram _____

10. -graphy _____

11. -lucent _____

12. -opaque _____

13. cine- _____

14. echo- _____

15. ultra- _____

Chapter Twenty
CROSSWORD PUZZLE

Name: _____

Fill in the crossword puzzle below using the clues listed underneath it.

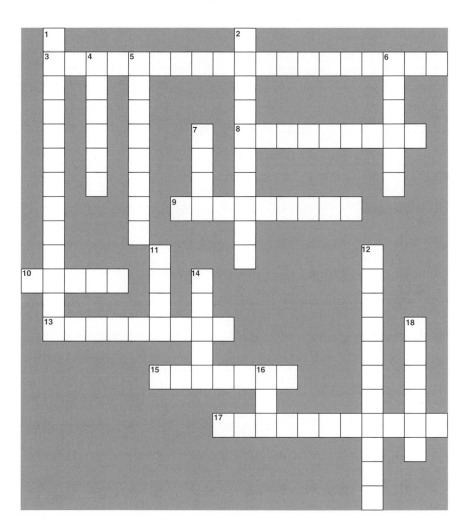

Across Clues

3. An x-ray record of the uterus and fallopian tubes to determine patency.
8. Moving a part of the body away from the midline.
9. Lying down; synonym of decubitus.
10. Lying on the belly.
13. An x-ray recording of the spinal cord.
15. -opaque means _____ .
17. Permitting the passage of most x-rays.

Down Clues

1. An x-ray recording of the bile vessels.
2. Diagnostic technique that projects and retrieves high-frequency sound waves.
4. Lying on the back.
5. Turning outward.
6. -gram means _____.
7. Viv/o means _____.
11. Pharmaceut/o means _____.
12. Process of using x-rays to produce a fluorescent image on a screen.
14. Vitr/o means _____.
16. Abbreviation for radiation absorbed dose is _____ .
18. Ultra means _____.

Chapter Twenty
PRACTICAL APPLICATIONS

Name: _____

A. Radiology Report

Mass Adjacent to Thyroid – Lt side on US done 5/5/06
EXAM: NECK W/WOUT CONTRAST
5/9/00

Initially scans were obtained throughout the neck without IV contrast. Following this, a bolus of IV contrast was given and rapid scans obtained through the region of interest in the neck, related to the left lobe of the thyroid. As demonstrated on the recent ultrasound, there is a well-defined oblong mass in the left neck measuring 2.2 × 3 × 1.8 cm in size. This lies posterolateral to the left thyroid lobe and is predominantly between the left common carotid artery, which is displaced posteromedially, and the left internal jugular vein, which is displaced laterally. No other adenopathy and the remainder of the thyroid appears unremarkable.

IMPRESSION: The mass appears to be extrinsic to the thyroid, possible even within the carotid sheath. The lesion appears to be relatively avascular. The differential diagnosis would include an unusually enlarged lymph node, a very atypical thyroid nodule, or a soft tissue tumor. The lesion is very easily accessible to needle biopsy and this would certainly be the easiest method of obtaining positive confirmation. This could be done using US guidance.

1. **What type of radiological test is described here?** .... ☐
   A. Ultrasound
   B. CT scans
   C. Pyelogram
   D. PET scan

2. **Where is the mass located?** .... ☐
   A. Within the left lobe of the thyroid gland
   B. Between the left and right carotid arteries
   C. Behind and to the side of the left lobe of the thyroid gland
   D. In front and to the side of the thyroid gland

3. **Which of the following is not a possible diagnosis?** .... ☐
   A. An unusual mass on the thyroid gland
   B. Lymphadenopathy
   C. Tumor mass adjacent to the thyroid gland
   D. Lesion composed of many blood vessels

4. **What procedure will help determine the diagnosis?** .... ☐
   A. Aspiration of tissue and pathological examination
   B. Removal of the thyroid gland
   C. Removal of thyroid tissue for biopsy
   D. Further scans with ultrasound guidance

B. Chart Note

The pt underwent a bone scan, which revealed irregular foci of tracer in lower T spine (T11-T12). consistent with compression fracture. There was also increased tracer in the posterior/lateral right ribs. On physical exam she was diffusely tender and in pain throughout her chest/ribs and spine. The pt also underwent chest CT, which demonstrated extensive parenchymal and pleural disease encasing the entire chest and involving vessels and bronchi. Her adrenals and liver, vertebral bodies, and R scapula were also involved with metastatic disease.

1. **What type of test is a bone scan?** .... ☐
   A. Chest x-ray of ribs and bones of back
   B. MRI of the skeleton
   C. Dye is injected and traced in blood vessels
   D. Radioisotope is injected and traced in bones

2. **What type of doctor administers this test?** .... ☐
   A. Diagnostic radiologist
   B. Nuclear medicine specialist
   C. Radiation oncologist
   D. Medical oncologist

3. **Extensive parenchymal and pleural disease means:** .... ☐
   A. Tumor is in the spinal cord
   B. Tumor is in the backbones
   C. Tumor is in the lungs and membranes around the lungs
   D. Tumor is in the abdominal, pelvic, and chest regions

4. **The bone scan revealed:** .... ☐
   A. Disease in the lungs
   B. Areas of tumor in the lower chest region and ribs
   C. Disease in the adrenals and liver
   D. Metastatic disease in the right shoulder bone

Chapter Twenty
ANSWERS TO THE QUIZZES

Multiple Choice Quiz

1. B	4. C	7. C	10. A	13. D	16. A	19. B	22. B		
2. D	5. B	8. B	11. D	14. C	17. A	20. D	23. C		
3. A	6. D	9. D	12. B	15. D	18. D	21. A			

Exercise Quiz

A

1. radiopaque
2. radiolucent
3. sonographer
4. radionuclide or radioisotope
5. radiopharmaceutical
6. ionization
7. radiologist
8. nuclear

B

9. contrast studies
10. cineradiography
11. positron emission tomography
12. ultrasonography
13. fluoroscopy
14. magnetic resonance imaging
15. computed tomography
16. interventional radiology

C

17. a test in which something is measured or observed outside a living organism
18. a test in which something is measured or observed in a living organism
19. a radioactive drug that is given safely for diagnostic and therapeutic purposes
20. radioisotope is administered and traced within the bones

D

21. B
22. G
23. D
24. A
25. E
26. H
27. F
28. C

E

29. magnetic resonance imaging
30. computed tomography
31. chest x-ray
32. ultrasound
33. posteroanterior
34. positron emission tomography
35. picture archival and communications system
36. digital image communication in medicine
37. anteroposterior
38. kidneys, ureters, bladder
39. lateral
40. radioactive iodine

Dictation and Comprehension

A

1. adduction
2. cholangiography
3. cineradiography
4. computed tomography
5. echocardiography
6. eversion
7. fluorescence
8. hysterosalpingogram
9. in vitro
10. in vivo
11. lateral decubitus
12. intravenous pyelogram
13. positron emission tomography
14. radioisotope
15. radiolucent
16. radiopaque
17. radiopharmaceutical
18. scintigraphy
19. therapeutic
20. uptake

B

6 Turning outward
3 Use of motion picture techniques to record a series of x-ray images using fluoroscopy
10 Measurement or observation within a living organism
15 Permitting the passage of most x-rays
20 Rate of absorption of a radionuclide into an organ or tissue
9 A procedure in which something is measured or observed outside a living organism
7 The emission of glowing light resulting from exposure to and absorption of radiation
14 A radioactive form of a substance
18 Process (two dimensional) used to detect radioactivity emitted in diagnostic imaging
8 X-ray record of the uterus and fallopian tubes
1 Movement toward the midline of the body
13 Radioactive substances produce cross-sectional images of regions of the body
17 Radioactive drug (radionuclide plus chemical) that is administered for diagnostic or therapeutic purposes
19 Pertaining to treatment
16 Obstructing the passage of x-rays
4 Diagnostic x-ray procedure in which cross-sectional images are made of specific body segments
12 X-ray record of the renal pelvis
2 Process of recording x-ray images of bile vessels
11 X-ray position; lying down and on one's side
5 Process of recording sound waves in order to produce an image of the heart

Spelling Quiz

A

1. fluoroscopy—using x-rays to produce fluorescent image
2. therapeutic—pertaining to treatment
3. cholangiography—x-ray record of the bile vessels
4. radionuclide—radioactive chemical that gives off energy in the form of radiation; radioisotope
5. radiolucent—permitting the passage of most x-rays
6. anteroposterior—pertaining to the front and back
7. transducer—device that sends and receives ultrasound signals
8. radiopharmaceutical—a radioactive drug that is given for diagnostic or therapeutic purposes
9. tracer studies—radionuclides are used as labels and traced within the body
10. in vitro—tests are done outside a living organism

B

11. myelogram
12. adduction
13. recumbent
14. supine
15. radiopaque
16. pyelogram
17. angiogram
18. radioisotope
19. prone
20. roentgenology

Pronunciation Quiz

A

1. radioisotope
2. ultrasonography

3. angiography
4. supine
5. recumbent
6. echocardiography
7. ionization
8. photopenic
9. lateral decubitus
10. fluoroscopy

B

1. C
2. G
3. B
4. H
5. D
6. A
7. I
8. J
9. E
10. F

C

1. urogram
2. cholangiogram
3. radiopharmaceutical
4. hysterosalpingogram
5. radiology or roentgenology
6. radiolucent
7. fluoroscopy

Vocabulary Quiz

A

1. half-life
2. fluorescence
3. gamma rays
4. cineradiography
5. interventional radiology
6. ionization
7. computed tomography (CT)
8. contrast studies
9. gamma camera
10. fluoroscopy

B

1. radiolucent
2. in vivo

3. positron emission tomography (PET)
4. in vitro
5. nuclear medicine
6. magnetic resonance (MR)
7. labeled compound
8. radioimmunoassay
9. radioisotope
10. radiology

C

1. uptake
2. scan
3. transducer
4. tagging
5. ventilation/perfusion studies
6. radiopaque
7. ultrasound
8. single-photon emission computed tomography
9. radiopharmaceutical
10. roentgenology

Review Sheet Quiz

A

1. luminous, fluorescence
2. same
3. drug
4. x-rays
5. sound
6. treatment
7. glass
8. life
9. record
10. process of recording
11. to shine
12. obscure
13. movement
14. a repeated sound
15. beyond

Crossword Puzzle

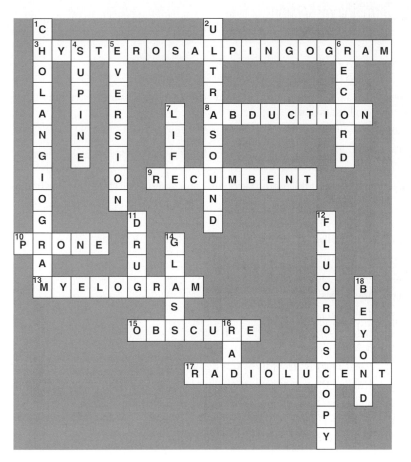

Practical Applications

A

1. B
2. C
3. D
4. A

B

1. D
2. B
3. C
4. B

Chapter Twenty
Answers to Combining Forms and Terminology Sections

(textbook pages 836–837)

Terminology	Meaning
fluoroscopy	Process of using x-rays to produce a fluorescent image on a screen.
radioisotope	A radioactive form of an element (radioisotopes of an element have similar structure but with different weights and charges).
radiopharmaceutical	Pertaining to the combination of a radioisotope and a drug.
radiographer	Aids physicians in administering diagnostic x-ray procedures.
roentgenology	The study of x-rays.
hysterosonogram	Record of sound waves within the uterus (after injection of fluid to distend the uterine cavity).
therapeutic	Pertaining to treatment (therapy).
in vitro	Experiments performed in a test tube (glass); outside of a living organism.
in vivo	Experiments performed within a living organism.
angiogram	Record (x-ray) of blood vessels.
hysterosalpingogram	Record (x-ray) of the uterus and fallopian tubes.
pyelogram	Record (x-ray) of the renal pelvis of the kidney.
computed tomography	Process of recording x-ray images of the body in a cross-sectional view; a computer is used and images taken all around a section of the body.
radiolucent	Permitting the passage of x-rays (rays shine through).
radiopaque	Obscuring or obstructing the passage of x-rays.
cineradiography	Process of using motion picture techniques to record a series of x-ray images.
echocardiography	Process of recording sound waves (echoes) as they bounce off the heart; a picture is produced that shows the sound waves as they are reflected from tissues of different densities.
ultrasonography	Process of using ultrasound waves in the body to produce sound echoes that are recorded as an image.

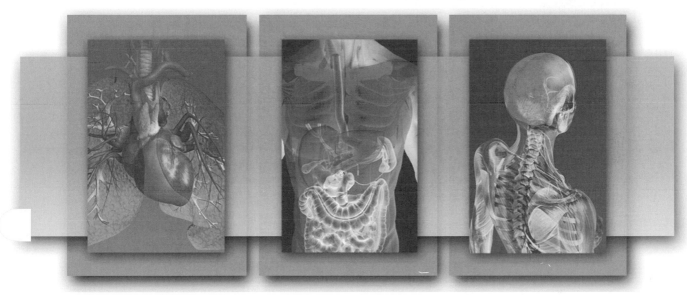

chapter 21

Chapter Twenty-One
MULTIPLE CHOICE QUIZ

Name: _____

In the box write the letter of the choice that is the definition of the term or best answers the question. There is only one correct answer for each question.

1. **Study of the interaction of drugs and subcellular entities such as enzymes and DNA is called:** .... ☐
   A. Medicinal chemistry
   B. Pharmacodynamics
   C. Chemotherapy
   D. Molecular pharmacology
   E. Pharmacokinetics

2. **Finding proper antidotes to the harmful effects of drugs is part of the specialty of:** .... ☐
   A. Molecular pharmacology
   B. Toxicology
   C. Medicinal chemistry
   D. Pharmacodynamics
   E. Pharmacokinetics

3. **Which of the following is a drug generic name?** .... ☐
   A. Omnipen
   B. Ampicillin
   C. Aminopenicillanic acid
   D. Polycillin
   E. Principen

4. **Which agency holds the legal responsibility for deciding whether a drug may be distributed and sold?** .... ☐
   A. PDR
   B. United States Pharmacopeia
   C. National Institutes of Health
   D. Hospital Formulary
   E. FDA

5. **The combination of two drugs can cause an effect that is greater than the sum of the individual effects of each:** .... ☐
   A. Iatrogenic
   B. Additive action
   C. Tolerance
   D. Synergism
   E. Idiosyncrasy

6. **Suppositories are inserted:** .... ☐
   A. Parenteral administration
   B. Rectal administration
   C. Inhalation
   D. Topical
   E. Oral

7. **Drugs are swallowed and absorbed through the intestinal tract:** .... ☐
   A. Parenteral administration
   B. Rectal administration
   C. Inhalation
   D. Topical
   E. Oral

8. **Drugs are injected through a syringe into a muscle, vein, or body cavity:** ..... ☐
   A. Parenteral administration
   B. Rectal administration
   C. Inhalation
   D. Topical
   E. Oral

9. **Aerosols are administered in this way:** .... ☐
   A. Parenteral administration
   B. Rectal administration
   C. Inhalation
   D. Topical
   E. Oral

10. **Drugs are applied on the skin:** .... ☐
    A. Parenteral administration
    B. Rectal administration
    C. Inhalation
    D. Topical
    E. Oral

11. **What is anaphylaxis?** .... ☐
    A. A type of hypersensitivity reaction
    B. Factors in the patient's condition that make the use of a drug dangerous
    C. A condition produced by the treatment
    D. Toxic effects that routinely result from use of a drug
    E. An antipruritic and antiseptic drug

12. **Drugs that block release of a substance that causes allergic reactions are called:** .... ☐
    A. Anticoagulants
    B. Antidiabetics
    C. Anticonvulsants
    D. Antihistamines
    E. Anesthetics

13. **Morphine:** .... ☐
   A. Endocrine drug
   B. Cardiovascular drug
   C. Analgesic drug
   D. Stimulant drug
   E. Anticoagulant drug

14. **Beta-blocker:** .... ☐
   A. Endocrine drug
   B. Cardiovascular drug
   C. Analgesic drug
   D. Stimulant drug
   E. Anticoagulant drug

15. **Heparin:** .... ☐
   A. Endocrine drug
   B. Cardiovascular drug
   C. Analgesic drug
   D. Stimulant drug
   E. Anticoagulant drug

16. **Estrogen:** .... ☐
   A. Endocrine drug
   B. Cardiovascular drug
   C. Analgesic drug
   D. Stimulant drug
   E. Anticoagulant drug

17. **Amphetamine and caffeine:** .... ☐
   A. Endocrine drug
   B. Cardiovascular drug
   C. Analgesic drug
   D. Stimulant drug
   E. Anticoagulant drug

18. **What is the effect of a diuretic?** .... ☐
   A. Lowers blood pressure by promoting fluid
      excretion from the kidney
   B. Widens blood vessels
   C. Stops blood clotting
   D. Lowers cholesterol
   E. Increases blood pressure by holding water
      in the body

19. **Penicillin is an example of which type
   of drug?** .... ☐
   A. Antihistamine
   B. Analgesic
   C. Antiemetic
   D. Antibiotic
   E. Hypnotic

20. **A drug that works against
   fever is:** .... ☐
   A. Antipruritic
   B. Antipyretic
   C. Anesthetic
   D. Anticoagulant
   E. Hypnotic

21. **Drugs that control anxiety and severe
   disturbances of behavior:** .... ☐
   A. Sedatives
   B. Anticonvulsants
   C. Analgesics
   D. Tranquilizers
   E. Anesthetics

22. **Drugs that relax without necessarily
   producing sleep:** .... ☐
   A. Sedatives
   B. Anticonvulsants
   C. Analgesics
   D. Tranquilizers
   E. Anesthetics

23. **Drugs used to relieve pain, induce
   sleep, and suppress cough:** .... ☐
   A. Sedatives
   B. Anticonvulsants
   C. Analgesics
   D. Tranquilizers
   E. Anesthetics

24. **Drugs that produce loss of sensation
   throughout the entire body:** .... ☐
   A. Sedatives
   B. Anticonvulsants
   C. Analgesics
   D. Tranquilizers
   E. Anesthetics

25. **Drugs used to treat epilepsy:** .... ☐
   A. Sedatives
   B. Anticonvulsants
   C. Analgesics
   D. Tranquilizers
   E. Anesthetics

Chapter Twenty-One
EXERCISE QUIZ

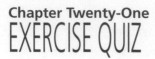

Name: _____

A. *Match the pharmacologic specialty with its description below:*

chemotherapy   pharmacodynamics   toxicology
molecular pharmacology   pharmacokinetics

1. study of how drugs interact with subcellular parts_____

2. use of drugs in the treatment of disease _____

3. study of the harmful effects of drugs_____

4. study of drug effects in the body _____

5. measurement of drug concentrations in tissues and in blood over time _____

B. *Name the route of drug administration from its description below:*

6. Drug is administered via suppository or fluid into the anus _____

7. Drug is administered via vapor or gas into the nose or mouth _____

8. Drug is administered under the tongue _____

9. Drug is applied locally on skin or mucous membrane _____

10. Drug is given by mouth and absorbed through the stomach or intestine_____

11. Drug is injected via syringe under the skin, or into a vein, muscle, or cavity_____

C. *Give meanings for the following terms:*

12. antipruritic _____

13. intrathecal_____

14. antiseptic_____

15. aerosol_____

16. subcutaneous _____

D. *Give the meaning for the following terms:*

17. cathartic _____

18. antiemetic_____

19. narcotic_____

20. beta-blocker _____

21. bronchodilator _____

E. Match the term in Column I with an associated term in Column II:

Column I

22. antihistamine _____
23. analgesic _____
24. stimulant _____
25. sedative _____
26. tranquilizer _____
27. antidiabetic _____
28. antibiotic _____

Column II

A. Relieves allergic symptoms
B. Penicillin or erythromycin
C. Barbiturate
D. Nonsteroidal anti-inflammatory drug
E. Phenothiazines
F. Caffeine or amphetamines
G. Insulin

F. Select from the following terms to complete the definitions below:

antianginal   cholesterol-lowering drug   vasoconstrictor
digoxin   vasodilator
antihypertensive   diuretic

29. drug that widens blood vessels_____

30. drug that reduces blood pressure _____

31. drug that strengthens the force and efficiency of the heartbeat _____

32. drug that narrows blood vessels_____

33. drug that prevents chest pain due to ischemia _____

34. drug that reduces lipids in blood_____

35. drug that promotes excretion of urine, lowering blood pressure_____

G. Match the drug or type of drug in Column I with the condition it treats in Column II:

Column I

36. anticonvulsant _____
37. anticoagulant _____
38. antacid _____
39. antibiotic _____
40. tranquilizer _____
41. analgesic _____
42. digoxin _____
43. antihistamine _____
44. antihypertensive _____
45. progestins _____

Column II

A. Myalgia
B. Epilepsy
C. Epigastric discomfort
D. Thrombosis
E. Bacterial pneumonia
F. Congestive heart failure
G. High blood pressure
H. Abnormal uterine bleeding due to hormonal imbalance
I. Severe behavior disturbances and anxiety
J. Anaphylaxis

Chapter Twenty-One

DICTATION AND COMPREHENSION QUIZ

Name: _____

A. *Dictation of Terms*

1. _____   11. _____

2. _____   12. _____

3. _____   13. _____

4. _____   14. _____

5. _____   15. _____

6. _____   16. _____

7. _____   17. _____

8. _____   18. _____

9. _____   19. _____

10. _____   20. _____

B. *Comprehension of Terms: Match the number of the above term with its meaning below.*

_____ An unexpected effect produced in a sensitive individual, but not seen in most patients

_____ An agent given to counteract an unwanted effect of a drug

_____ Harmful effects of a drug

_____ Drug action in which the combination of two drugs causes an effect that is greater than the sum of the individual effects of each drug alone

_____ A central nervous system stimulant

_____ Drug that relieves constipation

_____ Drug that stops the action of epinephrine at sites on receptors of heart muscle cells

_____ Drug that lowers body temperature

_____ An antibiotic substance

_____ Pertaining to delivery of a drug within the membranes lining the spinal cord

_____ A factor in the patient's condition that prevents the use of a drug or treatment

_____ Drug that acts as a sedative

_____ Pertaining to killing microorganisms

_____ Drug that prevents abnormal brain activity

_____ Drug that opens airways

_____ Particles of drug suspended in air

_____ Tube for introducing or withdrawing fluids

_____ Drug that prevents vomiting and nausea

_____ Pertaining to giving a drug by injection into the skin, muscles, or veins

_____ Drug that blocks the action of histamine and helps prevent symptoms of allergy

Chapter Twenty-One
SPELLING QUIZ

Name: _____

A. *Circle the term that is spelled correctly and write its meaning in the space provided.*

1. areolsol   aerosol _____

2. antacid   antiacid _____

3. antedote   antidote _____

4. antipyretic   antepyretic _____

5. cartharic   cathartic _____

6. hypnotic   hipnotic _____

7. iatrogenic   iatragenic _____

8. caffiene   caffeine _____

9. syringe   syrinje _____

10. tolerence   tolerance _____

B. *Circle the term that is spelled correctly. The meaning of each term is given.*

11. agent that excites and
promotes activity .... stimulent   stimulant   stimolent

12. drug that promotes vomiting .... emetic   enemetic   emetik

13. drug that relieves chest pain .... anteanginal   anteanjinal   antianginal

14. hypersensitivity reaction .... anaphilaxis   anaphylaxis   antiphylaxis

15. drug that is given by injection .... parenteral   parinteral   parentarol

16. legal, non-commercial name
for a drug .... genareic   generic   jeneric

17. harmful effects of a drug .... toxcity   toxicity   toxicitiy

18. drug that relieves pain .... analjesic   anesthetic   analgesic

19. drugs that are applied locally
on the skin .... topical   typoical   typical

20. drug that restores heart to a
regular cycle .... antirhhytmic   antiarrhythmic   antiarryhthmic

Chapter Twenty-One
PRONUNCIATION QUIZ

Name: _____

A. *Underline the accented syllable in the following words:*

1. antiarrhythmic
2. anaphylaxis
3. idiosyncrasy

4. synergistic
5. pharmacokinetics
6. antihistamine

7. cathartic
8. antidote
9. intrathecal

10. generic name

B. *Match the term in Column I with its meaning in Column II:*

Column I

1. amphetamine   _____

2. antiemetic   _____

3. diuretic   _____

4. narcotic   _____

5. hypodermic   _____

6. erythromycin   _____

7. laxative   _____

8. analgesic   _____

9. toxicity   _____

10. additive action   _____

Column II

A. The combination of two similar drugs is equal to the sum of the effects of each.

B. An agent that lowers blood pressure by increasing the release of urine.

C. A habit-forming drug that produces sleep and stupor.

D. A central nervous system stimulant.

E. A drug that relieves pain.

F. Pertaining to under the skin.

G. A drug that relieves constipation.

H. An agent that acts against vomiting.

I. Harmful effects of a drug.

J. An antibiotic.

C. *Complete the following medical terms from their definitions:*

1. anti _____   Pertaining to an agent that reduces fever.

2. anti _____   An agent that prevents or delays blood clotting.

3. par _____   Administration of drugs other than through the intestinal tract, such as into the skin, muscles, or veins.

4. gluco _____   Hormone from the adrenal cortex that raises blood sugar.

5. anti _____   Agent that lowers blood pressure.

6. _____ ology   Study of poisonous effects of drugs.

7. intra _____   Pertaining to within a sheath or within the membranes surrounding the spinal cord.

Chapter Twenty-One
VOCABULARY QUIZ

Name: _____

A. *Match the following terms with their descriptions below:*

addiction	antagonistic action	chemical name
additive action	antidote	contraindication
aerosol	brand name	generic name
anaphylaxis		

1. Commercial name for a drug; trademark or trade name _____

2. Exaggerated hypersensitivity reaction to a previously encountered drug or foreign protein _____

3. Physical and psychological dependence on and craving for a drug _____

4. Particles of a drug suspended in air _____

5. Chemical formula for a drug _____

6. Factor in the patient's condition that prevents the use of a particular drug or treatment _____

7. Legal, noncommercial name for a drug _____

8. Combination of two drugs gives less than an additive effect _____

9. Agent given to counteract an unwanted effect of a drug _____

10. Drug action in which the combination of two similar drugs is equal to the sum of the effects of each _____

B. *Match the following terms with their descriptions below:*

iatrogenic	molecular pharmacology	pharmacist
idiosyncrasy	oral administration	pharmacy
inhalation	parenteral administration	pharmacodynamics
medicinal chemistry		

1. Study of new drug synthesis; relationship between chemical structure and biological effects _____

2. Condition caused by treatment given by physicians or medical personnel _____

3. Drugs are given by mouth _____

4. Administration of drugs in gaseous or vapor form through the nose or mouth _____

5. Drugs are given by injection into the skin, muscles, or veins _____

6. Study of interaction of drugs and their target molecules, enzymes, or cell surface receptors _____

7. Location for preparing and dispensing drugs _____

8. Specialist in preparing and dispensing drugs _____

9. Unexpected effect produced in a particularly sensitive individual but
   not seen in most patients _____

10. Study of the effects and strength of a drug within the body _____

C. Match the following terms with their descriptions below:

Food and Drug Administration (FDA)   receptor   sublingual administration
pharmacokinetics   rectal administration   synergism
pharmacology   side effect   syringe
Physician's Desk Reference (PDR)

1. Drugs are inserted through the anus into the rectum _____

2. Study of the preparation, properties, uses, and actions of drugs _____

3. Target substance with which a drug interacts in the body _____

4. Instrument for introducing or withdrawing fluids from the body _____

5. Combination of two drugs causes an effect that is greater than the sum of the individual effects of
   each drug alone _____

6. Drug products are listed and described in this book _____

7. Calculation of drug concentration in tissues and body fluids over a period of time _____

8. Governmental agency having the legal responsibility for enforcing proper drug manufacture
   and clinical use _____

9. Drugs are given by placement under the tongue _____

10. Adverse reaction that routinely results from use of a drug _____

D. Match the following terms with their descriptions below:

ACE inhibitor   antacid   toxicity
amphetamine   tolerance   toxicology
analgesic   topical application   vitamin
anesthetic

1. Drug that relieves pain _____

2. Substance found in foods and essential in small quantities for growth
   and good health _____

3. Harmful effects of a drug _____

4. Larger and larger drug doses must be given to achieve the desired effect _____

5. Study of harmful chemicals and their effects on the body _____

6. Central nervous system stimulant _____

7. Drug that reduces or eliminates sensation _____

8. Drug that lowers blood pressure _____

9. Drug that neutralizes acid in the stomach _____

10. Drugs are applied locally on the skin or mucous membranes of the body _____

E. Match the following terms with their descriptions below:

antibiotic	calcium channel blocker	emetic
beta-blocker	cathartic	glucocorticoid
bisphosphonate	diuretic	hypnotic
caffeine		

1. Drug that promotes vomiting _____

2.   Drug that produces sleep or a trance-like state _____

3. Drug that prevents bone loss and osteopenia _____

4.   Drug that relieves constipation _____

5. Drug that is antiarrhythmic, antihypertensive, and antianginal;
    blocks receptors in blood vessels _____

6. Hormone from the adrenal cortex that raises blood sugar and reduces inflammation _____

7. Drug that increases production of urine and thus reduces the volume
    of blood in the body; lowers blood pressure _____

8. Central nervous system stimulant _____

9. Drug produced by a plant or microorganism, which has the ability to inhibit
    or destroy foreign organisms _____

10. Drug that blocks the entrance of calcium into heart muscle and lining of blood vessels;
    antihypertensive, antiarrhythmic, and antianginal drug _____

F. Match the following terms with their meanings below:

antihistamine   progestin   stimulant
antiplatelet   purgative   thyroid hormone
aromatase inhibitor   sedative   tranquilizer
narcotic

1. Reduces estrogen in the blood by blocking an enzyme _____

2. Reduces the ability of thrombocytes to stick together and form a clot _____

3. Drug that excites and promotes activity; caffeine and amphetamines are examples _____

4. Drug that controls anxiety and severe disturbances of behavior _____

5. Drug that relieves constipation; strong cathartic and laxative _____

6. Habit-forming drug that relieves pain by producing stupor or insensibility; morphine and opium are examples _____

7. Secretion from an endocrine gland in the neck; stimulates cellular metabolism _____

8. Female hormone that stimulates the uterine lining during pregnancy _____

9. A mildly hypnotic drug that relaxes without necessarily producing sleep _____

10. Drug that is effective in preventing symptoms of allergy _____

Chapter Twenty-One
REVIEW SHEET QUIZ

Name: _____

A. *Give meanings for the following combining forms:*

1. aer/o _____

2. alges/o _____

3. bronch/o _____

4. chem/o _____

5. cras/o _____

6. cutane/o _____

7. derm/o _____

8. erg/o _____

9. esthesi/o _____

B. *Give meanings for the following combining forms:*

1. hist/o _____

2. hypn/o _____

3. iatr/o _____

4. lingu/o _____

5. myc/o _____

6. narc/o _____

7. or/o _____

8. pharmac/o _____

9. prurit/o _____

10. pyret/o _____

11. thec/o _____

C. *Give meanings for the following combining forms, suffixes, and prefixes:*

1. tox/o _____

2. vas/o _____

3. ven/o _____

4. vit/o _____

5. -dote _____

6. -genic _____

7. -in _____

8. -phylaxis _____

9. ana- _____

10. anti- _____

11. contra- _____

12. syn- _____

13. par- _____

Chapter Twenty-One
CROSSWORD PUZZLE

Name: _____

Fill in the crossword puzzle below using the clues listed underneath it.

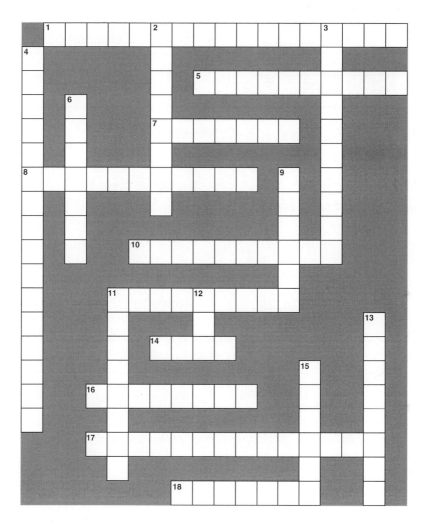

Across Clues

1. Factors in the patient's condition that prevent the use of a particular drug or treatment.
5. Administration of drugs in gaseous or vapor form through the nose or mouth.
7. Instrument for introducing or withdrawing fluids from the body.
8. Hypersensitive reaction of the body to a drug or foreign organism.
10. Drug that reduces or eliminates sensation.
11. Drug that relieves constipation.
14. Erg/o means _____; as in synergism.
16. Mildly hypnotic drug that relaxes without necessarily producing sleep.
17. Type of drug that prevents convulsions.
18. Cras/o means _____; as in blood dyscrasia.

Down Clues

2. Particles of drug suspended in the air.
3. Any adverse condition in a patient resulting from treatment by a physician.
4. Study of the effects of a drug within the body (including absorption, metabolism, and excretion).
6. Substance found in foods and essential in small quantities for growth and good health.
9. Drug that promotes vomiting.
11. Central nervous system stimulant; found in coffee.
12. Aer/o means _____.
13. An agent that produces sleep; from the Greek "hypnos", meaning sleep.
15. Hist/o means _____; as in anti<u>hista</u>mine.

Chapter Twenty-One
PRACTICAL APPLICATIONS

Name: _____

A. The following questions are based on the prescription information given below:

Fluoxetine (Prozac) 20 mg p.o. b.i.d.

Dimenhydrinate (Dramamine) 10 mg 2 tab q 4–6h.

Ondansetron (Zofran) 4 mg 1 tab/caps t.i.d. p.r.n. for nausea.

Ranitidine (Zantac) 300 mg 1 tab p.c. daily.

Pseudoephedrine (Sudafed) 60 mg 1 caps q.i.d. for 15 days.

Acetaminophen (300 mg) & codeine (30 mg) 1 tab q.i.d. p.r.n. for pain.

1. Which drug is given after meals to relieve the pain of ulcers? .... ☐
   A. Fluoxetine
   B. Dimenhydrinate
   C. Acetaminophen
   D. Ranitidine

2. Which drug is an antiemetic and prescribed three times a day as necessary? .... ☐
   A. Ranitidine
   B. Pseudoephedrine
   C. Ondansetron
   D. Dimenhydrinate

3. Which drug is an analgesic and prescribed four times a day as needed? .... ☐
   A. Fluoxetine
   B. Acetaminophen and codeine
   C. Dimenhydrinate
   D. Ranitidine

4. Which drug is used to treat depression and prescribed twice a day orally? .... ☐
   A. Ondansetron
   B. Pseudoephedrine
   C. Fluoxetine
   D. Acetaminophen

5. Which drug is an antihistamine, bronchodilator, and decongestant and prescribed four times a day for an extended period? .... ☐
   A. Pseudoephedrine
   B. Dimenhydrinate
   C. Fluoxetine
   D. Acetaminophen

6. Which drug is an antihistamine and antinauseant, used to prevent motion sickness, and prescribed every few hours (up to six times a day)? .... ☐
   A. Ranitidine
   B. Dimenhydrinate
   C. Pseudoephedrine
   D. Ondansetron

B. FYI

Drugs taken by a mother during pregnancy may have harmful effects on the fetus or newborn. Some examples are analgesics (heroin, morphine) that produce respiratory depression, addiction, and neonatal mortality; anesthetics that produce fetal bradycardia; anticoagulants that lead to hemorrhage and fetal death; hormones (androgens and estrogens) that produce masculinization or clitoromegaly.

1. **What drug can produce slow heartbeat in the fetus?** .... ☐

    A. Testosterone
    B. Morphine
    C. Anesthetic
    D. Anticoagulant

2. **What drug, taken by the mother, puts the fetus at risk for bleeding?** .... ☐

    A. Estrogen
    B. Anticoagulant
    C. Heroin
    D. Anesthetic

C. Drug Identifications

Match the following drugs with a description that fits it below. Write the name of the drug in the space provided.

Bactrim (sulfamethoxazole/trimethoprim)

Benadryl (diphenhydramine)

BuSpar (buspirone)

Fosamax (alendronate sodium)

Lasix (furosemide)

Lovenox (enoxaparin sodium)

Motrin (ibuprofen)

Nolvadex (tamoxifen)

Prevacid (lansoprazole)

Vasotec (enalapril)

1. This is a nonsteroidal antiestrogen medication indicated for the treatment of breast cancer in postmenopausal women. It is used when tumor cells are estrogen-receptor positive. It can be used to prevent breast cancer in women at high risk. _____

2. This is a potent diuretic to treat edema associated with congestive heart failure. _____

3. This is a nonsteroidal anti-inflammatory drug (NSAID) used to relieve the pain and inflammation of arthritis. It is also indicated for use to treat fever, dysmenorrhea, and mild to moderate pain. _____

4. This is a nonprescription antihistamine often used for severe allergic reactions (bee stings or poison ivy) and nasal allergy symptoms. It may also be used as an antipruritic (cream or lotion), sleep aid, or cough suppressant. _____

5. This antibiotic medication is prescribed to treat urinary tract infections, acute otitis media, and respiratory infections. _____

6. This medication is indicated for the treatment and prevention of osteoporosis in postmenopausal women. It increases bone mass to help reduce the incidence of fractures, such as in the wrist and spine. _____

7. This tranquilizer is prescribed for a patient with diagnosed general anxiety disorder. _____

8. This medication is commonly prescribed to treat duodenal and gastric ulcers. _____

9. This angiotensin-converting enzyme (ACE) inhibitor is indicated for the treatment of hypertension and heart failure, and in patients after MI, when the function of the left ventricle of the heart has been affected. _____

10. This is a low molecular weight heparin, indicated for the prevention of deep vein thrombosis, which may lead to pulmonary embolism in patients undergoing surgery (e.g., hip or knee replacement). It is usually administered by injection. _____

Chapter Twenty-One
ANSWERS TO THE QUIZZES

Multiple Choice Quiz

1. D	4. E	7. E	10. D	13. C	16. A	19. D	22. A	25. B
2. B	5. D	8. A	11. A	14. B	17. D	20. B	23. C	
3. B	6. B	9. C	12. D	15. E	18. A	21. D	24. E	

Exercise Quiz

A
1. molecular pharmacology
2. chemotherapy
3. toxicology
4. pharmacodynamics
5. pharmacokinetics

B
6. rectal
7. inhalation
8. sublingual
9. topical
10. oral
11. parenteral

C
12. against itching
13. within the membranes around the spinal cord
14. against infection
15. particles suspended in air
16. under the skin

D
17. drug that relieves constipation
18. drug that prevents nausea and vomiting
19. potent analgesic that relieves pain
20. drug that lowers blood pressure, restores heart rhythm
21. drug that opens bronchial tubes

E
22. A
23. D
24. F
25. C
26. E
27. G
28. B

F
29. vasodilator
30. antihypertensive
31. digoxin
32. vasoconstrictor

33. antianginal
34. cholesterol-lowering drug
35. diuretic

G
36. B
37. D
38. C
39. E
40. I
41. A
42. F
43. J
44. G
45. H

Dictation and Comprehension Quiz

A
1. aerosol
2. amphetamine
3. anticonvulsant
4. antidote
5. antihistamine
6. antinauseant
7. antipyretic
8. bactericidal
9. benzodiazepine
10. beta-blocker
11. bronchodilator
12. cathartic
13. contraindication
14. erythromycin
15. idiosyncrasy
16. intrathecal
17. parenteral
18. synergism
19. syringe
20. toxicity

B
15 An unexpected effect produced in a sensitive individual, but not seen in most patients
4 An agent given to counteract an unwanted effect of a drug
20 Harmful effects of a drug
18 Drug action in which the combination of two drugs causes an effect that is greater than the sum of the individual effects of each drug alone
2 A central nervous system stimulant
12 Drug that relieves constipation
10 Drug that stops the action of epinephrine at sites on receptors of heart muscle cells
7 Drug that lowers body temperature
14 An antibiotic substance
16 Pertaining to delivery of a drug within the membranes lining the spinal cord
13 A factor in the patient's condition that prevents the use of a drug or treatment
9 Drug that acts as a sedative
8 Pertaining to killing microorganisms
3 Drug that prevents abnormal brain activity (as in epilepsy)
11 Drug that opens airways
1 Particles of drug suspended in air
19 Tube for introducing or withdrawing fluids
6 Drug that prevents vomiting and nausea
17 Pertaining to giving a drug by injection into the skin, muscles, or veins
5 Drug that blocks the action of histamine and helps prevent symptoms of allergy

Spelling Quiz

A
1. aerosol—particles of drug suspended in air
2. antacid—drug that neutralizes acid in the stomach
3. antidote—agent given to counteract an unwanted effect of a drug

4. antipyretic—drug given against fever
5. cathartic—drug that relieves constipation
6. hypnotic—agent that produces sleep
7. iatrogenic—an effect that is produced as a result of mistakes in drug use or of individual sensitivity to a drug
8. caffeine—central nervous system stimulant
9. syringe—instrument for introducing or withdrawing fluid
10. tolerance—drug action in which larger and larger doses must be given to achieve the desired effect

B

11. stimulant
12. emetic
13. antianginal
14. anaphylaxis
15. parenteral
16. generic
17. toxicity
18. analgesic
19. topical
20. antiarrhythmic

Pronunciation Quiz

A

1. antiar**rhy**thmic
2. ana**phy**laxis
3. idio**syn**crasy
4. syner**gis**tic
5. pharmacoki**ne**tics
6. anti**his**tamine
7. ca**thar**tic
8. **an**tidote
9. intra**the**cal
10. ge**ne**ric name

B

1. D
2. H
3. B
4. C
5. F
6. J
7. G
8. E
9. I
10. A

C

1. antipyretic
2. anticoagulant
3. parenteral
4. glucocorticoid
5. antihypertensive
6. toxicology
7. intrathecal

Vocabulary Quiz

A

1. brand name
2. anaphylaxis
3. addiction
4. aerosol
5. chemical name
6. contraindication
7. generic name
8. antagonistic action
9. antidote
10. additive effect

B

1. medicinal chemistry
2. iatrogenic
3. oral administration
4. inhalation
5. parenteral administration
6. molecular pharmacology
7. pharmacy
8. pharmacist
9. idiosyncrasy
10. pharmacodynamics

C

1. rectal administration
2. pharmacology
3. receptor
4. syringe
5. synergism
6. Physician's Desk Reference (PDR)
7. pharmacokinetics
8. Food and Drug Administration (FDA)
9. sublingual administration
10. side effect

D

1. analgesic
2. vitamin
3. toxicity
4. tolerance
5. toxicology
6. amphetamine
7. anesthetic

8. ACE inhibitor
9. antacid
10. topical application

E

1. emetic
2. hypnotic
3. bisphosphonate
4. cathartic
5. beta-blocker
6. glucocorticoid
7. diuretic
8. caffeine
9. antibiotic
10. calcium channel blocker

F

1. aromatase inhibitor
2. antiplatelet
3. stimulant
4. tranquilizer
5. purgative
6. narcotic
7. thyroid hormone
8. progestin
9. sedative
10. antihistamine

Review Sheet Quiz

A

1. air
2. sensitivity to pain
3. bronchial tube
4. drug
5. mixture
6. skin
7. skin
8. work
9. feeling, sensation

B

1. tissue
2. sleep
3. physician, treatment
4. tongue
5. mold, fungus
6. stupor
7. mouth
8. drug
9. itching
10. fever
11. sheath (of brain and spinal cord)

C

1. poison
2. vessel
3. vein
4. life
5. what is given
6. pertaining to producing
7. substance
8. protection
9. upward, excessive, again
10. against
11. against, opposite
12. together, with
13. other than, apart from

Practical Applications

A

1. D
2. C
3. B
4. C
5. A
6. B

B

1. C
2. B

C

1. Nolvadex (tamoxifen)
2. Lasix (furosemide)
3. Motrin (ibuprofen)
4. Benadryl (diphenhydramine)
5. Bactrim (sulfamethoxazole/ trimethoprim)
6. Fosamax (alendronate sodium)
7. BuSpar (buspirone)
8. Prevacid (lansoprazole)
9. Vasotec (enalapril)
10. Lovenox (enoxaparin sodium)

Crossword Puzzle

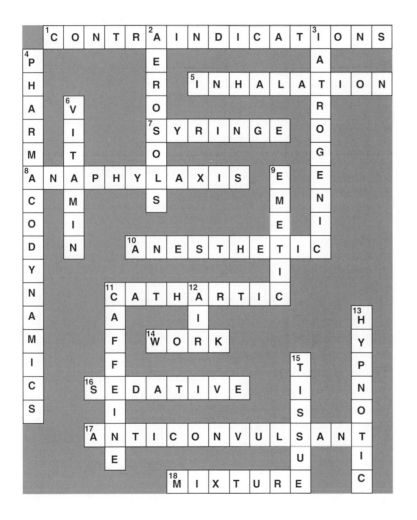

Chapter Twenty-One
Answers to Combining Forms and Terminology Sections

(textbook pages 871–873)

Terminology	Meaning
aerosol	Particles of drug (in solution) suspended in air.
analgesic	Pertaining to without sensitivity to pain.
bronchodilator	Drug that relaxes the smooth muscle lining bronchial tubes and is used to treat asthma, emphysema, and chronic bronchitis.
chemotherapy	Treatment using drugs.
idiosyncrasy	An unexpected effect of a drug that is peculiar to an individual.
subcutaneous	Pertaining to under the skin.
hypodermic	Pertaining to under the skin.
synergism	Condition of working together; the drug action in which the combination of two drugs causes an effect that is greater than the sum of the individual effects of each drug alone.
anesthesia	Condition of being without nervous sensation.
antihistamine	An agent that acts against histamine production in the body. Histamine is released as a result of an allergic reaction.
hypnotic	Pertaining to a condition of sleep (a trance-like state).
iatrogenic	Pertaining to an adverse condition that is caused or produced by a physician or a specific treatment.
sublingual	Pertaining to under the tongue.
erythromycin	An antibiotic that is produced from a red (erythr/o) mold (myc/o).
narcotic	Pertaining to a substance that produces stupor (has a morphine or opium-like action).
oral	Pertaining to the mouth
pharmacology	Study of drugs.
antipruritic	Pertaining to an agent that acts to relieve itching.
antipyretic	Pertaining to an agent that acts to relieve fever.
intrathecal	Pertaining to within the sheath of membranes surrounding the spinal cord.
toxic	Pertaining to poison.
toxicology	Study of poisons and the harmful effects of drugs.
vasodilator	Substance that causes blood vessels to widen.
intravenous	Pertaining to within a vein.
vitamin	A substance in foods that is essential in small quantities for growth and good health (life-giving amines).

Prefixes

anaphylaxis	A hypersensitive state of the body to a foreign protein (antigen) or drug. Can produce severe symptoms and shock.
antidote	An agent given to counteract unwanted effect of a drug.
antibiotic	A substance that acts against microorganisms, such as bacteria.
contraindication	Factor in the patient's condition that prevents the use of a drug or treatment.
parenteral	Pertaining to injection of drugs other than through the intestines.
synergistic	Pertaining to synergism (the drug action in which the sum of the effects of giving two drugs together is greater than that of giving each drug lone).

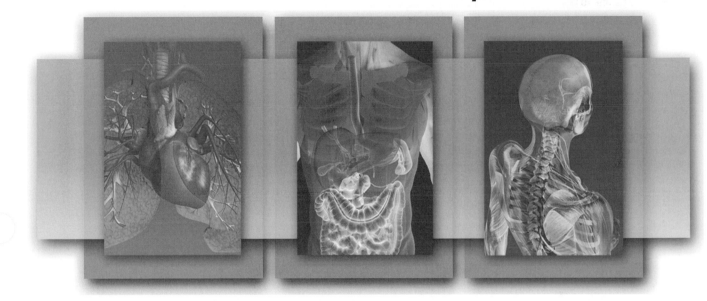

chapter 22

Chapter Twenty-Two

MULTIPLE CHOICE QUIZ

Name: _____

In the box write the letter of the choice that is the definition of the term or best answers the question. There is only one correct answer for each question.

1. **A forensic psychiatrist specializes in:** .... ☐
   A. Educational psychology
   B. Psychoanalysis
   C. Child psychiatry
   D. Experimental psychiatry
   E. Legal aspects of psychiatry

2. **Which of the following best describes one of the roles of a clinical psychologist?** .... ☐
   A. Uses tests to measure mental health and intelligence
   B. Uses drug therapy to treat mental illness
   C. Treats only adults
   D. Uses electroconvulsive therapy to treat mental illness

3. **Which of the following is a mood disorder?** .... ☐
   A. Phobia
   B. Panic attack
   C. Obsessive-compulsive behavior
   D. Psychogenic amnesia
   E. Manic-depressive illness

4. **A term that describes an exaggerated feeling of well-being is:** .... ☐
   A. Autism
   B. Paranoia
   C. Labile
   D. Euphoria
   E. Delusion

5. **An uncontrollable urge to perform an act repeatedly is a(an):** .... ☐
   A. Conversion
   B. Compulsion
   C. Hypochondriasis
   D. Mania
   E. Paranoia

6. **Preoccupation with one's self and lack of responsiveness to others is a characteristic of:** .... ☐
   A. Dissociation
   B. Dysphoria
   C. Delusion
   D. Apathy
   E. Autism

7. **False or unreal sensory perceptions are called:** .... ☐
   A. Obsessions
   B. Dissociations
   C. Hallucinations
   D. Phobias
   E. Panic disorders

8. **What best describes repression?** .... ☐
   A. Defense mechanism in which unacceptable thoughts are pushed into the unconscious
   B. A mild depression
   C. Repetitive acts
   D. An involuntary, persistent idea, emotion, or urge
   E. Delusions of persecution

9. **Fear of leaving one's home is:** .... ☐
   A. Acrophobia
   B. Agoraphobia
   C. Claustrophobia
   D. Necrophobia
   E. Social phobia

10. **Which of the following psychotherapies uses free association and transference?** .... ☐
    A. Hypnosis
    B. Behavior therapy
    C. Psychodrama
    D. Psychoanalysis
    E. Sex therapy

11. **Alternating moods of exalted feelings and excitement with moods of extreme sadness and decreased activity:** ....
    A. Major depression
    B. Cyclothymic disorder
    C. Bipolar disorder
    D. Hypomania
    E. Dysthymic disorder

12. **Short depressive periods and moods with no psychotic features:** ....
    A. Major depression
    B. Cyclothymic disorder
    C. Bipolar disorder
    D. Hypomania
    E. Dysthymic disorder

13. **Numerous periods of mania and depression, but not of long duration; no psychotic features:** ....
    A. Major depression
    B. Cyclothymic disorder
    C. Bipolar disorder
    D. Hypomania
    E. Dysthymic disorder

14. **Resembling mania, but not as severe:** ....
    A. Major depression
    B. Cyclothymic disorder
    C. Bipolar disorder
    D. Hypomania
    E. Dysthymic disorder

15. **Severe dysphoric mood with psychotic features:** ....
    A. Major depression
    B. Cyclothymic disorder
    C. Bipolar disorder
    D. Hypomania
    E. Dysthymic disorder

16. **Grandiose sense of self-importance and preoccupation with fantasies of success and power:** ....
    A. Antisocial
    B. Paranoid
    C. Histrionic
    D. Narcissistic
    E. Schizoid

17. **Continually suspicious and mistrustful of other people:** ....
    A. Antisocial
    B. Paranoid
    C. Histrionic
    D. Narcissistic
    E. Schizoid

18. **No loyalty or concern for others; without moral standards:** ....
    A. Antisocial
    B. Paranoid
    C. Histrionic
    D. Narcissistic
    E. Schizoid

19. **Emotionally cold and aloof; indifferent to praise or criticism and to the feelings of others:** ....
    A. Antisocial
    B. Paranoid
    C. Histrionic
    D. Narcissistic
    E. Schizoid

20. **Emotional, immature, and dependent; irrational outbursts and flamboyant behavior:** ....
    A. Antisocial
    B. Paranoid
    C. Histrionic
    D. Narcissistic
    E. Schizoid

21. **Mental symptoms such as amnesia hide the pain and anxiety of unconscious conflicts:** ....
    A. Hypochondriasis
    B. Conversion disorder
    C. Anorexia nervosa
    D. Bulimia nervosa
    E. Dissociative disorder

22. **Physical symptoms appear as a defense against overwhelming anxiety:** ....
    A. Hypochondriasis
    B. Conversion disorder
    C. Anorexia nervosa
    D. Bulimia nervosa
    E. Dissociative disorder

23. **General preoccupation with bodily aches and pains and irrational fear about one's health:** ....
    A. Hypochondriasis
    B. Conversion disorder
    C. Anorexia nervosa
    D. Bulimia nervosa
    E. Dissociative disorder

24. **Psychological factors such as anxiety, anger, and fear produce unrealistic body image and reluctance to eat:**.........
    A. Hypochondriasis
    B. Conversion disorder
    C. Anorexia nervosa
    D. Bulimia nervosa
    E. Dissociative disorder

25. **Fear of obesity in which binge eating is followed by induced vomiting:** ....
    A. Hypochondriasis
    B. Conversion disorder
    C. Anorexia nervosa
    D. Bulimia nervosa
    E. Dissociative disorder

Chapter Twenty-Two
EXERCISE QUIZ

Name: _____

The questions on this quiz have all been taken from the exercises at the end of this chapter.

A. *Match the following psychiatric symptoms with their meanings below:*

anxiety	autism	delusion	mania
amnesia	compulsion	dissociation	mutism
apathy	conversion	hallucination	obsession

  1. Loss of memory _____

  2. State of excessive excitability; agitation _____

  3. A non-reactive state; stupor _____

  4. Persistent idea, emotion, or urge _____

  5. Uncontrollable urge to perform an act repeatedly _____

  6. Feelings of apprehension, uneasiness, dread _____

  7. Uncomfortable feelings are separated from their real object and redirected _____

  8. Anxiety becomes a bodily symptom that has no organic basis _____

  9. Lack of responsiveness to others; preoccupied with self _____

 10. Absence of emotions _____

 11. False or unreal sensory perception _____

 12. Fixed, false belief that cannot be changed by logical reasoning or evidence _____

B. *Give meanings for the following terms:*

 13. dysphoria _____

 14. euphoria _____

 15. agoraphobia _____

 16. labile _____

 17. affect _____

 18. paranoia _____

 19. bipolar disorder _____

 20. dementia _____

C. *Select from the following terms to complete the sentences below:*

anxiety disorders   eating disorder   somatoform disorders
delirium   mood disorders   substance-related disorders
dementia   personality disorder
dissociative disorders   sexual disorders

21. Disorders involving paraphilias are _____

22. Mental symptoms (loss of memory and identity) that hide unconscious conflicts are _____

23. Troubled feelings, unpleasant tensions, distress, and avoidance behavior are hallmarks of _____

24. Illnesses related to regular use of drugs and alcohol are _____

25. Bulimia nervosa is an example of a (an) _____

26. Illnesses marked by prolonged emotions (mania or depression) are _____

27. Mental disorders in which physical symptoms cannot be explained by a known physical problem are _____

28. A lifelong personality pattern that is inflexible and causes impairment of social functioning is a _____

29. Loss of intellectual abilities with impairment of memory, judgment, and reasoning are known as a (an) _____

30. Confusion in thinking with faulty perceptions and irrational behavior is a (an) _____

D. *Identify the personality disorder from its description below:*

31. Fantasies of success and power and grandiose sense of self importance _____

32. Flamboyant, theatrical, emotionally immature _____

33. No loyalty or concern for others; does not tolerate frustration and blames others when he or she is at fault _____

34. Pervasive, unwarranted suspiciousness and mistrust of people _____

35. Emotionally cold, aloof, indifferent to praise or criticism or feelings of others _____

E. *Identify the psychotherapeutic technique from its description below:*

36. A trance is used to help the patient recover deeply repressed feelings _____

37. Patients express feelings by acting out roles with other patients _____

38. Long-term and intense exploration of unconscious feelings, using techniques such as transference and free association _____

39. Toys are used to help children express conflict and feelings _____

40. Conditioning is used to relieve anxiety and improve symptoms of illness _____

41. Neuroleptic substances are used to relieve symptoms
    of psychiatric disorders _____

42. Electric current is applied to the brain to produce convulsions and reverse
    major depression _____

43. Techniques are used to help patients overcome sexual dysfunction _____

F. *Select from the following terms to complete the sentences below:*

agoraphobia	kleptomania	pyromania
amphetamines	MAO inhibitors	tricyclic antidepressants
cyclothymia	minor tranquilizers and sedatives	xenophobia
dysthymia	phenothiazines	

44. Fear of strangers is _____

45. Obsessive preoccupation with stealing is _____

46. Antidepressant agents that work by blocking the action of
    a specific enzyme are _____

47. A mood disorder marked by depressive periods that are milder than
    major depression is _____

48. Fear of being left alone in unfamiliar surroundings is _____

49. Anxiolytic agents used to reduce tension are _____

50. Antipsychotic tranquilizers such as Thorazine are _____

Chapter Twenty-Two
DICTATION AND COMPREHENSION QUIZ

Name: _____

A. Dictation of Terms

1. _____   11. _____

2. _____   12. _____

3. _____   13. _____

4. _____   14. _____

5. _____   15. _____

6. _____   16. _____

7. _____   17. _____

8. _____   18. _____

9. _____   19. _____

10. _____   20. _____

B. Comprehension of Terms: Match the number of the above term with its meaning below.

_____ Confusion in thinking; faulty perceptions and irrational behavior

_____ Drug used as a mild tranquilizer

_____ Unstable, undergoing rapid emotional change

_____ Loss of memory

_____ Tranquilizers used to treat psychoses

_____ Withdrawal from reality into an inner world of disorganized thinking and conflict; a psychosis

_____ Internalized conscience and moral part of the personality

_____ Fear of strangers

_____ Treatment that allows the patient to explore inner emotions and conflicts; transference, free association, and dream analysis are elements of the therapy

_____ Drugs that produce a state of CNS excitement, hyperactivity, and mood change

_____ The use of nonliving objects as substitutes for a human sexual love object

_____ Sexual gratification is gained by being humiliated, beaten, or made to suffer by another person

_____ The outward expression of emotion, or emotional response

_____ An anxiety disorder in which recurrent thoughts and repetitive acts dominate behavior

_____ Loss of intellectual abilities with impairment of memory, identity, and reasoning

_____ Fear of closed places

_____ Study of drugs and their effect on the mind and mental illness

_____ Sadness, hopelessness, worry, discouragement (literally, "bad feeling")

_____ Preoccupation with bodily aches, pains, and discomforts in the absence of real illness

_____ Eating disorder marked by refusal to maintain minimally normal body weight

Chapter Twenty-Two
SPELLING QUIZ
Name: _____

A. *Circle the term that is spelled correctly and write its meaning in the space provided:*

1. masochism   maschoschism _____

2. dilerium   delirium _____

3. bulemia nervosa   bulimia nervosa _____

4. physchoanalysis   psychoanalysis _____

5. schizophrenia   shizophrenia _____

6. paranoid   paraniod _____

7. dimentia   dementia _____

8. eufouria   euphoria _____

9. narsicissm   narcissism _____

10. bipoler disorder   bipolar disorder _____

B. *Circle the term that is spelled correctly. The meaning of each term is given.*

11. troubled feelings, distress, and
    avoidance behavior .... anxeity   anxiety   angsiety

12. stimulant drug that causes
    euphoria and hallucinations .... cocaine   cokaine   cociane

13. external emotion or emotional
    response of a person .... effect   effact   affect

14. severe lack of response to
    other people .... autism   aughtism   autoism

15. amnesia with fleeing from
    customary surroundings .... feuge   fugue   fugeue

16. depressive episodes but not of
    intensity of major depression .... dysthimia   disthymia   dysthymia

17. dried leaves and flowers of the hemp
    plant; causes euphoria .... maryjuana   marijana   marijuana

18. sexual arousal that requires
    unusual and bizarre fantasies .... paraphilia   paraphillia   parephilia

19. absence of emotion .... apethy   apathy   apathe

20. fear of strangers .... xerophobia   xerophobea   xenophobia

Chapter Twenty-Two
PRONUNCIATION QUIZ

Name: _____

A. *Underline the accented syllable in the following terms:*

1. narcissism   4. dementia   7. voyeurism   10. euphoria
2. opioid   5. catatonic stupor   8. psychoanalysis
3. agoraphobia   6. dysthymia   9. autism

B. *Match the term in Column I with its meaning in Column II:*

Column I

1. affect   _____
2. dementia   _____
3. delirium   _____
4. delusion   _____
5. labile   _____
6. sadism   _____
7. mutism   _____
8. mania   _____
9. amnesia   _____
10. conversion   _____

Column II

A. Loss of memory.

B. A false belief or idea that cannot be changed by logical reasoning.

C. Pervasive lack of responsiveness to other people; stupor.

D. Unstable; undergoing rapid emotional change.

E. The emotional reaction of a patient.

F. Pleasure received from inflicting pain on others.

G. Loss of higher mental functioning.

H. A defense mechanism in which anxiety is converted into a bodily symptom.

I. State of excessive excitability and agitation.

J. Confusion in thinking; faulty perceptions and irrational behavior.

C. *Complete the following medical terms from their definitions:*

1. _____ nervosa   Eating disorder marked by excessive dieting.

2. pheno _____   Antipsychotic tranquilizers.

3. cyclo _____   Pertaining to exhibiting cycles of depression and exhilaration.

4. _____ phrenia   A psychosis involving delusions, hallucinations, bizarre and illogical thinking.

5. psycho _____   Pertaining to the interrelationship of mind and body.

6. _____ phobia   Fear of strangers.

7. hypo _____   Exaggerated concern with one's health.

8. _____ phobia   Fear of heights.

Chapter Twenty-Two
VOCABULARY QUIZ

Name: _____

A. *Match the following terms with their descriptions below:*

affect	autistic thought	cannabis
amnesia	bipolar disorder	compulsion
anxiety disorders	bulimia nervosa	conversion disorder
apathy		

1. A disorder marked by physical symptoms, with no organic basis, appearing as a result of anxiety and unconscious inner conflict _____

2. Eating disorder of binge eating followed by vomiting, purging, and depression _____

3. Absence of emotions; lack of interest or emotional involvement_____

4. External expression of emotion or emotional response _____

5. Mood disorder with alternating periods of mania and depression _____

6. Thinking is internally stimulated and ideas have a private meaning; fantasy is thought of as reality _____

7. Loss of memory _____

8. Active substance in marijuana _____

9. Characterized by unpleasant tension, distress, and avoidance behavior; phobias, obsessive-compulsive disorder, and post-traumatic stress disorder _____

10. Uncontrollable urge to perform an act repeatedly _____

B. *Match the following terms with their descriptions below:*

anorexia nervosa	dementia	ego
defense mechanism	depression	fugue
delusion	dissociative disorder	gender identity disorder
delirium		

1. Major mood disorder with chronic sadness, loss of energy, hopelessness, worry, discouragement _____

2. Unconscious technique (coping mechanism) that a person uses to resolve or conceal conflict and anxiety _____

3. Chronic or sudden disturbance of memory, identity or consciousness; multiple-personality disorder is an example _____

4. Central coordinating branch of the personality or mind _____

5. False sensory perception (hearing "voices" and seeing "things") _____

6. Loss of intellectual abilities with impairment of memory,
   judgment, and reasoning _____

7. Strong and persistent cross-gender identification with the opposite sex _____

8. Flight from customary surroundings _____

9. Eating disorder of excessive dieting and refusal to maintain a
   normal body weight _____

10. Confusion in thinking; faulty perceptions and irrational behavior _____

C. *Match the following terms with their descriptions below:*

hallucination	mood disorders	obsessive-compulsive disorder
id	mutism	paranoia
labile	neurosis	paraphilia
mania		

1. Overly suspicious system of thinking with fixed delusions that one is being
   harassed, persecuted, or unfairly treated _____

2. Unstable, undergoing rapid emotional change _____

3. Non-reactive state; stupor _____

4. Major unconscious part of the personality; instinctual drives and desires _____

5. Repressed conflicts leading to mental symptoms such as anxiety and fears;
   less severe than a psychosis _____

6. Extreme excitement; hyperactive elation and agitation _____

7. False sensory perception _____

8. Anxiety disorder in which recurrent thoughts and repetitive acts
   dominate behavior _____

9. Recurrent intense sexual urge, fantasy, or behavior that involves unusual
   objects, activities, or situations _____

10. Prolonged emotion dominates a person's life; bipolar and depressive disorders _____

D. *Match the following terms with their meanings below:*

personality disorders	projective test	psychosis
pervasive developmental disorders	psychiatrist	reality testing
phobia	psychologist	repression
post-traumatic stress disorder		

1. Defense mechanism by which unacceptable thoughts, feelings, and impulses
   are automatically pushed into the unconscious _____

2. Diagnostic, personality test using unstructured stimuli to evoke responses
   that reflect aspects of an individual's personality _____

3. Medical doctor trained in diagnosis, prevention and treatment of mental disorders _____

4. Irrational or disabling fear of an object or situation _____

5. Childhood disorders characterized by delays in socialization and communication skills (autism and Asperger syndrome) _____

6. Anxiety related symptoms appear following exposure to personal experience of a distressing event _____

7. A Ph.D or Ed.D specializing in mental processes and how the brain functions in health and disease _____

8. Disorder marked by loss of contact with reality; often with delusions and hallucinations _____

9. Ability to perceive fact from fantasy _____

10. Life-long personality patterns marked by inflexibility and impairment of social functioning _____

E. Match the following terms with their descriptions below:

amphetamines   family therapy   somatoform disorders
benzodiazepines   free association   substance-related disorders
cognitive behavioral therapy   schizophrenia   superego
electroconvulsive therapy

1. Physical symptoms occur and cannot be explained by actual physical disorders or mental illness _____

2. Drugs that lessen anxiety, tension, agitation, and panic attacks _____

3. Psychoanalytic technique in which the patient verbalizes, without censorship, the passing contents of his or her mind _____

4. Central nervous system stimulants that are used to treat depression and attention-deficit hyperactivity disorder (ADHD) _____

5. Treatment of an entire family to resolve and understand conflicts _____

6. Psychosis marked by withdrawal from reality into an inner world of disorganized thinking and conflict _____

7. Internalized conscience and moral part of the personality _____

8. Regular overuse of psychoactive materials (alcohol, cannabis, cocaine) that affect the CNS _____

9. Electric current used to produce convulsions in the treatment of depression _____

10. Conditioning is used to relieve anxiety and improve symptoms of mental illness _____

F. Match the following terms with their descriptions below:

group therapy
hypnosis
phenothiazines
psychoanalysis

psychodrama
psychopharmacology
sedatives

supportive psychotherapy
transference
tricyclic antidepressants

1. Antipsychotic drugs (neuroleptics) used to treat severe psychoses, such as schizophrenia _____

2. Treatment of psychiatric disorders with drugs _____

3. Drugs that lessen anxiety _____

4. Trance state is used to increase the pace of psychotherapy _____

5. Treatment that allows the patient to explore inner emotions and conflicts so as to understand and change current behavior _____

6. Offering encouragement and hope to patients facing difficult life transitions and events _____

7. Psychoanalytic process in which the patient relates to the therapist as though the therapist was a prominent childhood figure _____

8. Therapy that allows a patient to express feelings by acting out roles with other patients _____

9. Drugs used to treat severe depression; three-ringed fused structure _____

10. Patients with similar problems gain insight into their personalities through discussion and interaction with each other _____

Chapter Twenty-Two
REVIEW SHEET QUIZ

Name: _____

A. *Give meanings for the following combining forms:*

1. anxi/o _____   6. neur/o _____

2. hypn/o _____   7. phren/o _____

3. iatr/o _____   8. psych/o _____

4. klept/o _____   9. pyr/o _____

5. ment/o _____   10. schiz/o _____

B. *Give meanings for the following combining forms and suffixes:*

1. somat/o _____   6. -leptic _____

2. xen/o _____   7. -mania _____

3. aut/o _____   8. -phobia _____

4. phil/o _____   9. -thymia _____

5. -genic _____   10. -phoria _____

Chapter Twenty-Two
ANSWERS TO THE QUIZZES

Multiple Choice Quiz

1. E	4. D	7. C	10. D	13. B	16. D	19. E	22. B	25. D
2. A	5. B	8. A	11. C	14. D	17. B	20. C	23. A	
3. E	6. E	9. B	12. E	15. A	18. A	21. E	24. C	

Exercise Quiz

A

1. amnesia
2. mania
3. mutism
4. obsession
5. compulsion
6. anxiety
7. dissociation
8. conversion
9. autism
10. apathy
11. hallucination
12. delusion

B

13. sadness, hopelessness
14. exaggerated good feeling
15. fear of being alone in open, crowded places
16. unstable, undergoing rapid emotional change
17. external emotion or emotional response of a person
18. delusions of persecution or grandeur
19. intermixed periods of mania and depression
20. loss of higher mental functioning

C

21. sexual disorders
22. dissociative disorders
23. anxiety disorders
24. substance-related disorders
25. eating disorder
26. mood disorders
27. somatoform disorders
28. personality disorder
29. dementia
30. delirium

D

31. narcissistic
32. histrionic
33. antisocial
34. paranoid
35. schizoid

E

36. hypnosis
37. psychodrama
38. psychoanalysis
39. play therapy
40. behavior therapy
41. drug therapy
42. electroconvulsive therapy
43. sex therapy

F

44. xenophobia
45. kleptomania
46. MAO inhibitors
47. dysthymia
48. agoraphobia
49. minor tranquilizers and sedatives
50. phenothiazines

Dictation and Comprehension Quiz

A

1. affect
2. amnesia
3. anorexia nervosa
4. anxiolytic
5. claustrophobia
6. delirium
7. dementia
8. dysphoria
9. fetishism
10. hallucinogens
11. hypochondriasis
12. labile
13. obsessive-compulsive disorder
14. phenothiazines
15. psychoanalysis
16. psychopharmacology
17. schizophrenia
18. sexual masochism
19. superego
20. xenophobia

B

6 Confusion in thinking; faulty perceptions and irrational behavior
4 Drug used as a mild tranquilizer
12 Unstable, undergoing rapid emotional change
2 Loss of memory
14 Tranquilizers used to treat psychoses
17 Withdrawal from reality into an inner world of disorganized thinking and conflict; a psychosis
19 Internalized conscience and moral part of the personality
20 Fear of strangers
15 Treatment that allows the patient to explore inner emotions and conflicts; transference, free association and dream analysis are elements of the therapy
10 Drugs that produce a state of CNS excitement, hyperactivity, and mood change
9 The use of nonliving objects as substitutes for a human sexual love object
18 Sexual gratification is gained by being humiliated, beaten, or made to suffer by another person
1 The outward expression of emotion, or emotional response
13 An anxiety disorder in which recurrent thoughts and repetitive acts dominate behavior
7 Loss of intellectual abilities with impairment of memory, identity, and reasoning
5 Fear of closed places
16 Study of drugs and their effect on the mind and mental illness

8 Sadness, hopelessness, worry, discouragement (literally, "bad feeling")

11 Preoccupation with bodily aches, pains, and discomforts in the absence of real illness

3 Eating disorder marked by refusal to maintain minimally normal body weight

Spelling Quiz

A

1. masochism—gratification gained by being humiliated
2. delirium—confusion in thinking; faulty perceptions and irrational behavior
3. bulimia nervosa—binge eating followed by vomiting and depression
4. psychoanalysis—treatment that allows the patient to explore unconscious emotions and conflicts
5. schizophrenia—psychosis involving withdrawal from reality into an inner world of disorganized thinking and conflict
6. paranoid—delusions of persecution or grandeur
7. dementia—loss of higher mental functioning
8. euphoria—exaggerated good feeling; "high"
9. narcissism—pervasive interest in one's self
10. bipolar disorder—alternating periods of mania and depression

B

11. anxiety
12. cocaine
13. affect
14. autism
15. fugue
16. dysthymia
17. marijuana
18. paraphilia
19. apathy
20. xenophobia

Pronunciation Quiz

A

1. narcissism
2. opioid
3. agoraphobia
4. dementia

5. catatonic stupor
6. dysthymia
7. voyeurism
8. psychoanalysis
9. autism
10. euphoria

B

1. E
2. G
3. J
4. B
5. D
6. F
7. C
8. I
9. A
10. H

C

1. anorexia
2. phenothiazines
3. cyclothymia
4. schizophrenia
5. psychosomatic
6. xenophobia
7. hypochondriasis
8. acrophobia

Vocabulary Quiz

A

1. conversion disorder
2. bulimia nervosa
3. apathy
4. affect
5. bipolar disorder
6. autistic thought
7. amnesia
8. cannabis
9. anxiety disorders
10. compulsion

B

1. depression
2. defense mechanism
3. dissociative disorder
4. ego
5. delusion
6. dementia
7. gender identity disorder
8. fugue
9. anorexia nervosa
10. delirium

C

1. paranoia
2. labile
3. mutism
4. id

5. neurosis
6. mania
7. hallucination
8. obsessive-compulsive disorder
9. paraphilia
10. mood disorders

D

1. repression
2. projective test
3. psychiatrist
4. phobia
5. pervasive developmental disorders
6. post-traumatic stress disorder
7. psychologist
8. psychosis
9. reality testing
10. personality disorders

E

1. somatoform disorders
2. benzodiazepines
3. free association
4. amphetamines
5. family therapy
6. schizophrenia
7. superego
8. substance-related disorders
9. electroconvulsive therapy
10. cognitive behavioral therapy

F

1. phenothiazines
2. psychopharmacology
3. sedatives
4. hypnosis
5. psychoanalysis
6. supportive psychotherapy
7. transference
8. psychodrama
9. tricyclic antidepressants
10. group therapy

Review Sheet Quiz

A

1. uneasy, anxious, distressed
2. sleep
3. treatment
4. to steal
5. mind
6. nerve
7. mind
8. mind
9. fire
10. split

_B_

1. body
2. stranger
3. self
4. attraction to, love
5. produced by
6. to seize hold of
7. obsessive preoccupation
8. fear
9. mind
10. feeling, bearing

Practical Applications

_A_

1. C
2. A
3. D
4. C

_B_

1. D
2. C

Crossword Puzzle

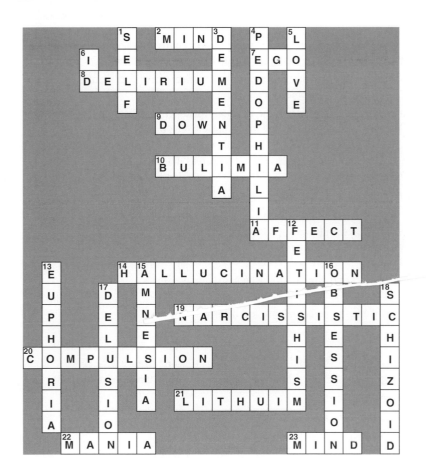

Chapter Twenty-Two
Answers to Combining Forms and Terminology Sections

(textbook pages 911–914)

Terminology	Meaning
anxiolytic	A drug that is used for relief of anxiety; a mild tranquilizer.
autism	Disorder marked by difficulties in verbal and nonverbal communication and in social and play interactions.
hallucinogen	A substance that causes hallucinations (false sensory perceptions).
hypnosis	Condition or state of altered consciousness in which there is increased responsiveness to commands and suggestions.
psychiatrist	One who specializes in the treatment of the mind.
mental	Pertaining to the mind.
neurosis	An emotional disorder that can interfere with a person's ability to lead a normal life, but is milder than a psychosis. Examples are anxiety states and phobias.
paraphilia	A psychosexual disorder in which sexual arousal is dependent on bizarre fantasies or acts involving use of a nonhuman object or suffering and humiliation of a human.
schizophrenia	A psychosis involving withdrawal from the external world with a disturbed sense of self; includes delusions, hallucinations, and inappropriate affect. Literally means "split mind."
psychosis	Significant impairment of reality with symptoms such as delusions, hallucinations, and bizarre behavior.
psychopharmacology	Study of the effect of drugs on the mind.
psychotherapy	Treatment of the mind.
schizoid	Traits of shyness, social withdrawal, and introversion that characterize the schizoid personality. Also, can refer to schizophrenia-like traits that indicate a predisposition to schizophrenia.
psychosomatic	Pertaining to the effect of the mind on the body in causing illness.
somatoform disorders	Mental disorders that are characterized by symptoms that suggest a physical disorder but can't be explained by an actual physical disorder.

Suffixes

psychogenic	Pertaining to produced by the mind.
neuroleptic drugs	Drugs that modify psychotic behavior and symptoms (phenothiazines are examples).
kleptomania	Madness or compulsion to steal.
pyromania	Madness for setting fires or seeing them.
agoraphobia	Fear of being alone in open or public places.
xenophobia	Fear of strangers.
euphoria	Exaggerated feeling of well-being; "high."
dysphoria	Depressed mood; sadness and hopelessness.
cyclothymia	Mania alternating with depression; mild form of bipolar (manic-depressive) disorder.
dysthymia	Depressed mood that is not as severe as major depression.

Prefixes

apathy	Lack of feeling; indifference, without emotion.
catatonia	A state of diminished responsiveness to stimuli associated with schizophrenia.
hypomania	A mood disorder that resembles mania, but is of lesser intensity.
hypochondriasis	Condition marked by exaggerated concern for one's physical health and exaggeration of minor complaints and normal sensations.
paranoia	Delusions of grandeur or persecution. Literal meaning is "abnormal mind."

MORE PRACTICAL APPLICATIONS

On the next pages you will find additional examples of medical terminology in context. Here are paragraphs about disease conditions, case reports, research reports, and a wide variety of examples of medical writing. Medical terms are underlined to draw attention to terminology that students may define. I use paragraphs like this for dictation or discussion in class. Sometimes I include a paragraph on a quiz as a bonus question, asking the students to explain the meaning of the sentences in their own words. Many of the paragraphs on diseases were written by me in response to questions that came up in class that were not covered in *The Language of Medicine* or that needed further explanation.

As I have indicated previously, the possessive of eponyms has been omitted for clarity and consistency. If you are uncomfortable with this change, you may continue to be guided by *Dorland's Medical Dictionary, Mosby's Dental Dictionary,* or other references.

I have noted the chapter in *The Language of Medicine* with which you may choose to use each of the following.

1. Chapter 4

    Reye syndrome. This is an acute disease of childhood, characterized by severe edema of the brain, and increased intracranial pressure, hypoglycemia, and fatty infiltration and dysfunction of the liver.

    The etiology of Reye syndrome is unknown, but it is almost always associated with a previous viral infection. In the U.S., the most frequently reported viral diseases present prior to development of Reye syndrome are influenza type B and varicella (chickenpox). There is an association between the administration of aspirin for these illnesses and the subsequent occurrence of Reye syndrome, so children should not be given aspirin for such infections.

    Symptoms of Reye syndrome are persistent emesis, fatigue, increased agitation and delirium, convulsions, and coma. Treatment is aimed at correcting hypoglycemia and reducing intracranial pressure.

2. Chapter 5

    Mr. Smith's hemoglobin was normal and his leukocyte count was 16,000 cu/mm, showing slight neutrophilia. Physical examination of the abdomen revealed a mass, and a histological examination disclosed it to be a pancreatic adenocarcinoma. His condition progressively worsened and he died after 23 hospital days. Autopsy revealed carcinoma of the pancreas with metastatic hepatic and peritoneal lesions as well as peritonitis.

3. Chapter 5 or 6

    Colic is acute, paroxysmal abdominal pain. It is marked by spasmodic contractions of the intestine, most commonly during the first three months of life. The infant may pull up his or her arms and legs, cry loudly, turn red-faced, and expel gas from the anus or belch it up from the stomach. Etiology is not known, but several factors may contribute to its occurrence.

These include excessive <u>aerophagia</u>, too rapid feeding or overfeeding, overexcitement, and occasionally allergy to milk.

4. Chapter 5

<u>Colonoscopy</u>. The patient had a <u>colonoscopic polypectomy</u> in 1988 and now presents for follow-up interval examination. She has some rectal bleeding that has been attributed to <u>hemorrhoids</u>.

The scope was introduced without difficulty and advanced through the rectosigmoid. Bowel preparation was adequate, and there was good visualization throughout. Scattered <u>diverticula</u> were seen, particularly in the sigmoid area and around the <u>hepatic flexure</u>. The instrument was advanced through the <u>descending</u>, <u>transverse</u>, and <u>ascending colon</u> to the <u>cecum</u>. There was no evidence for any recurrent mass lesion. On withdrawal of the instrument, small internal hemorrhoids were seen.

5. Chapter 5 or Chapter 16

<u>Thrush</u> is an infection of the <u>oral mucous membrane</u> by a <u>fungus</u> (<u>Candida albicans</u>). It is characterized by white patches on a red, moist inflamed surface, occurring anywhere in the mouth, including <u>lingual</u> and <u>buccal</u> surfaces. The patches are occasionally accompanied by pain and fever. Thrush is treated with <u>antibiotics</u> and <u>fungicidal</u> drugs. The best preventive measures are good general health, a well-balanced diet, and good oral hygiene.

6. Chapter 6

Ms. Jones had been taking birth control pills for several years. Lower abdominal pain and non-bloody <u>diarrhea</u> made her seek a doctor's advice after experiencing <u>postprandial</u> nausea and <u>emesis</u>, <u>epigastric</u> pain, and weight loss. <u>Cholecystography</u> and <u>barium swallow</u> were reported as normal. Laparotomy revealed massive gangrene of the <u>sigmoid colon</u> and almost the entire <u>ileum</u> and <u>jejunum</u>. She underwent extensive excision and <u>anastomosis</u>, but she never fully recovered. She finally succumbed to <u>septicemia</u>. On autopsy, it was revealed that her <u>celiac</u> and <u>mesenteric</u> arteries were <u>thrombosed</u>. She had premature atherosclerosis in the common iliac arteries as well.

7. Chapter 6

The patient, a 53-year-old male, had been well until 3 weeks before hospital admission. At that time, he noted <u>anorexia</u>, <u>malaise</u>, and <u>epigastric</u> discomfort. On the day of admission he had <u>hematemesis</u> but had observed no sign of melena or change in bowel habits. He had previously undergone <u>cholecystectomy</u> for <u>calculi</u> and partial <u>colectomy</u> for <u>diverticulitis</u>.

8. Chapter 6

Barrett esophagus is a <u>premalignant</u> condition that should be suspected in any patient presenting with signs and symptoms of <u>chronic reflux esophagitis</u>. The condition itself is <u>asymptomatic</u> but can be diagnosed by <u>barium swallow</u>, which reveals esophageal <u>strictures</u> or <u>ulcerations</u> with a <u>hiatal hernia</u>.

9. Chapter 6

<u>Fatigue</u> is often an important symptom of underlying <u>hepatic</u> disease. Intense <u>pruritus</u> and other <u>dermatologic</u> changes in the presence of elevated <u>bilirubin</u> and <u>alkaline phosphatase</u> suggest <u>cholestasis</u>. Transaminase elevations generally signify hepatocellular inflammation or necrosis. <u>Hepatomegaly</u> and elevated alkaline phosphatase may be the only signs of <u>infiltrative</u> disease and mass lesions. Bilirubin exceeding 10 mg/dl is more often associated with <u>carcinoma</u> than with <u>cholecystitis</u> or stones.

10. Chapter 6

Bilirubin is classified as indirect ("free" or unconjugated) when it is en route to the liver from the spleen, where erythrocytes are destroyed. Bilirubin is classified as direct (bilirubin diglucuronide) after its conjugation (combination) in the liver with glucuronic acid. Elevation of indirect bilirubin means prehepatic jaundice such as in hemolytic jaundice or inability to conjugate bilirubin.

Elevation of direct bilirubin indicates other types of hepatic jaundice such as in viral or alcoholic hepatitis or posthepatic jaundice as in biliary obstruction.

Total bilirubin is the sum of direct and indirect bilirubin in blood.

11. Chapter 7

Persons suffering from nephrotic syndrome have been known to occasionally develop as much as 40 liters of excess fluid, and 15 liters of this is ascites. In addition, joints swell and pleural and pericardial cavities can become partially filled with fluid. Intravenous infusion of large quantities of plasma proteins can be of only temporary benefit since enough protein can be lost in the urine in a day to return the person to his or her original predicament.

12. Chapter 7

Peritoneal dialysis versus hemodialysis. Peritoneal dialysis is more quickly initiated since no dialysis machine is needed; anticoagulants are not necessary and there is no need for vascular cannulation (a cannula is a tube or sheath). Also, there is less stress on internal organs since chemicals and fluid exchanges occur more slowly. Hemodialysis is used in cases of severe abdominal trauma, multiple abdominal surgical procedures and adhesions, diffuse peritonitis, and paralytic ileus. It is also used in patients with severe coagulation defects and is more effective in removing toxins from the blood.

13. Chapter 7

A 65-year-old man with a two-month history of weakness, gross hematuria, and intermittent hemoptysis was admitted to the hospital. Past history included alcohol abuse, asbestos exposure, and heavy smoking (two packs a day for 42 years). A cystoscopy with retrograde pyelography showed a filling defect in the base of the bladder. Transurethral biopsy of the bladder revealed a transitional-cell carcinoma, grade IV. Chest x-ray showed a right lower lobe lesion, and CT scan confirmed the presence of the abnormality. Biopsy of the lung mass revealed a metastatic bladder carcinoma.

14. Chapter 8

Much of the focus of neonatology now is on improving survival of premature infants, and nutrition is important for optimum outcome. Total parenteral nutrition (TPN) is used extensively to provide caloric and protein needs to these infants, especially those who have intestinal disease and chronic respiratory distress syndrome. Intrahepatic cholestasis occurring during TPN has surfaced as a major clinical problem and is second only to catheter complications as a reason for discontinuing therapy.

15. Chapter 8

A 28-year-old premenopausal woman, G0 P0, presented with an upper outer quadrant breast mass of three months' duration. Modified radical mastectomy was performed; none of the 33 nodes was positive for metastasis. Tumor size 3.7 cm; pathology report indicated infiltrating ductal carcinoma, grade IV. The tumor is estrogen receptor positive. Bone scan and chest x-ray are negative and liver enzymes are normal.

16. Chapter 8

    <u>Ovarian cancer</u>. The ovary is the second most common site of cancer in the female reproductive organs (<u>endometrial carcinoma</u> is the first). Unlike endometrial cancer there is no obvious warning sign (bleeding) and unlike <u>cervical</u> cancer there is no routine diagnostic test (like the <u>Pap smear</u>) that will detect early or <u>occult</u> disease of the ovary.

    The common malignancies of the ovary are believed to arise from the <u>surface epithelium</u> of the ovary. The names of the common epithelial tumors are <u>serous</u>, <u>mucinous</u>, <u>endometrioid</u>, <u>clear-cell</u>, and <u>undifferentiated</u> tumors. These tumors can be benign, in which case they are treated by simple <u>excision</u>.

    When the ovarian cancer is confined to the ovaries (Stage 1), the patient is usually treated by a <u>total abdominal hysterectomy</u> and <u>bilateral salpingo-oophorectomy</u>. An <u>omentectomy</u> (the omentum is a part of the <u>peritoneum</u> that hangs over the intestines) is performed to be certain that occult disease is not present in the upper abdomen. In addition, any nodules, <u>retroperitoneal</u> or <u>intraperitoneal</u>, are removed and the diaphragm is inspected for metastatic carcinoma. <u>Para-aortic lymph node biopsies</u> are performed and <u>cytologic washings</u> are obtained from the pelvis and <u>paracolic spaces</u>. A <u>bowel resection</u> may be necessary with <u>anastomoses</u>.

    The cancer seems to spread by direct extension and not <u>hematogenously</u>, so that <u>debulking</u> surgery is important. <u>Adjuvant therapy</u> for Stage 1 disease may be either <u>cytotoxic chemotherapy</u> or <u>radiation therapy</u> (whole abdominal irradiation using <u>external beam irradiation</u> or <u>intraperitoneal radioactive isotopes</u>).

17. Chapter 8

    <u>Kegel exercises</u>, named after Dr. Arnold Kegel, a gynecologist who first developed the exercises to strengthen <u>pelvic-vaginal</u> muscles, are used to control <u>stress incontinence</u>. Patients are taught awareness of the <u>pubococcygeus</u> muscle, a <u>sphincteric</u> muscle that surrounds the <u>vagina</u>, and how to control it. Once the muscle has been strengthened it tends to maintain its strength and is in a state of partial contraction at all times.

18. Chapter 8 or Chapter 19

    <u>Alpha-fetoprotein</u> (AFP) is a <u>globulin</u> present in the <u>serum</u> of the <u>fetus</u>, infant, and normal pregnant female. High concentrations are often diagnostic of <u>hepatocellular carcinoma</u> in adults. Although they often do not reach the levels found in association with hepatocellular carcinoma, elevated concentrations of AFP are found in association with a variety of <u>malignant neoplasms</u> and inflammatory conditions.

    In fetuses with open <u>spina bifida</u> or <u>anencephaly</u>, AFP leaks into the <u>amniotic fluid</u> and maternal serum, and its measurement is of significant diagnostic value.

19. Chapter 9

    <u>Chlamydial infections</u>. Chlamydia is a type of bacteria. Chlamydia infections have replaced <u>gonorrhea</u> as the most prevalent <u>STD</u> in the United States. Symptoms may be very mild and those affected may not be aware that they have the disease. Often they do not seek treatment until a serious complication occurs. In males, the symptoms, when they do occur, are <u>dysuria</u> and watery discharge from the penis. Women may suffer <u>pruritus</u> and burning sensation in the <u>genital</u> area; an odorless, thick <u>leukorrhea</u>; dull abdominal pain; and <u>metrorrhagia</u>.

    One type of Chlamydia (trachomatis) causes about half of all PID. Symptoms can appear from 1 to 5 weeks after exposure to the bacteria and almost all sexual contacts become infected.

In pregnancy, chlamydial infection can increase the risk of stillbirth or premature birth. The newborns suffer from <u>conjunctivitis</u> that may have serious complications. Chlamydial infection also leads to <u>pneumonia</u> some weeks after birth, probably because of infectious material in the eye draining through the ducts between the eye and the nose and then passing into the lungs.

The infection is treated with an <u>antibiotic</u> such as <u>tetracycline</u>. As in the case of all STDs, both partners should be treated at the same time to prevent reinfection. If left untreated, chlamydial infection can cause scar tissue to form in the <u>fallopian</u> tubes and lead to <u>infertility</u> and <u>ectopic pregnancies</u>. In the male, it can lead to <u>epididymitis</u> and <u>sterility</u>.

20. Chapter 9

I saw Mr. John Smith for symptoms of <u>prostatism</u> (lessening of force of urinary flow, hesitancy in initiating <u>voiding</u>, inability to end <u>micturition</u> abruptly, <u>urinary retention</u>) in 1988. At that time he underwent <u>TURP</u> of a clinically benign prostate, and pathology report confirmed <u>benign prostatic hyperplasia</u>. In September of 1992 he was found to have a <u>PSA</u> of 10 ng/ml (elevated). <u>Biopsies</u> were obtained that revealed an <u>adenocarcinoma</u> involving the left lobe of the prostate.

Patient elected to proceed with a <u>radical prostatectomy</u>. Pathology report confirmed the presence of an adenocarcinoma with <u>perineural</u> and left <u>seminal vesicle</u> invasion and <u>transcapsular</u> extension into the left <u>periprostatic</u> fat. <u>Adjuvant</u> radiation therapy was advised.

21. Chapter 10, Chapter 16

<u>Neurofibromatosis</u> (also called von Recklinghausen disease) is an inherited disorder marked by pigmented skin lesions, multiple tumors of <u>spinal</u> and <u>cranial</u> nerves, tumors of the skin, and brain tumors. There is an increased association with <u>adrenal gland</u> tumors (<u>pheochromocytomas</u>), kidney <u>vascular</u> disease (causing <u>hypertension</u>), fibrous tissue <u>dysplasia</u>, and tumors in the <u>gastrointestinal</u> tract.

The main feature of this disease is the occurrence of many tumors composed of nerve and fibrous tissue (<u>neurofibromas</u>). The tumors can press on nerves, resulting in facial weakness, deafness, and vision loss. Many tumors that appear together can result in <u>elephantiasis</u> (blockage of lymphatic vessels in the lower extremities leads to enlargement of the legs) along with <u>hypertrophy</u> of skin and <u>subcutaneous</u> tissues of the head, neck, and trunk of the body. The spinal cord can become compressed by tumor and <u>hydrocephalus</u> can develop.

The condition is diagnosed readily by the presence of characteristic neurofibromas and skin-pigmented lesions (light brown marks that are smooth with sharp, regular borders found over the trunk and in the <u>axilla</u>). There is no treatment for neurofibromatosis other than <u>resection</u> of tumors that are causing symptoms and decompression of hydrocephalus if that occurs.

22. Chapter 10, Chapter 16

Leprosy is a <u>chronic</u> infectious disease caused by a <u>bacillus</u>, which is a rod-shaped <u>bacterium</u>. The bacillus attacks the <u>skin</u>, <u>mucous membranes</u>, and <u>peripheral nerves</u> (nerves that are outside the brain and spinal cord). Transmission occurs most often through infected <u>nasal</u> discharges.

Only about 5% of contacts acquire the disease; others appear to be immune. Leprosy is found mainly around the equator, in Southeast Asia, Africa, and South America. Of the estimated 12 to 20 million cases, about 2000 are in the USA; areas of leprosy occurrence are in Texas, Louisiana, and Hawaii. The disease is also seen in California, Florida, and New York City, primarily among immigrants.

In all forms of leprosy the bacillus invades the peripheral nerves, producing anesthesia of the skin. <u>Paralysis</u>, <u>ulcers</u>, and secondary infections are common. Nasal stuffiness and <u>epistaxis</u> occur early; later, ulceration and <u>necrosis</u> destroy supporting <u>cartilages</u>, causing <u>nasal</u> deformity and collapse. Earlobe enlargement and loss of eyebrows are common. Isolated lesions of the lip, tongue, and <u>palate</u> can occur and must be differentiated from malignancy.

Drug treatment (sulfur drugs) is successful and must be given until two years after the disease becomes inactive.

23. Chapter 10

<u>Bacterial meningitis</u>. Common etiological agents are <u>meningococcus</u>, <u>streptococcus</u>, <u>pneumococcus</u>, and tubercle bacillus.

The <u>streptococcal</u> and <u>pneumococcal</u> types reach the meninges from the middle ear or frontal sinus, but they may be carried by the bloodstream from the lungs as well. The <u>meningococcal</u> type comes from the nose or throat.

The meningococcus is usually the type causing epidemics. The infection is spread by carriers, who harbor the organisms in their throat but do not themselves develop the infection.

Examination of the <u>cerebrospinal fluid</u> by <u>lumbar puncture</u> gives the final diagnosis, including the type of bacterial infection. When normal CSF is removed by LP it is as clear as water, and the pressure is so low that it flows out drop by drop. In meningitis due to <u>pyogenic</u> bacteria, the fluid is <u>turbid</u> because of pus accumulation and the pressure is raised to such a degree that it may spurt from the needle. The fluid contains <u>polymorphonuclear leukocytes</u> and bacteria.

Treatment is with <u>antibiotics</u>; the fatality rate of acute bacterial meningitis is below 10% if recognized early.

24. Chapter 10

<u>Viral meningitis</u> (<u>encephalitis</u> or <u>aseptic</u> meningitis). In this type of inflammation, no <u>pyogenic</u> organisms can be found in the <u>cerebrospinal fluid</u>. The illness may appear following viral infections such as in chickenpox, measles, smallpox vaccination, and others.

Even desperately ill patients can recover completely. Treatment is supportive and symptomatic (symptoms include fever, headache, stiffness of the neck, and a high <u>lymphocyte</u> count in the <u>CSF</u>), and the disease is self-limiting.

25. Chapter 10

<u>Pain</u>. Receptors for pain <u>stimuli</u> are the <u>dendrites</u> of <u>neurons</u> distributed in the superficial layers of the skin and in certain deeper tissues such as the <u>periosteum</u>, joint surfaces, and arterial walls. The gastrointestinal <u>mucosa</u> is also quite sensitive to irritation and painful stimuli. The <u>parenchymal</u> tissues of the liver and the lung (air sacs) are insensitive to pain, while the bile ducts and associated liver tissue, <u>bronchi</u>, and <u>parietal pleura</u> are extremely sensitive.

Some stimuli that excite the pain receptors are mechanical stress of trauma, extremes of heat and cold, and chemical substances such as acids, histamine, and prostaglandins.

A lack of oxygen supply to tissues can also produce pain by causing the release of chemicals from ischemic tissue. Muscle spasm is another cause of pain because it can cause ischemia and stimulate chemosensitive pain receptors.

When superficial pain receptors are excited, the impulses are transmitted to synapses in the gray matter of the spinal cord. They then travel upward through sensory neurons to the thalamus, which is the main sensory relay station of the brain. The thalamus is probably where the conscious perception of pain takes place. Impulses are then transmitted to the cortex of the brain (frontal lobe) where the interpretation of the quality of the pain takes place.

Referred pain occurs in a part of the body distinct from where the cause that produced the pain is situated. Thus, pain originates in a visceral organ but is felt in the skin or another area of the body. Referred pain probably occurs because pain signals from the viscera travel along the same neural pathways used by pain signals from the skin. The person perceives the pain but interprets it as having originated in the skin rather than in a deep-seated visceral organ. An example of this type of pain is radiating pain in the left arm that is felt when a person has heart muscle damage (myocardial infarction) due to ischemia and necrosis.

Analgesics are agents that relieve pain. Aspirin is an example of a non-narcotic analgesic. It relieves pain by blocking the production of prostaglandins.

26. Chapter 10

    Migraine. Migraine is a paroxysmal disorder characterized by recurrent attacks of cephalgia, with or without associated visual and GI disturbances.

    Etiology is idiopathic, but evidence suggests a disturbance of cranial circulation. Prodromal symptoms (for example, flashes of light, paresthesias, hemianopia) are probably due to intracerebral vasoconstriction, and the actual head pain to dilation of scalp arteries.

    Headache may be preceded by a short period of depression, irritability, restlessness, or anorexia. These symptoms may disappear shortly before the headache appears or may merge with it. Pain is either unilateral or generalized. Nausea, emesis, and photophobia are common.

    Aspirin or codeine may help in mild attacks. In severe attacks, only codeine or stronger analgesics offer relief and only if taken before the headache has lasted two hours.

27. Chapter 11

    Angelo Payne, a 70-year-old house painter, noticed chest discomfort in the form of a substernal ache with radiation to the left arm brought on by exertion and relieved by rest. He had undergone repair surgery of an abdominal aortic aneurysm five years earlier. His only cardiovascular risk factor was a long history of cigarette smoking; he had no history of diabetes, hypertension, or hyperlipidemia and the family history was not remarkable for premature atherosclerosis.

28. Chapter 11

    A 35-year-old female with an eight-year history of heroin abuse was admitted to the hospital confused, agitated, and with a right hemiparesis of two days' duration. A left common carotid arteriogram demonstrated an aneurysm of the left parietal region involving one of the distal branches of the middle cerebral artery. The patient had subacute bacterial endocarditis and a septic embolus from the heart lodged in this parietal vessel, with the resulting aneurysm brain abscess. The endocarditis was secondary to repeated bouts of septicemia resulting from the unsterile techniques used by the patient for injecting drugs.

29. Chapter 11

    Beta-blockers are drugs that block the action of epinephrine at the beta-adrenergic receptors on cells of certain organs. There are two types of these receptors: beta receptors in the myocardium and beta receptors in the bronchial and vascular smooth muscle cells.

    Normally, if the beta receptors in the myocardium are stimulated by the secretion of epinephrine, they will cause the heart to beat more rapidly. Beta-blockers counter this effect and are used to treat angina pectoris, hypertension, and cardiac arrhythmias. By decreasing the workload of the heart, they are effective in reducing the long-term risk of mortality and reinfarction after recovery from the acute phase of a myocardial infarction.

    They are also used as prophylaxis for migraine headaches because they constrict the dilated vessels that are associated with migraines.

    Examples of beta-blockers are propranolol (Inderal), nadolol (Corgard), and timolol (Timoptic), an ophthalmic preparation used to treat glaucoma.

30. Chapter 11

    An apolipoprotein (apo- is a prefix used in biochemistry to denote the protein portion of a complex molecule) is a protein associated with lipids (such as triglycerides, phospholipids, and cholesterol) to form the various lipoproteins found in plasma and tissues. These proteins transport cholesterol, triglycerides, and phospholipids between tissues, and possess specific binding sites that are recognized by tissues. Apolipoprotein A-I and A-II are components of high-density lipoproteins (HDLs), which transport cholesterol to the liver to be metabolized.

31. Chapter 11

    Poisonous chicken soup. A 70-year-old man presented with profound weakness of 3 days' duration. He had a 2-year history of congestive heart failure following a myocardial infarction. His wife had gone out of town and his daughter had been preparing his meals. She made his favorite foods using a salt substitute (the patient was careful to weigh himself daily and watch his salt intake). On the day of admission he had eaten a large bowl of chicken soup to "treat a cold." The patient was found to have hyperkalemia resulting from an overdose of potassium chloride found in the salt substitute. Consumption of a large amount led to depression of the SA node and bradyarrhythmia. A transvenous pacemaker was inserted and hyperkalemia controlled with drugs. Patients with congestive heart failure and renal impairment should be warned about the hazards of using salt substitutes.

32. Chapter 12

    Patients with non-small cell lung cancer are candidates for palliative therapy only if they have any one or more of the following:
    - Distant metastatic disease
    - Supraclavicular adenopathy
    - Contralateral pulmonary metastasis
    - Recurrent laryngeal nerve paralysis
    - Weight loss and anorexia
    - Recurrent local disease following surgery or radiotherapy
    - Severe coexisting cardiac or pulmonary disease

33. Chapter 12 or Chapter 14

    Sarcoidosis is a chronic disorder in which the lymph nodes in many parts of the body are enlarged, and small, fleshy nodules called granulomas develop in the lungs, liver, and spleen. The skin, eyes, nervous system, muscles and bones, and salivary glands also can be affected.

    Etiology is unknown, and it is likely that the disease results from an abnormal immune response. In the United States, it is 10 to 20 times more frequent in blacks than in whites, but in Europe it affects mostly whites. Females are slightly more susceptible than males. Most people are between 20 and 40 when they are diagnosed with the illness, but it can occur in children and the elderly.

    Symptoms include fever, fatigue, malaise, anorexia, or weight loss. Many people have coughs and discomfort in their chest.

    Overall, the prognosis in sarcoidosis is good. Most people recover completely without medication, but others require corticosteroid therapy.

    Smoking is harmful because it aggravates impaired lung function, and prolonged exposure to sunlight should be avoided because vitamin D aids absorption of calcium, which can lead to kidney stones.

34. Chapter 12

    Tonsils. The tissue usually referred to as tonsils are the palatine tonsils, a pair of oval shaped structures about the size of small almonds, partially embedded in the mucous membrane, one on each side of the oropharynx. Below them, at the base of the tongue, are the lingual tonsils. On the upper rear wall of the mouth cavity are the pharyngeal tonsils, or adenoids, which are of fair size in childhood but usually shrink after puberty.

35. Chapter 12

    Chronic obstructive pulmonary disease. This is a term applied to a group of disorders of lung function that share an element of irreversible expiratory airflow obstruction. The three disorders commonly included are emphysema, chronic bronchitis, and chronic asthma in adults.

    Emphysema is destruction of alveolar spaces, usually accompanied by the loss of the natural elastic recoil of the lung and weakening of the walls of the bronchiolar airways.

    Chronic bronchitis is defined as daily production of sputum for a continuous period of 3 months. Pathologically, there is hypertrophy of mucous glands in the bronchial wall and chronic bronchial inflammation. Emphysema and chronic bronchitis frequently coexist in varying degrees.

    Asthma is marked by recurrent attacks of dyspnea with wheezing due to spasmodic constriction of bronchi.

    The single most important cause of COPD is smoking, which impairs the lungs' natural defenses against infection. Almost all chronic smokers demonstrate some impairment of pulmonary function. Other causes that frequently coexist with tobacco exposure include exposure to fumes and dust.

    In addition to dyspnea, an individual may demonstrate labored breathing, often with halting speech, weight loss, and cyanosis. Rales and rhonchi may be present.

    Diagnosis is based on clinical presentation and the results of spirometry, which show reduction in expiratory flow rates and volumes. The main complications of COPD are respiratory failure, overwhelming infections, and right-sided heart failure. When symptoms are present chronically at rest, the prognosis is poor.

36. Chapter 12 or Chapter 15

    Case Report:

    A 29-year-old man with complaints of pain in the low back and mid-epigastrium was found to have vertebral osteomyelitis. Mediastinal abscess was also diagnosed on the basis of findings on chest x-ray film, thoracic ultrasonography, thoracentesis, and cultures of the pleural fluid. Antibiotic therapy was begun, and after six weeks of treatment the patient was free of symptoms.

37. Chapter 12

    Nosocomial pneumonia accounts for about 10 to 17 percent of hospital-acquired infections. The rate of acquiring pneumonias in the hospital is 6 to 20 times higher in patients receiving mechanical ventilation, but the disease is most common in elderly intubated patients with chronic underlying disease.

38. Chapter 12

    Pleurodesis induces scarring of the pleura to prevent fluid accumulation in the pleural space. An irritant is injected into the pleural space through a thoracotomy or in a more extensive procedure that involves scraping the lungs.

39. Chapter 12

    A 67-year-old man had a 10-year history of COPD from heavy cigarette smoking. When he was hospitalized the first time, his major complaints included a 3-year history of increasing cough, SOB, fever, and weight loss. The occurrence of gross hemoptysis set off the alarm for any of several diagnoses: tuberculous pneumonia, pneumonia, acute and chronic bronchitis, bronchiectasis, trauma, pulmonary embolism, and lung cancer.

40. Chapter 13

    In summary, this 68-year-old man had diffuse histiocytic lymphoma for seven years and is currently in clinical remission. His current diagnosis is fungal pneumonitis. His ischemic colitis remains of uncertain etiology, but may result from the presence of numerous intestinal adhesions and recurrent hypotension.

41. Chapter 13

    G6PD is glucose-6-phosphate dehydrogenase. It is an enzyme normally found in erythrocytes. Deficiency of this enzyme can lead to hemolysis. Several forms of genetic deficiencies of the enzyme are recognized, affecting some black males, people of Chinese origin, Sephardic (from Spain) Jews, and other persons of Mediterranean origin. Deficiencies of G6PD cause hemolysis when affected people are treated with antimalarial or sulfa drugs or eat certain types of fava beans.

    About 10% of black American males suffer from a mild form of G6PD deficiency and only occasionally have symptoms in early infancy. Asians and some groups of Mediterranean origin develop a more severe form, with hemolysis.

42. Chapter 14

Parasitic infections are caused by small plants or animals that live on or within another living organism at whose expense they obtain some advantage. Some examples of these infections are:

acariasis	Infection with mites or ticks. Mange and scabies are examples.
candidiasis	Infection by fungus. Most commonly affects skin, oral mucosa (thrush), respiratory tract and vagina. The most prominent symptom of vaginitis due to Candida infection is severe pruritus. Candidiasis is often associated with AIDS infection.
filariasis	Infection with filariae, a type of worm. Most often found in Africa, the South Pacific and Asia, and tropical countries. It is transmitted by a mosquito or by mites (tiny organisms with jointed legs) or flies. Small worms invade lymph tissues and grow to adult worms. Resulting obstruction of the lymphatic vessels causes swelling, lymphadenitis, and pain. Repeated infections with impaired circulation and formation of excess connective tissue may cause enlargement of the affected part of the body (arm, leg, or scrotum), leading to elephantiasis.
giardiasis	Infection with Giardia, a type of tiny enteric organism (protozoa), is spread by contaminated food and water or by direct person-to-person contact. Symptoms are diarrhea, nausea, malaise, anorexia, and weight loss.
leishmaniasis	Infection with a type of protozoa (one-celled organism) called leishmania (after Sir William B. Leishman). Disease is transmitted by the sandfly and marked by cutaneous papules that form nodules and break down to form ulcers. The ulcers heal to form scars. Found in the tropics and subtropics; also called Aleppo boil, Delhi sore, Baghdad sore, and oriental sore.

43. Chapter 14

Kaposi sarcoma. Kaposi (named for Morris Kaposi, Austrian dermatologist, 1837–1902) sarcoma (KS) is a rare malignancy that consists of multiple lymph node tumors and angiosarcomas. These lesions appear on the legs or toes as purple or dark brown nodules. It is multifocal and metastasizing, involving chiefly the skin. This is an opportunistic neoplasm associated with AIDS. With metastatic lymphadenopathy, prognosis for a patient with Kaposi sarcoma may not be more than 3 years. Patients often have prodromal symptoms such as fever, diarrhea, weight loss, malaise, thrush (fungal infection), and wasting (cachexia). Lymphadenopathy may occur and then skin lesions characteristic of KS appear. As many as one-third of KS patients develop other malignancies such as lymphoma and squamous cell carcinomas.

Treatment of KS is difficult, but chemotherapy is tried and some patients have positive remissions.

44. Chapter 15 or Chapter 16

Systemic lupus erythematosus (SLE) is a chronic inflammatory disease of connective tissue. It also affects the skin and internal organs. Typically, there is an erythematous, scaly rash on the face, around the nose and the cheeks, and in the shape of a butterfly. Other characteristics of the disease are arthritis and nephropathy.

Although the etiology is unknown, it is thought to be an autoimmune disease and can be diagnosed by the presence of abnormal antibodies in the bloodstream. Another test shows characteristic white blood cells, called LE cells.

Common symptoms of SLE are fatigue, malaise, pyrexia, weight loss, and arthralgias. In addition to arthropathy, myositis can occur as well; alopecia may be present in some patients. Cardiac symptoms include pericarditis and myocarditis.

SLE predominantly afflicts women, one in 700 females between the ages of 15 and 64. It also occurs more often in blacks than in whites. Although there is no cure for SLE, treatment involves administration of non-steroidal anti-inflammatory drugs (NSAIDs) for management of mild symptoms (arthralgias, fever, myalgia) and corticosteroids for life-threatening and severely disabling complications.

45. Chapter 15

Scleroderma. This connective tissue and skin disorder is about four times more common in women than in men; it is rare in children. It may be an autoimmune disorder, meaning that the body produces antibodies against its own good tissue. Common initial complaints are Raynaud phenomenon and swelling of the fingers and toes with gradual thickening of the fingers. Induration (hardening) of the skin is symmetric and may be confined to the fingers or affect most of the body. As the disease progresses, the skin becomes taut, shiny, and hyperpigmented; the face becomes masklike, and telangiectases appear on the fingers, face, lips, and tongue. Esophageal dysfunction is the most frequent internal disturbance and eventually occurs in the majority of patients. The course of scleroderma is variable and unpredictable. It is often slowly progressive. Most, if not all, patients eventually show evidence of visceral involvement. Prognosis is poor if cardiac, pulmonary, or renal manifestations are present at diagnosis. However, the disease may remain limited in extent and nonprogressive for long periods of time.

Corticosteroids are often helpful in patients with disabling muscle involvement. Immunosuppressive agents are under trial for use in scleroderma. Palliative (relieving symptoms, but not curing) treatment is used for esophageal problems and nephropathy.

46. Chapter 15 or Chapter 16

Researchers conducted a study to determine the incidence of bacteremia in association with decubitus ulcers in a general hospital population. The incidence was higher in men, and 46% of the cases of bacteremia in association with decubitus ulcers occurred in paraplegics or in individuals with neurological defects.

The most common location of decubitus ulcers was the sacrum, followed by the ischial tuberosities, the heels, and the buttocks. Patients with multiple decubitus ulcers were more likely to develop bacteremia.

47. Chapter 16

Hexachlorophene is an antibacterial substance used in soaps and detergents to inhibit bacterial growth. It is contained in pHisoHex. The pH of pHisoHex is slightly acid (5.0–6.0). It has a bacteriostatic action against staphylococci and other bacteria.

Infants, especially premature infants or those with dermatoses, are particularly susceptible to absorption of hexachlorophene through the skin. Systemic toxicity may be manifested by signs of stimulation (irritation) of the central nervous system (brain and spinal cord), sometimes with convulsions. Infants have developed dermatitis, irritability, generalized muscle contractions, and rigidity following application of a 6 percent hexachlorophene powder.

48. Chapter 16 or Chapter 19

Progress Notes

This 50-year-old patient has had a progressively worsening headache for 6 months, and episodic weakness of his R leg for the past several months. These episodes last 5–10 minutes and are described as "numbness" or clumsiness of gait, with inability to walk or lift the leg. Has noted a dark mole that progressively enlarged on the upper tip of the R ear lobe over the past 3 yr. Suspected a melanoma but did not consult a physician.

FH/SH: denies sun exposure. No fam. hx of cancer. Works as a clerk. No children. Unmarried.

ROS: Smoker (30 pack yr) but not known to have COPD. Heart—no known disease. Had total colectomy for ulcerative colitis at age 12. No Sx since. Has lost about 10 pounds in past few months.

CT and MRI demonstrate R and L cerebral lesions. Chest: multiple 1 cm nodules.

PE: Pale, asthenic, bearded man in NAD (no apparent distress). Conversation appropriate. Large, 1 cm long bluish mole on R earlobe.

No other susp. Lesions. No nodes.

      Chest: clear to A&P

      Abd: no hepatomegaly or splenomegaly

      Extr: no edema, tenderness

      Neurol: Oriented and knows president and candidates

         No apparent motor defect.

         Touch intact

         Reflexes good in knees and ankles

Impression:
1. Likely melanoma met. to brain and lung. Bx results pending.
2. COPD

Suggest:
1. RT for brain lesions (no role for surgery)
2. Consult melanoma service
3. Social service evaluation
4. ?HIV status

49. Chapter 18

    Cushing syndrome (named for Dr. Harvey Cushing, who first described it in 1932) is a group of symptoms produced by an excess of cortisol from the adrenal gland. This can be caused by hyperplasia of the gland (due to increased stimulation from the pituitary gland and ACTH), ectopic production of ACTH from tumors in the lung or thyroid gland, and iatrogenically by too much administration of corticosteroids by physicians.

    Diagnosis is made by laboratory findings indicating a continuous elevation of plasma cortisol. The condition is characterized by increase in adipose tissue (especially between the shoulder blades), moon face, distention of the abdomen, ecchymoses following even minor trauma, acne, hypertension, and amenorrhea and hirsutism in females. If these symptoms are associated with an adenoma of the pituitary gland, the condition is known as Cushing disease.

    Treatment of the condition is by surgical removal of any neoplasm or with radiation using cobalt. Drug therapy using adrenocorticolytic agents may be used as an adjunct to surgery and radiation.

50. Chapter 22

    Alcoholism. Alcohol is a toxic drug, harmful to all body tissues. Chronic use can lead to pathological changes in the CNS, liver, heart, kidney, and gastrointestinal tract. Cirrhosis is the most recognized complication of alcoholism, but dementia and brain damage can also occur in the early stages of the disease. Fetal alcohol syndrome with growth deficiency, mental retardation, irritability in infancy, hyperactivity in childhood, and heart defects occurs in newborn infants of mothers who drink heavily throughout their pregnancy.

    Alcohol affects the liver by direct hepatotoxic effects as well as from malnutrition associated with chronic alcohol abuse. Gastritis, excessive peristalsis, and esophageal varices are further complications.

    Hypertension and coronary artery disease are related to intake of alcohol because alcohol elevates triglycerides in the blood. Alcohol abusers have an increased risk of oral and esophageal carcinoma. Immunosuppression may occur and result in lower resistance to infection. Alcohol has also been associated with sexual impotence by suppressing the production of testosterone.

MEDICAL FORMS

These are a collection of medical forms that I use in class with my students. They contain many terms that are taught in chapters of *The Language of Medicine*. I suggest that you use them as they pertain to the terminology you are teaching. For example, in Chapter 3, when I introduce the different types of blood cells, I hand out a laboratory form and show students the section pertaining to the different types of white blood cells, red blood cells (cell morphology), and platelets. Students see the terms in their actual context on a laboratory sheet.

You can also use the forms as a quiz by creating questions and asking students to find specific terms or abbreviations on the form that answer the questions. Please let me know (*Meddavi@aol.com*) if you find these helpful, and please share any interesting ways of using them in your classes. Also, please let me know if you have other forms that you include in your teaching.

The medical forms included here are:

1. **Health Laboratories** sheet

2. **Laboratory Diagnostics** (This form shows laboratory results from Sarah Smith, who is an 84-year-old patient who has been increasingly lethargic and gaining weight. After obtaining these laboratory results, the physician at her nursing home realized that Ms. Smith had been given only half the prescribed dose of thyroid hormone.)

3. **Review of Systems**

4. **Otolaryngology Associates**

5. **GYN Women's Health Encounter Form**

6. **Attending Physician's Statement with diagnostics codes**

7. **Center for Women's Cancers: Check-Out Sheet**

8. **Request for EKG**

9. **Lung Cancer Staging Sheet**

10. **Visit Sheet**

HEALTH LABORATORIES

DATE _____

PATIENT NAME _____   ACCESSION # _____   DOCTOR _____

CHEMISTRIES

GLUCOSE (65-110)	___	mg/dl	CALCIUM (8.5-11.0)	___	mg/dl
BUN (10-25)	___	mg/dl	PHOSPHATE (2.5-4.5)	___	mg/dl
CREATININE (0.7-1.4)	___	mg/dl	CHOLESTEROL (150-300)	___	mg/dl
NA$^+$ (135-145)	___	meq./1	TRIGLYCERIDES (30-200)	___	mg/dl
K$^+$ (3.5-5.0)	___	meq./1	ALK. PHOS. (30-115)	___	U./1
CI (98-109)	___	meq./1	AST (SGOT) (0-40)	___	U./1
CO$_2$ (24-32)	___	meq./1	ALT (SGPT) (0-40)	___	U./1
URIC ACID (2.5-8.0)	___	mg/dl	LDH (100-225)	___	U./1
PROTEIN-TOT. (6.0-8.0)	___	g/dl	BILIRUBIN-TOT. (0.2-1.5)	___	mg/dl
ALBUMIN (3.5-5.0)	___	g/dl	IRON (40-150)	___	mcg/dl
GLOBULIN (2.0-3.6)	___	g/dl			
A/G (0.9-2.3)	___				

THYROID CHEMISTRIES
T-4 ___ mcg/dl (4.5-13.5)
T-3 ___ % (25-35%)

SYPHILIS SEROLOGY
___ REACTIVE
___ NON REACTIVE

PROTHROMBIN TIME
PATIENT ___ sec ___ %act.
CONTROL ___ sec

DIGOXIN ___ ng/ml (0.8-2.0)
PREGNANCY TEST ___

ORGANISM (S)

ANTIBIOTICS
			900 AMPICILLIN
			902 CARBENICILLIN
			904 CEPHALOTHIN
			906 CHLOPAMPHENICOL
			908 CLINDAMYCIN
			910 COLISTIN
			912 ERYTHROMYCIN
			914 GENTAMICIN
			916 KANAMYCIN
			918 METHICILLIN
			920 NAFCILLIN
			922 NALIDIXIC ACID
			924 NEOMYCIN
			926 NITROFURANTOIN
			928 PENICILLIN
			930 POLYMYXIN B
			932 SULFONAMIDES
			934 TETRACYCLINE
			936 TOBRAMYCIN

TECHNOLOGIST COMMENTS:

URINALYSIS
COLOR ___
APPEARANCE ___
REACTION ___
SPEC. GRAVITY ___
GLUCOSE ___
PROTEIN ___
ACETONE ___
WBC/HPF ___
RBC/HPF ___
EPITH. CELLS ___
BACTERIA ___
CRYSTALS ___
CASTS ___
OTHER: ___

COMPLETE BLOOD COUNT

			MALE	FEMALE				MALE	FEMALE
WHITE BLOOD COUNT	___	x10^3/mm^3	4-11	4-11	LYMPH ___	%		20-40	20-40
RED BLOOD COUNT	___	x10^6/mm^3	4.7-6.0	4.0-5.4	SEG. ___	%		50-70	50-70
HEMOGLOBIN	___	g/dl	14-18	12-16	MONO ___	%		0-10	0-10
HEMATOCRIT	___	vol. %	42-52	37-47	EOSIN ___	%		0-5	0-5
MCV	___	cu. microns	80-94	81-91	BASO ___	%		0-1	0-1
MCH	___	pg	27-33	27-33	BANDS ___	%		0-5	0-5
MCHC	___	%	31.5-36	31.5-36	JUVEN ___	%		0-1	0-1
					%ATYP. ___	%		0	0

ADDITIONAL TESTS RESULTS:

CELL MORPHOLOGY: ___
HYPOCROMIA ___
ANISOCYTOSIS ___
POIKILOCYTOSIS ___
POLYCHROMIA ___
OTHER: ___

Laboratory Diagnostics

PATIENT: SARAH SMITH FINAL

WBC	RBC	HGB	HCT	MCV	MCH	MCHC	RDW	MPV	PLAT	BAND	NEUT	LYMP	MONO	EOS	BASO	ATYP L	MORPH
4.9	4.27	12.3	37	86	29	34	13.4	9.0	196	0	63	22	13	2	0	0	
3.8-10.8 1000/uL	3.80-5.10 mil/uL	11.7-15.5 g/dL	35-45 %	80-100 fL	27-33 pg	32-36 g/dL	11.0-15.0 %	7.5-11.5 fL	140-400 thou/uL	0-5 %	48-75 %	17-40 %	0-14 %	0-5 %	0-3 %	0-5 %	

Ca	PO4	GLU	BUN	CREAT	BUN/CR	URIC	CHOL	TRIG	HDL	TP	ALB	GLOB	A/G	ALKP	LDH	SGOT	SGPT
8.7		105	24	1.1						7.0	3.9	3.1	1.3	88	161	20	13
8.5-10.4 mg/dL		65-109 mg/dL	7-25 mg/dL	0.5-1.2 mg/dL						6.0-8.3 g/dL	3.2-4.6 g/dL	2.2-4.2 g/dL	0.8-2.0	20-125 U/L	100-250 U/L	2-35 U/L	2-40 U/L

BILI	BILI D	BILI I	Na	K	Cl	CO2	ANION	Fe	TIBC	GGT	T3U	T4	FTI	TSH	T4 F	B12	
0.3	0.1	0.2	146	4.4	104	29				15				17.9 HI			
0.2-1.3 mg/dL	0-0.3 mg/dL	0.0-1.3 mg/dL	135-146 mmol/L	3.5-5.3 mmol/L	98-110 mmol/L	21-33 mmol/L				2-60 U/L				0.3-5.5 uIU/mL			

Urinalysis

COLOR	APP	SPGR	PH	ALB	GLU	KET	BILI	BLOOD	LEU	NIT
Yellow	Clear	1.028	6.0	NEG	NEG	NEG	NEG	NEG	NEG	NEG
Yellow	Clear		5.0-8.0	NEG	NEG	NEG	NEG	NEG	NEG	NEG

Test Name	Result		Reference
Differential (absolute count)			
Absolute Band Count	0		0-500 /uL
Absolute Neutrophil Count	3087		1500-7800 /uL
Absolute Lymphocyte Count	1078		850-3900 /uL
Absolute Monocyte Count	637		200-950 /uL
Absolute Eosinophil Count	98		50-550 /uL
Absolute Basophil Count	0		0-200 /uL
Absolute Atypical Lymphocytes	0		/uL
Cardiac Risk Profile			
Cholesterol	267	HI	100-199 mg/dL
Triglycerides	151	HI	30-149 mg/dL
HDL-Cholesterol	56		40-77 mg/dL
LDL-Cholesterol	181	HI	62-130 mg/dL
Cholesterol/HDL Risk Factor	4.77		
Relative Risk	1.2 times average		1.0 is average risk for CHD

Comments

Risk Category: LDL-Cholesterol Goal
CHD and CHD Risk equivalents: <100
Multiple (2+) factors: <130
Zero to one risk factor: <160

Review of Systems

MR#:_____
Name: _____
Date:_____

Circle positives, cross out negatives, leave blank items not discussed

GENERAL: fatigue, malaise, chills, fever, night sweats, change in appetite, change in weight, amount of change in weight _____.
History of heat injury; History of radiation therapy.
_____
_____.

EYES: visual changes. diplopia, scotomata_____
_____
last eye exam_____

EARS/NOSE/THROAT: tinnitus; hearing loss, epistaxis, sinusitis; post-nasal drip, hay fever, sneezing, nasal stuffiness, sore tongue, gum bleeding, poor dentition; hoarseness_____

last dental visit _____

RESPIRATORY: SOB, DOE, wheezing, cough, sputum production, hemoptysis, asthma; exposure to TB or history of TB_____
_____

CARDIOVASCULAR: chest pain, SOB, DOE, orthopnea, edema, palpitations, dizziness, syncope, claudication, heart murmurs, DVT or PE, hypertension, history of heart attack, last cholesterol level_____
_____

GI: difficulty swallowing, nausea, vomiting, abdominal pain, diarrhea, indigestion, antacid use, constipation, change in stool, melena, rectal bleeding, laxative use; history of polyps; history of ulcerative colitis or Crohn disease_____
last flexible sigmoidoscopy and results:_____
_____

GENITOURINARY: dysuria, urgency, frequency, polyuria, nocturia, hesitancy, incontinence, foul urine, hematuria, history of STIs: number of sexual partners _____.
Last HIV test date_____Result_____
_____.

Male: discharge from penis; lump or skin change of the penis: lump on scrotum, impotence; history of undescended testicle_____
_____

Female: abnormal vaginal bleeding, regular periods, irregular periods, dysmenorrhea, last menstrual period _____.
vaginal discharge; age of menarche_____;
last pap smear_____and results _____.
method of contraception_____.

MUSCULOSKELETAL: joint pain, redness, swelling, stiffness, muscle pain, muscle weakness, decreased ROM; fracture, sprain, dislocation, history of osteoporosis_____
_____

SKIN: color changes, rash, photosensitivity, itching, mole changes; History of skin cancer, history of sun exposure on daily basis or sunburns
_____

CNS: headache, seizures, paralysis, incoordination, unsteadiness, abnormal sensations, decreasing mentation, tremor, confusion, pinched nerves; temporary blindness; history of stroke or TIA_____
_____

PSYCHIATRIC: depression. high stress, anxiety, sleep disturbances, suicidal thoughts, homicidal thoughts_____

ENDOCRINE: breast masses or discharge, heat or cold intolerance, nervousness, increased thirst, polyphagia; hair changes, last mammogram and result_____

HEMATOLOGY: anemia, bleeding problems, easy bruisability, lymph node enlargement_____
_____

SAFETY: guns in home, domestic violence, HIV risk factors, smoke detectors_____

Otolaryngology Associates

S/C	SERVICE	CHG.	S/C	SERVICE	CHG.	S/C	SERVICE	CHG.	S/C	SERVICE	CHG.	S/C	SERVICE	CHG.
1	Comprehen., New Pt.		36	Myringotomy, Bilat.		112	I & D Subling. Abscess		244	Spont. Nystagmus			**LABORATORY**	
2	Intermed., New Pt.		37	Removal Tube		113	Frenulectomy		245	Posit. Nystagmus		270	Allergy Injection	
3	Limited, New Pt.		38	Removal, Foreign Bdy.		114	Uvulectomy					271	Prist	
4	Consult., Ref. Dr.			**NOSE**		115	Dilation, Salivary Duct		247	Optokinetic Nystagmus		272	Rast, up to 5 All.	
5	Comprehen., Est. Pt.		60	I&D Intra-Nasal Abscess		116	Steroid Inj. TMJ		248	Oscillating Tracking Tst		273	Rast, 6 or more All.	
6	Intermed., Est. Pt.		61	I&D Septal Abscess			**AUDIOLOGY**			**X-RAY**		274	Allergy Serum	
7	Limited, Est. Pt.		62	Excision Polyps, Unila.		230	Air Only		251	Mandible		275	Eosinophil Count	
8	Brief, Est. Pt.		63	Excision Polyps, Bilat.		231	Air and Bone		252	Mastoid		276	Nasal Smear	
9	Consult., Est. Pt.		64	Cautery Nasal Septum		232	Comp. Audiometry		253	Facial Bones		277	CBC	
10	Pre-Op Visit		65	Cautery Turbinates					254	Nasal Bones		278	Mono Spot	
11	Post-Op Visit		66	Antral Punct., Unilat.		237	Speech Audiometry, Threshold only		255	Sinuses		279	Ear Culture	
12	Emerg. Visit, Ext.		67	Antral Punct., Bilat.		235	Ear Mold Fitting		256	Skull		280	Nose Culture	
13	Emerg. Visit, Limited		68	Reduction Nasal Fract.		236	Hearing Aid Consult.		257	Temporal, Mand. Jt.		281	Throat Culture	
	EAR		69	Repair N.S. Perf.					258	Neck, Soft Tissue		282	Sensitivity Studies	
31	I&D Abscess Auricle		70	Inj. Turbinates		239	Tone Decay		259	Sialography				
32	I&D Hematoma Auricle		71	Removal, Foreign Bdy.					260	Int. Auditory Meati				
33	I&D Abscess Ext. Auditory Canal			**THROAT**		241	Stenger Puretone							
34	Pierce Ears		110	I & D Perit. Abscess		242	Acoustic Reflex					221	Removal of Sutures	
35	Myringotomy, Unilat.		111	Direct Fiberoptic Laryngoscopy								222	Medical Report	

D/C	DIAGNOSIS	D/C	DIAGNOSIS	D/C	DIAGNOSIS	D/C	DIAGNOSIS	D/C	DIAGNOSIS
1	External Otitis	13	Perforated Tymp. Memb.	41	Tonsillitis	48	Sialadenitis	55	Laryngeal Polyps
2	Otitis Media, Acute	20	Rhinitis	42	Laryngitis	49	Dysphagia	56	Foreign Body, Throat
3	Otitis Media, Chronic	21	Allergic Rhinitis	43	Stomatitis	50	Hoarseness	57	Peritonsillar Abscess
4	Serous Otitis Media	22	Sinusitis, Acute	44	Adenitis	51	Cephalgia	58	Meniere Syndrome
5	Sensorineural Hear. Loss	23	Sinusitis, Chronic	45	Cough, Chronic	52	Upper Resp. Infection	59	Bronchitis, Acute
6	Impacted Cerumen	24	Maxillary Sinusitis	46	Adenoiditis	53	T.M. Joint Dysfunction	60	Hypertrophic Tonsils
7	Vertigo	25	Epistaxis	47	Salivary Calculus	54	Vocal Cord Nodules	61	Hypertrophic Adenoids
8	Labyrinthitis	26	Nasal Polyps		**DIAGNOSIS**				**CODE**
9	Eustach. Salpingitis	27	Nasal Fracture	1.					
10	Tinnitus	28	Foreign Body, Nose	2.					
11	Otalgia	29	Deviated Nasal Septum	Instructions/Remarks:					
12	Foreign Body, Ear	40	Pharyngitis						
	Date of Injury or Illness		Date Dr. First Saw Patient						

**GYN Women's Health
Encounter Form**

Physician_____
Time_____
Date_____

Referral #:   Yes
                Not Needed

Authorized for: _____

PLAN:

IN OFFICE PROCEDURES

Uterus

☐ 7950058	Endometrial +/or endocervical	
	sampling (biopsy)	58100
		58120

Vaginal-Vulva

☐ 7950140	Bx vaginal mucosa, extensive	
	with suture	57105
☐ 7950033	Bx vag.mucosa,simple	57100
☐ 7950157	Destr vag lesion(s), ext	57065
☐ 7950165	Destr vag lesion(s) simple	57061
☐ 7950173	Destr vulvar lesion(s), ext	56515
☐ 7950181	Destr vulv lesion(s) simple	56501
☐ 7950116	I+D Bartholin's abscess	56420
☐ 7950199	I+D vulva or perineal abscess	56405
☐ 7950207	Marsup of Barth..gland	56440
☐ 7950041	Bx vulva, one lesion	56605
☐ 7950371	Bx vulva, each add'l lesion	
	Number of Units ____	56606
☐ 7950074	Pessary Insertion	57160
☐	Postcoital Test	89300

Contraception

☐ 7950108	Diaphragm/cervical cap fitting	
	w/ instructions	57170
☐ 7950082	IUD Insertion	58300
☐ 7950090	IUD removal	58301

Skin

☐ 7950215	Biopsy, skin, single	11100
☐ 7950223	Biopsy, skin,each add'l lesion	11101
☐ 7950231	Destruct flat warts	17110
☐ 795044	Excision Skin Tag <16	11200
☐ 795045	Excision Benign Lesion	
	<.5cm	11420
☐ 795046	Excision Benign Lesion	
	.6-1 cm	11421
☐ 795047	I+D wound infection	10180

Breast

☐ 7950124	Breast Aspiration	19000

Cervix

☐ 7950066	Bx, or local exc of lesions	
	w/wo fulguration	57500
☐ 7950322	Colposcopy	57452
☐ 7950330	Colpo w/cervical bx +/or endo	57454
☐ 7950363	Conization/loop excision	57522
☐ 7950025	Cryocautery cervix	57511
☐ 7950389	Dilation cervical canal	57800
☐ 7950397	Endocervical curettage	57505

Misc/Supplies

☐	Cath Supplies/Materials	99070
☐	IUD/Paragard	1234Z
☐	IUD/Progestasert	1234Y
☐ 7950256	KOH	87220
☐ 7950272	Pessary supply	A4560
☐ 7950280	Stool Occult Blood	82270
☐ 7950264	Urinanalysis dipstick	81002
☐ 7950249	Wet Mount	87210
☐ 7950413	Breast and Pelvic Screening	G0101
☐ 7950421	Pap screening,obtaining,	
	preparing for lab	Q0091
☐	OTHER	

Injections

☐ 7950306	Injection of Med-subQ/IM	90782
	Substance _____	

Urodynamics

☐ 7950298	Catheterization, simple	53670
☐ 795043	Cystometrics - simple	51725
☐ 795049	Cystometrogram, complex	51726
☐ 795050	Urethral Pressure Profile	51772
☐ 795048	Uroflowmetry	51741

ATTENDING PHYSICIAN'S STATEMENT
MEDICAL GROUP LTD.

37991

Patient No.		DR. _____			
Account No.	Patient Name			Date of Birth	Sex
Date	Insurance Company		Policy No.–Cert. No.	Soc. Sec. No.	Employer

THIS SUPERBILL IS YOUR INSURANCE CLAIM - SUBMIT DIRECTLY TO YOUR INSURANCE COMPANY FOR PAYMENT OF BENEFITS DUE.

DIAGNOSIS CODES

789.00	Abd Pain	185	Cancer Prostate	250.03	DM, Insul. Dep., Uncont.	729.5	Limb Pain	582.9	Renal Disease Ch
794.8	Abn Liver Funct.	427.9	Cardic Arryth.	787.91	Diarrhea	272.9	Lipid Disorder	398.90	Rheumatic Heart Dis.
790.6	Abn. Blood Chem.	425.4	Cardiomyopathy	562.11	Diverticulitis	710.0	Lupus	V70.0	Routine Med. Exam
042	AIDS	366.9	Cataracts	562.10	Diverticulosis	V58.61	Medication Monitoring Anti Coag	786.05	Shortness of Breath
477.9	Allergic Rhinitis	682.9	Cellulitis	782.3	Edema	V58.69	Medication Monitoring High Risk	427.81	Sick Sinus Syndrome
280.9	Anemia-Iron Def.	437.0	Cerebral Arterio.	530.10	Esophagitis, Unspec.	627.9	Menopausal Syn.	461.9	Sinusitis, Acute
285.9	Anemia Unspec.	786.50	Chest Pain	780.79	Fatigue	346.90	Migraine	848.9	Sprain-Strain
413.9	Angina	428.0	CHF	610.1	Fibrocystic Breast	424.0	Mitral Valve Disorder	780.2	Syncope
424.1	Aortic Valve Disorder	571.5	Cirrhosis	729.1	Fibromyalgia	410.90	Myocardial Infarct.	726.90	Tendinitis
719.40	Arthralgia, Site Unspec.	558.9	Colitis	780.6	Fever	443.9	Occ Peri Vas Dis	435.9	TIA
714.0	Arthritis RH	211.3	Colon Polyps	530.81	GE Reflux	715.90	Osteoarthritis	465.9	URI
414.00	ASHD	564.0	Constipation	578.9	GI Bleed	733.00	Osteoporosis	788.41	Urinary Frequency
493.90	Asthma	496	COPD	241.1	Goiter-M N	785.1	Palpitations	599.0	UTI
427.31	Atrial Fib.	414.9	Coronary Artery Dis.	V72.3	Gynecological Exam	782.0	Paresthesia	454.9	Varicose Veins
300.00	Anxiety	786.2	Cough	784.0	Headache	462.	Pharyngitis	447.6	Vasculitis
724.5	Back Pain	555.9	Crohn's Dis.	455.6	Hemorrhoids	511.9	Pleural Effusion	386.11	Vertigo
600.0	BPH	436	CVA	053.9	Herpes Zoster	486	Pneumonia	079.99	Viral Illness
466.0	Bronchitis Acute	595.0	Cystitis Acute	553.3	Hiatus Hernia	V72.83	Pre-Op Exam, Other Spec.	787.01	Vomiting-Nausea
491.9	Bronchitis Ch	451.11	DVT, Lower Extrem.	272.4	Hyperlipidemia	601.0	Prostatitis, Acute		
727.3	Bursitis	692.9	Dermatitis	401.9	Hypertension	415.19	Pulmonary Emboli		
174.9	Cancer Breast, female	250.00	Diabetes Mellitus	244.9	Hypothyroidism	569.3	Rectal Bleed		
154.0	Cancer Colon	250.02	DM, Uncontrolled	564.1	IBS	530.11	Reflux Esophagitis		
162.9	Cancer-Lung	250.01	Diabetes Insul. Dep.						

PREVIOUS BALANCE	
TODAY'S CHARGES	
PAID	
NEW BALANCE	

This is your Standard Insurance Report Form. Unless so stated, patient's claim is not related to pregnancy or occupation. An additional charge will be made for further information.

Signature of Doctor _____

Center for Women's Cancers
Check-Out Sheet

Next Appointment Information

Type		Time Period		Provider Name		
Cancer F/U	☐	PRN	☐	Multi. Session	☐	_____
Cancer Post-Op	☐	10+ day post proced.	☐	Med. Onc.	☐	_____
Post-Op, Bx	☐	2 mos.	☐	Rad. Onc.	☐	_____
Benign F/U	☐	3 mos.	☐	Surg. Onc.	☐	_____
		6 mos.	☐	Plastic Surgery	☐	_____
		1 year	☐	Nurse Praction.	☐	_____
		Other	☐ _____			

Blood	ASAP	Before Next Appt.	Next Appt.	Comments
CBC, Diff	☐	☐	☐	_____
Hematocrit	☐	☐	☐	_____
Blood cultures	☐	☐	☐	_____
Lytes, BUN, Creat.	☐	☐	☐	_____
LFT's	☐	☐	☐	_____
PT, PTT	☐	☐	☐	_____
Sed rate (ESR)	☐	☐	☐	_____
Basic Metabolic	☐	☐	☐	_____
Cal, Phos, Mg	☐	☐	☐	_____
Glucose	☐	☐	☐	_____
LDH	☐	☐	☐	_____
Total protein	☐	☐	☐	_____
Thyroid	☐	☐	☐	_____
Ca 125	☐	☐	☐	_____
CA 27-29	☐	☐	☐	_____
CEA	☐	☐	☐	_____
Beta HCG	☐	☐	☐	_____
Type and Cross	☐	☐	☐	_____
Panels	☐	☐	☐	_____
Other	☐	☐	☐	_____

Miscellaneous

EKG	_____	Urinalysis	_____
Beta strep test	_____	Urine culture	_____
Echocardiogram	_____	Port-a-cath P/R	_____

Radiology
Breast Imaging:

Mammo. Side: ☐ R ☐ L ☐ B
Sched: ☐ ASAP ☐ 6 mo. ☐ 1 yr ☐ Other _____
Locat: ☐ Zero Emer. ☐ ACC
Mag Views ☐

Ultrasound	☐	
U/S guided cyst asp.	☐	Side: ☐ R ☐ L ☐ B
U/S guided core bx	☐	
Stereotactic core bx	☐	
Breast MRI	☐	

Comments: _____
_____

Radiology	ASAP	Bef. Next Apt.	N. Appt.	Comments
Bone Density	☐	☐	☐	_____
Bone Films	☐	☐	☐	_____
Bone Scan	☐	☐	☐	_____
CT Abd/Pel. +/-	☐	☐	☐	_____
CT Chest +/-	☐	☐	☐	_____
CT Neck/Head	☐	☐	☐	_____
CXR PA/LAT R/L	☐	☐	☐	_____
Gallium scan	☐	☐	☐	_____
Gated heart scan	☐	☐	☐	_____
MRI _____	☐	☐	☐	_____
Pulmonary function test	☐	☐	☐	_____
+/- DLCO +/- O2 Sat.				
Vascular Studies	☐	☐	☐	_____
Other (please specify)			_____	

Surgery	L/R	Comments	Anesthesia
Lump + SN Bx	☐	_____	O Local
Lump ax.	☐	_____	O IV Sed
Sentinel Node BX	☐	_____	O MAC
ALND	☐	_____	O General
Re-excision	☐	_____	
MRM	☐	_____	
Simple Mastectomy	☐	_____	
Reconstruction	☐	_____	
Open Bx.	☐	_____	
Needle loc'd Bx.	☐	_____	
FNA	☐	_____	
Site-Select	☐	_____	
Other	☐	_____	

Comments: _____

Chemo scheduling

____ AC	____ CAF ____ CMF
____ Docetaxel	____ Doxorubicin Liposomal
____ Doxorubicin	____ Doxorubicin High Dose
____ Gemcitabine	____ Paclitaxel 100
____ Paclitaxel 175	____ Paclitaxel weekly/Trastuzumb
____ Trastuzumab	____ Vinorelbine (30)
____ Paclitaxel/Trastuzumab	____ Vinorelbine/Trastuzumb

_____
_____

XRT scheduling

☐ Yes if yes: O ASAP O Other ☐ No

Clinician Sign [_____]

REQUEST FOR EKG

DIAGNOSIS CODES *(Check off those that apply)*

Preopertative Exam/Post Op Status
___ V72.81   Pre-operative cardiovascular exam
___ V42.1   Heart transplant status
___ V43.3   Heart valve replacement

Signs and Symptoms
___ 786.50   Chest pain NOS
___ 786.59   Other chest pain
___ 729.5   Pain in limb
___ 780.09   Somnolence/Stupor
___ 780.2   Syncope and collapse
___ 780.4   Dizziness and Giddiness
___ 780.79   Malaise and fatigue, other than chronic
___ 782.3   Edema
___ 785.1   Palpitations
___ 785.2   Undiagnosed cardiac mummurs
___ 786.09   Respiratory distress/insufficiency
___ 789.00   Abdominal pain, unspecified site
___ 789.06   Abdominal pain, epigastric
___ 789.07   Abdominal pain, generalized
___ 799.0   Asphyxia

Coronary Athersclerosis
___ 414.00   CAD of unspecified vessel
___ 414.01   of native coronary vessel
___ 414.02   of autologous vein bypass graft
___ 414.03   of nonautologous biological bypass graft
___ 414.04   of artery bypass graft (IMA)
___ 414.05   of unspecified type of bypass graft
___ 440.9   Atherosclerosis, generalized & unspecified

Acute Myocardial Infarction- Initial
___ 410.01   Anterolateral wall, initial
___ 410.11   Other anterior wall, initial
___ 410.21   Inferolateral wall, initial
___ 410.31   Inferoposterior wall, initial
___ 410.41   Other inferior wall, initial
___ 410.51   Other lateral wall, initial
___ 410.61   True posterior wall, initial
___ 410.71   Subendocardial infarct, initial
___ 410.81   Papillary muscle infarct, initial

Acute MI, Subsequent Care Within 8 wks
___ 410.02   Anterolateral wall, w/in 8 wks
___ 410.12   Other anterior wall, w/in 8 wks
___ 410.22   Inferolateral wall, w/in 8 wks
___ 410.32   Inferoposterior wall, w/in 8 wks
___ 410.42   Other inferior wall, w/in 8 wks
___ 410.52   Other Lateral wall, w/in 8 wks
___ 410.62   True posterior wall, w/in 8 wks
___ 410.72   Subendocardial infarct, w/in 8 wks
___ 410.82   Papillary muscle infarct, w/in 8 wks

Acute Myocardial Infarction, Unspecified
___ 410.90   Acute myocardial infarct, unspecified site

Digestive Disorders
___ 575.0   Acute cholecystitis
___ 575.10   Cholecystitis, unspecified
___ 575.12   Acute and chronic cholecystitis

IF DIAGNOSIS IS NOT IDENTIFIED EKG WILL NOT BE DONE

Heart Disease
___ 411.1   Intermediate coronary syndrome
___ 423.9   Pericardial disease, unspecified
___ 424.90   Endocarditis, valve unspecified
___ 425.9   Secondary cardiomyopathy, unspecified
___ 427.0   Paroxysmal supaventricular tachycardia
___ 427.2   Paroxysmal tachycardia, unspecified
___ 427.31   Atrial fibrillation
___ 427.32   Atrial flutter
___ 427.41   Ventricular fibrillation
___ 427.42   Ventricular flutter
___ 427.5   Cardiac arrest
___ 427.60   Premature beats, unspecified
___ 427.81   Sino-atrial node dysfunction
___ 427.89   Other cardiac dysrhythmias NEC
___ 427.9   Cardiac dysrhythmias, unspecified
___ 428.0   Congestive heart failure
___ 428.9   Heart failure, unspecified
___ 429.1   Myocardial degeneration
___ 429.3   Cardiomegaly
___ 429.9   Heart disease, unspecified

Other Circulatory Diseases
___ 415.19   Pulmonary embolism and infarction other than iatrogenic
___ 416.9   Chronic pulmonary heart disease, unspecified
___ 435.9   Transient cerebral ischemia, unspecified
___ 436   Acute, but ill-definied CVA
___ 441.00   Dissecting aortic aneurysm, unspecified site
___ 441.01   Dissecting aortic aneurysm, thoracic
___ 441.02   Dissecting aortic aneurysm, abdominal
___ 441.1   Thoracic aneurysm, ruptured
___ 441.2   Thoracic aneurysm, without mention of rupture
___ 441.3   Abdominal aneurysm, ruptured
___ 441.4   Abdominal aneurysm, without mention of rupture
___ 441.6   Thoracoabdominal aneurysm, ruptured
___ 441.7   Thoracoabdominal aneurysm, w/out mention of rupture
___ 441.5   Aortic aneurysm of unspecified site, ruptured
___ 441.9   Aortic aneurysm of unspecified site w/out mention of ruputre
___ 401.9   Essential hypertension, unspecified
___ 458.9   Hypotension, unspecified

Respiratory Disorders
___ 492.8   Emphysema other than emphysematous bleb
___ 493.90   Asthma w/o status asthmaticus
___ 511.0   Pleurisy w/out mention of effusion or tuberculous
___ 511.9   Pleural effusion, unspecified
___ 518.81   Acute respiratory failure
___ 518.82   Acute respiratory insufficiency
___ 518.83   Chronic respiratory failure
___ 518.84   Acute and chronic respiratory failure

Other
___ 038.9   Septicemia, unspecified
___ 276.1   Hyposmolality and/or hyponatremia
___ 276.5   Hypovolemia/dehydration
___ 276.7   Hyperpotassemia
___ 276.8   Hypopotassemia
___ 959.1   Trunk injury, other and unspecified
___ V72.85   Other specified exam

_____ (Other)

HAS PATIENT HAD DIGITALIS ☐ **YES**   **QUINIDINE** ☐ **YES**   ☐ **PACEMAKER CHECK WITH, AND WITHOUT MAGNET**

SPECIAL BILLING INSTRUCTIONS *(If you checked off "OTHER" at top of form, complete applicable field.)*

BILL TO	FUND NUMBER	COST CENTER	OTHER *(Name of Institution)*

LUNG CANCER STAGING SHEET

Name:_____ Hosp #_____ JCRT #_____

PAST HISTORY

___ age at dx

y/n Smoking hx; if y, ___ ppd ___ #yrs;
      ___ yrs since quit (<1yr = 0)

y/n Asbestos exposure

y/n Comorbid lung ds; if y, ___ COPD,
__ emphysema, ___ asthma, __ other:_____

y/n History of steroid use;
  if y, reason_____, duration _____,
  drug _____, date last use_____

SIGNS / SYMPTOMS AT DX

y/n > 10 % Wt loss over 6 mos prior to dx
      from ___ to ___ lbs; ___%

check all applicable:

__ no sx   __ hoarseness

__ hemoptysis   __ cough

__ chest pain   __ phrenic n. palsy

__ dysphagia   __ recent pneumonia

__ fever   __ SVC compromise

__ dyspnea; __ at rest __ w/ min. exertion
        __ w/ signif. exertion

__ atelectasis; ___ segmental ___ lobar
        ___ whole lung

__ pleural effusion

PFTs (pre-treat): date_____, hosp _____
  FEV$_1$ ___l (___ %); FVC ___l (___ %)
  ___ not done

STAGING EVALUATIONS

y/n **CXR**, date_____ Hosp _____
  __ positve, __ negative, __ equivocal

y/n **Chest CT**, date_____ Hosp_____
  ___ (cm) primary tumor size (max diam)
  ___ solitary   ___ multiple lesions
  hilar nodes: __ pos __ neg __ equiv
  ipsilat med nodes: __ pos __ neg __ equiv
  contralat med: __ pos __ neg __ equiv

y/n **liver/adr. CT**, date _____ Hosp ____
  __ pos __ neg __ equiv

y/n **bone scan**, date _____ Hosp _____
  __ pos __ neg __ equiv

y/n **head CT /MR**,date _____ Hosp ____
  __ pos __ neg __ equiv

PATH FINDINGS

Mediastinoscopy

Date :_____, Hosp: _____

Type: ___ cervical, ___ Chamberlain (ant.)
    ___ med dissection at resection

lymph nodes: [for LN diagram, see over]

station #	pos	neg
_____	_____	_____
_____	_____	_____
_____	_____	_____
_____	_____	_____
_____	_____	_____

Surgery

__ bx only, __wedge, __ segment,
__ lobectomy, __ pneumonectomy

Date surgery:_____, Hosp: _____

Path # _____

size of primary (max dimension): ____ cm

bronchial margin: __ pos __ ≤ 2mm __neg

other margin: __ pos __ ≤ 2mm __neg

positive nodes at surgery: _____

Histology: __ adenoca, ___ squamous cell,
   ___ large cell, ___ non-small cell, NOS,
   ___ bronchoalveolar, ___ small cell,
   ___ other, specify: _____

Differentiation: __ well, __ mod., __ poor

Vessel inv.: __ yes, __ no, __ no comment

Lymphatic inv.: __ y, __ n, __ no comment

STAGE [for staging system, see over]

clinical

T ___ N ___ M ___   STAGE ____

pathologic

T ___ N ___ M ___   STAGE ____

If SMALL CELL, ___ limited stage
          ___ extensive stage

PROPOSED TREATMENT

Local Rx:
  ___ surgery, specify:_____
  ___ RT,
  ___ both, give sequence:_____

Systemic Rx (list agents): _____

Sequencing: _____

PHYSICIAN completing form_____ **DATE _____**

Visit Sheet

Date: _____

Schedule return appointment with Dr. _____

Patient:

(and Fellow)_____

Nurse Practitioner _____

in ____ Day(s) ____ Week(s) ____ Month(s)

DX: _____   Chemo Regimen: _____

SCHEDULE:	Today	ASAP	Before Next Appointment	Next Appointment	Clinical Data
CBC, Diff					**CENTRAL VENOUS ACCESS**
Lytes, BUN, Creat					Port: single _____
Bili total ALK p'tase Bili Direct SGOT Total Protein LDH					double _____
ALB/GLOB					PICC: single _____
Glucose					double _____
Cal, Phos, Mg					Other: _____
PT, PTT					
Sed Rate					Continuous Infusion for Chemo _____
CEA					Consult Dr. _____
Type & Cross					Reason:
OrderX-rays					Procedures:
CXR					Reason:
Chest CT					
Abd CT, Pelvic CT					
Cranial CT					
Neck CT					
Bone Scan					
Gallium Scan					
Gated Heart Scan					
Mammogram Bilateral Unilateral (L, R)					
Vascular Studies					
Ultrasound of:					
MRI (cranial)					
MRI of:					
EKG					
Echocardiogram					
PFT with DLCO with O2 Sat.					

TEACHER TO TEACHER

This section contains selected responses of medical terminology teachers to a questionnaire about methods and activities they use in their classrooms. I hope that this will be a springboard for you to communicate with each other and share ideas about teaching. The questions are listed below, and following is an alphabetical list of teachers who responded and included their name and address. I want to thank all of you who took the time to share. Hopefully, you will continue to send comments and suggestions to me via my e-mail (*MedDavi@aol.com*) or our new website for teachers and students (*http://evolve.elsevier.com/chabner/language*).

Questionnaire

1. What activities or teaching aids have you developed to use in your classroom to make the subject come alive?
2. Have you developed any interesting quiz formats that your students find helpful?
3. Have you developed any supplemental handouts that are helpful to students?
4. What do you do to help students who have poor English skills?
5. What is your method of grading and evaluating students' work, and how do you encourage and praise their efforts?
6. What do you do to help students with pronunciation and spelling of medical terms?
7. Do you have any special hints to teach medical terminology to handicapped (visually impaired or hearing-impaired) students?
8. What lessons have you developed to teach various sections in *The Language of Medicine?*
9. Can you suggest ways of teaching terminology to a heterogenous group of students (various backgrounds and abilities)?
10. Do you have any humorous handouts to share with other teachers? (These are included in the following section of the teacher's manual, entitled "Medical Terminology Bloopers and Jokes.)"

Teachers

Mary Lu Albee
Biology Department
Lewis & Clark Community College
Godfrey, Illinois

Jeanne Christen
Phoenix College
Phoenix, Arizona

Carol Conti
School of Nursing
Elizabeth General Medical Center
Elizabeth, New Jersey

Brenda Erickson
John A. Logon College
Carterville, Illinois

Peggy G. Fuller
Bossier Parish Community College
Bossier City, Louisiana

Brenda Haueisen
Mason Lake ISD Technical Preparation
    Partnership
West Shore Community College
Scottville, Michigan

Linda Howe
Roper School of Nursing
Charleston, South Carolina

Trudi James-Parks
Radiologic Technology
Lorain County Community College
Elyria, Ohio

Janet Leitheiser
St. Paul Technical College
St. Paul, Minnesota

Thomas W. Owen
Billings Business College
Billings, Montana

Lu Ann Reicks
Iowa Central Community College
Fort Dodge, Iowa

Joy Renfro
Eastern Kentucky University
Richmond, Kentucky

Connie M. Schoon
Alpena Community College
Alpena, Michigan

Mary Schrader
Southwest Wisconsin Technical College
Fennimore, Wisconsin

Scott Sechrist
Nuclear Medicine
Old Dominion University
Norfolk, Virginia

David Tate
Medical Technology Program
Purdue University School of Health Sciences
West Lafayette, Indiana

Connie Taylor
Department of Biology
Southeastern Oklahoma State University
Durant, Oklahoma

Dottie Tolson
Edgecombe Community College
Tarboro, North Carolina

Susan J. Webb
Victoria, British Columbia
Canada

QUESTION ONE

What activities or teaching aids have you developed to use in your classroom to make the subject come alive?

Albee: I require students to find one article/week with at least 20 medical terms that they define and then summarize the article in common language.

Erickson: (1) Transparencies (color) for some sections; (2) made our own cassette tapes dictating words at the end of each chapter; (3) flash cards.

Fuller: I have included speakers: oncologist, ophthalmologist, physical therapist, x-ray technician, ER physician, and others.

Haueisen: When I teach body planes, positions and cavities, I use E.L. Fudge cookies and colored toothpicks to help the students see each body area. Each student gets two cookies and one each of red, blue, yellow and green toothpicks. After using overheads and model torsos to show all the areas then I have the students "put the blue toothpick in the anatomical left lateral portion of the cookie" and "put the yellow toothpick in the anatomical right lateral of the cookie." They are also instructed to "put the green toothpick in the superior aspect and red toothpick in the inferior aspect." Students then compare their toothpick placement to their partner's and if they don't match they check their text to see why not. We continue the activity with "divide the cookie along the coronal plane and break the anterior aspect along the transverse plane." I continue with various instructions until we have covered all body planes and directions. We get a lot of mileage out of two cookies and the students have fun and get a treat. Gummy bears work too and I'm sure some other cookies might be suitable. I have used it with high school and college groups and they all seemed to enjoy it.

Howe: I use A&P films with each unit and play <u>Jeopardy</u> or <u>Family Feud</u> as a review.

Leitheiser: Do some lab - microscope work; anatomical models, crossword puzzles, short work sheets to do at the end of each lecture.

Owen: Video tapes of operations. Check with doctors' offices for this type of material.

Schoon: Students are required to make their own flash cards and then with a partner, they flash the cards and test each other. I photocopied the diagram of the heart with the identified parts omitted. This was used to make a transparency, reduced to fit their flash cards and then became a question on the test. Having the diagram without answers is an excellent study aid for students.

Schrader: I have prepared a telecourse based on *The Language of Medicine*. I also teach a medical terminology course over ITV for students in our district and have prepared TV-ready visuals. I demonstrate the use of flash cards, student-prepared audiotapes, and other teaching tools over the television. Computer-enhanced video has helped emphasize words as I pronounce them.

Sechrist: I use lots of x-rays, scans, other medical images to bring the words "alive." There's nothing like an ultrasound to help demonstrate cholelithiasis! I assign diseases to each student, have another student define the term, and a third student give a second opinion or act as an attorney. I also use history sheets from actual patient files.

Tate: I occasionally break students into small groups. Each group has an MD, lab director/pathologist, and med tech. They are each given a paper with diagnostic requests on it. For example, the MD fills out a lab test and this is run through the pathologist and MT. Each segment requires the student to understand the abbreviation and terminology before moving to the next segment. This helps in that they must explain to me what the tests are asking for. We have fun and results then indicate quality of patient care.

Taylor:	Students must <u>make</u> their own flash cards—especially for word parts.
Tolson:	I use personal experiences as well as those that have been shared with me by others.
Webb:	I encourage students to study with a friend and it works! I also encourage the use of flashcards and tapes, and bring in guest speakers.
Anonymous:	Guest speakers, physician speakers, videos, illustrations of procedures (found in physician's library at local hospital).
Anonymous:	I use a lot of stories—having worked in healthcare for 20+ years.
Anonymous:	Team Jeopardy for large classes or individual Jeopardy for smaller ones. Group discussions of case studies.
Anonymous:	For a class on the respiratory system, I take the class outside and ask them to turn their heads upward to the sky to feel the sun and breeze on their faces. Then I ask that they feel air coursing through their air passages. I want them to feel the freedom of exchanging air. Next, I get them to take a finger and close one side of their nose. By closing a nare, the student understands words such as obstruction, anxiety, panic—many of the symptoms that a client with a compromised respiratory system feels. Positive feedback has been given by the students.
Anonymous:	Patient records. Approach from a clinical perspective.
Anonymous:	I usually write case studies that go along with each chapter—to encourage students to describe in "lay" terms.
Anonymous:	I use CIBA slides.

QUESTION TWO

Have you developed any interesting quiz formats that your students find helpful?

Albee:	I select 2–3 paragraphs containing medical terminology and highlight 10–20 terms which the students define. If time permits, they summarize the articles in common language.
James-Parks:	My final exam is comprehensive, but it is done by the student outside the classroom. Students are asked to select an article from a medical journal and rewrite a portion of it by changing the medical terms into lay terms. This has proven to be an interesting exercise which takes some thought and skill at interpretation of terms.
Owen:	Take selections from source documents and have students write out in common terms to ascertain understanding.
Schoon:	Use crosswords and word searches as quizzes.
Sechrist:	I give a 50–100 question exam every week (course meets for 2-1/2 hours—14 weeks long).
Taylor:	I give 100 point tests each week—mostly matching, but they must define word parts as well.

Webb: Each class begins with 10 minutes to do a crossword puzzle regarding the exam for that night. We then do a 25-word spelling test. Then they do the exam for that night. I use the flow charts and diagrams on the exam if there is one in the chapter.

Anonymous: I tell my students that I feel that their quiz grades are a grade for me and my abilities as a teacher. Seems to relax them when I stress this.

Anonymous: The students grade one another in oral quizzes, listening to see if the term is spelled correctly.

QUESTION THREE

Have you developed any supplemental handouts that are helpful to students?

Albee: I use crosswords or word searches for classroom and homework activities.

Erickson: (1) Supplemental drug (including new and unusual) and abbreviations handouts, (2) health articles found in local newspaper's health section, (3) handouts made from appendices from healthcare reference books.

Leitheiser: I have developed a more in-depth diagram of the kidney, and I use pictures of cells (WBCs and RBCs).

Schrader: I have prepared a student packet that informs students in all 3 medical terminology courses as to what and how to cover each unit.

Sechrist: I have used diagrams, photos, scanned images, even myself as a model during class. I also bring in used or discarded equipment to demonstrate medical technology terms (i.e., ophthalmoscope).

QUESTION FOUR

What do you do to help students who have poor English skills?

Christen: One-on-one tutoring-referral to learning center. It should be noted that medical terminology is approached like learning any second language.

Erickson: I have prepared cassette tapes where I dictate the terms at end of the chapter, pause so students can write the word, then spell the word so students can immediately check their spelling. Some of our adult learners who have difficulty spelling have found this to be very helpful.

Fuller: I encourage the use of the tape machine—if English is their second language they do very well. If they have non-standard English with no skills, I refer them to the developmental student's office.

Schrader: We have a special skills department. Students have each and every word pronounced and used on an individual card that has the word written on it. Students can see the word and run it through the machine—one at a time.

Sechrist: The English as a second language students I have had over the past 7 years have typically done better than the "traditional students." My theory is they work harder at memorization and pronouncing the terms.

Anonymous: I go down the row (line) and ask each student to give the answer and spell the term.

Anonymous: We have special tutors for these students. Students must pass an examination for English skills prior to admission to class.

Anonymous: Emphasize adjectival, adverbial endings and noun forms of terms.

Anonymous: Individual tutoring if needed. Place in group with students who can assist them.

Anonymous: One-to-one tutoring is offered; all students participate in test reviews and read the questions and answers (reading aloud helps everyone).

QUESTION FIVE

What is your method of grading and evaluating students' work, and how do you encourage and praise their efforts?

Anonymous: Any word misspelled is wrong; every term they get wrong I have them write 5 times correctly and then I give them 1/2 of the points they miss.

Albee: 20% of grade is weekly chapter quiz
20% of grade is based on the articles they bring in
40% of grade is 4 unit exams (4–6 chapters each)
20% of grade is comprehensive final

Quizzes and exams concentrate on testing knowledge of terms (70%) and anatomy and physiology (30%). Knowing that this will be the format for at least 50% of each quiz instills confidence. I encourage students individually and verbally and on returned papers. Student papers are corrected carefully.

Format for quizzes—5 sections are the core of all quizzes and exams: (1) matching word parts and definitions; (2) defining terms; (3) building terms; (4) defining abbreviations; (5) abbreviating terms.

Christen: Weekly quizzes with quarterly exams and final comprehensive exam. Students may elect to remove one quiz score and "A" Students do not have to count the final.

Erickson: Each exam (7) worth from 350–500 pts. Each exam consists of spelling, roots, suffixes, prefixes, definitions, matching, diagrams and multiple choice. Final is only multiple choice and is comprehensive. Scale: 94+ A, 85–93 B, 75–84 C, 69–74 D.

Fuller: 75% of grade comprises chapter examinations, 25% is comprehensive final. Lowest grade is dropped. Final comprehensive exam is not dropped.

James-Parks: Unit exams equal 2/3 of the final grade, and the final is 1/3 of the grade.

Owen: Always put number correct over total number/never use red to correct/believe it or not, hand-drawn comical smiley faces for perfect papers work well.

Schoon: Personal talks and short notes on quizzes. First quiz is a no-brainer—everyone gets 100%—a real morale booster at the beginning of semester.

Schrader: You might enjoy reading "The Teaching Professor." There are often methods shared by other faculty. I try very hard to give feedback. I use a system of name cards to encourage students. As I call on a student with a question, I check the student name card in my hand. If the student had difficulty with several questions over the past week (identified by a mark on my card that only I see), I address an easy, memorization-type question—maybe 2 or 3 in a row—and then indicate with another mark if the student is successful. This makes all students comfortable in asking/answering questions. It works.

Sechrist:	I keep a seating chart, keep notes on who is up to date and ready to answer each week. Students may elect to "pass" on an oral question twice, then I meet with them one on one.
Taylor:	Give 100-point test each week, but drop two grades. Final is comprehensive.
Tolson:	I give a test on each chapter and a separate spelling test on each chapter. A comprehensive exam is also given.
Anonymous:	I always mark 1/2 pt off for spelling and 1 pt off for wrong answer.
Anonymous:	Much verbal and written praise.
Anonymous:	Weekly quiz plus written note on papers; partial credit if term is known. As many of my students are older—"Refrigerator papers" for excellence.
Anonymous:	Students are given take-home quizzes and crossword puzzles.
Anonymous:	Listen, listen, listen. Most, if not all, students know their weak areas and know what to do about it. For the most part, students want to bounce off their ideas with faculty to see if they are on the right track.

QUESTION SIX

What do you do to help students with pronunciation and spelling of medical terms?

Albee:	We go over the word parts and examples together. Students take turns pronouncing and defining the terms to get practice. I point out spelling difficulties with certain terms as they come up.
Christen:	Tapes are used, along with verbal sharing in class. Spelling is incorporated in quizzes.
Fuller:	Have them listen to tapes and pronounce words in class.
Schoon:	Pronounce each term and they repeat after me. Then, divide into groups, have them practice as groups while I stroll among them to make corrections and answer questions. I usually pronounce words for students the class period before they are assigned (i.e., on last day of Chapter 3, I take a few minutes and pronounce all words for Chapter 4).
Tate:	We do group pronunciation and I randomly select students to pronounce words. I also bring in MDs and Med Techs.
Taylor:	We pronounce the terms out loud. I pronounce first and students then pronounce terms. We go through the list at the back of each chapter. Then we go around the room with each student pronouncing a term. They become used to using and saying terms out loud and in front of each other.
Tolson:	I pronounce the words and have the students repeat the terms after me. Students are allowed to tape the classes.
Anonymous:	Pronunciation drills are a part of each class. Spelling is a part of each weekly quiz. Hints are given to prompt correct spelling as each word is introduced in lecture.
Anonymous:	I have taped a total of 60 minutes of words for each section; students can have a copy for their own use.

QUESTION SEVEN

Do you have any special hints to teach medical terminology to handicapped (visually impaired or hearing-impaired) students?

Chabner:	One of my students had multiple sclerosis. I found that if I designed the exams for all matching and multiple choice questions she could easily circle items or put numbers in answer spaces.
Christen:	Taped lectures for review. I tape quizzes and exams. We have a learning center with special equipment for enlarging type.
Erickson:	Hearing-impaired individuals can easily be accommodated with written materials. Also, if they can read lips, we dictate every term every class. Also, we provide a signer for the hearing-impaired.
Schrader:	I had a visually impaired student in the class and have used single-word audio cards to spell and pronounce the term.
Sechrist:	I allowed the one visually impaired student I had to sit closer to me and to the board.

QUESTION EIGHT

What lessons have you developed to teach various sections in *The Language of Medicine?*

Albee:	I also teach A and P and bring in models and transparencies to illustrate.
Schoon:	We do most of this sort of thing with games, crosswords, word searches, regular classroom drill, use of skeletons and models, group work, etc.
Taylor:	I use overheads and give lectures—mostly work on definitions.
Anonymous:	Hands-on with a skeleton—oral and written questioning pertaining to practical applications boxes. I usually have some form of abbreviations on oral and written questions.
Anonymous:	For practical applications, I use actual history and physicals and let the students decipher them.

QUESTION NINE

Can you suggest ways of teaching terminology to a heterogenous group of students (various backgrounds and abilities)?

Albee:	I use group work in class—having students work on defining terms in the practical applications section in pairs or in small groups.
Christen:	Utilization of increased student interaction. Increased use of humor and relation to real-life situations.
Howe:	I teach on at least three levels. I reinforce using personal experience or equate to things they know. Also, they work together on teams.
James-Parks:	I have developed a method of teaching medical terminology based on a method called PSI (Personalized System of Instruction). It is a method of mastery learning. Each student progresses through the course (using *The Language of Medicine*) at their own pace and takes exams as they complete each unit. If they are unsuccessful in a unit, they have a second opportunity for mastery. This is one way I have dealt with students of various backgrounds and abilities.

Owen: Treat them as individuals/Give them immediate success/Relate to their own body—use it as a reference.

Schoon: This is my regular class population. I usually treat all the same but use those who have had anatomy and physiology as group leaders.

Schrader: I work hard every semester to be sensitive to individuals.

Anonymous: I have students with less background as leaders in group sessions. Pride makes them try harder!

Anonymous: The more advanced students help the slower ones. Study groups.

Anonymous: I bring the backgrounds of different types of students into the discussion in class.

Anonymous: Give examples of lay terms where the word parts are used. Common words can be identified with and the background of the student doesn't matter.

QUESTION TEN

Do you have any humorous handouts to share with other teachers?

(I have put together some of these handouts and included them in the next sections, "Common Usage Terms" and "Medical Terminology Bloopers and Jokes.")

Erickson: Besides a few assorted cartoons, I have a collection of Frank & Ernest cartoons that make fun of situations in healthcare. The dry sense of humor is well received with my adult learners.

Schrader: The students get to know me as their teacher and I use jokes—at least one a class period to keep their attention and interest up. Humor works in the standard classroom quite well, but does not work as well on TV.

Anonymous: I use personal experience.

COMMON USAGE TERMS

The following are common terms used by patients to describe symptoms and disorders.

1. "asleep" .... Paresthesias (of an extremity); numbness and tingling.
2. "bad blood" .... Syphilis or STD.
3. "blackout" .... Syncope (fainting).
4. "bowels" .... Intestines, colon.
5. "bug" .... (1) Insect or spider
   .... (2) Infectious disease.
6. "charley horse" .... Injury to a leg causing pain and limping; cause is usually pulled muscle or tendon.
7. "clap" .... Gonorrhea.
8. "clog" .... Clot of blood.
9. "crabs" .... Infestation with lice.
10. "crick" .... Painful spasm in a muscle; often in the neck.
11. "dry heaves" .... Retching, gagging without vomiting.
12. "game" .... Disabled by disease or injury (of an extremity).
13. "gimpy" .... Lame.
14. "goose egg" .... Swelling due to trauma (hematoma).
15. "heaves" .... Vomiting.
16. "irregularity" .... Constipation.
17. "mouse" .... Hematoma around the eye; "black eye."
18. "nature" .... Male sexual potency.
19. "oyster" .... Mass of mucus coughed up from the lungs.
20. "passage" .... Defecation.
21. "physic" .... Laxative.
22. "piles" .... Hemorrhoids.
23. "pins and needles" .... Paresthesias; see "asleep."
24. "plumbing" .... (1) Male or female urinary system
    .... (2) Penis.
25. "queasy" .... Faint or nauseated.
26. "runs" .... Diarrhea.
27. "sand" .... Encrusted secretions around the eye.
28. "shin splints" .... Pain in the anterior muscles of the lower leg caused by running.
29. "shiner" .... Hematoma around the eye; see "mouse."
30. "stitch" .... Sudden, sharp pain.
31. "strain" .... Urethral discharge in the male.
32. "sugar" .... Diabetes mellitus.
33. "sun poisoning" .... Used to indicate severe form of sunburn.
34. "trick" .... Unstable (of a joint).

35. "walking pneumonia" ..... Viral or other pneumonia that does not cause severe symptoms.
36. "water" .... (1)Urine
     .... (2)Edema.
37. "zit" .... Blackhead (comedo).

MEDICAL TERMINOLOGY BLOOPERS AND JOKES

Transcription Bloopers

The correct term is in parentheses.

1. "Bilingual" (inguinal) hernias.
2. Marital "discharge" (discord).
3. Bilateral "Cadillacs" (cataracts).
4. "Sick as hell" (sickle-cell) anemia.
5. Medication "regime" (regimen).
6. "April" (atrial) fibrillation.
7. There are no other palpable "nerds" (nodes).
8. BuSpar 10 mg, two p.o. b.i.d. #80, no "refunds" (refills).
9. Patient had a "Pabst beer" (Pap smear) today.
10. This was a case of "old timers" disease (Alzheimer's disease).
11. Pelvic ultrasound revealed "firebirds in the Eucharist" (fibroids in the uterus).
12. There was a recent outbreak of chicken "pops" (pox).
13. The colonoscope was passed into the "assending" (ascending) colon.
14. The term visceral means internal "orgasm" (organs).
15. The patient finally had a hysterectomy and "Singapore-roofectomy" (salpingo-oophorectomy).

Patient Malaprops

1. A doctor reported that during an interview with a patient—a middle aged woman—she reported that she had had her "ovary's sister" (ovarian cyst) removed.
2. A man walked into an ER complaining that he had taken "all six of those explositories" (suppositories) and still wasn't getting any relief.
3. While giving her history, a new patient related that there was a time when she thought she had "hog's skin disease" (Hodgkin's disease), but thankfully was proven wrong.
4. A patient presented at rounds with a complaint of "leakage from the micro-valve" (mitral valve). The doctor thought of recommending a plumber.
5. A patient reported being unable to "decaffeinate" (defecate).
6. Recently a patient appeared in a New York City ER complaining of "toxic sock syndrome" (toxic shock syndrome).

7. A patient informed her doctor that she had diverticulosis and had increased the amount of "fabric" (fiber) in her diet.

8. A man was admitted to the CCU complaining of chest pain. The family history was positive for heart disease, but the physician wasn't sure since the patient reported that his mother had "digestive" (congestive) heart failure.

9. One patient wasn't sure he believed his neurologist when he told him performing a "lumber puncture" (lumbar) wouldn't hurt.

10. One little boy volunteered that he knew his brother had his "independence" (appendix) cut out last year.

11. A patient always refers to her condition as "room of toys" (rheumatoid) arthritis.

Unusual Definitions for Medical Terms

(Humorous definitions of medical terms circulate freely throughout the medical community. This is just a sample of what can be found.)

Aorta	A statement of something you should do.
Artery	The study of fine paintings.
Bacteria	The back door of a cafeteria.
Barium	What you do when CPR fails.
Benign	What you are after you are eight.
Bowel	A letter like A, E, I, O, or U.
Bunion	Paul's surname.
Carpal	Someone with whom you drive to work.
Cat scan	Searching for kitty.
Cauterize	Made eye contact with her.
Cesarean section	A district in Rome.
Chiropractor	An Egyptian doctor.
Colic	A sheep dog.
Coma	A punctuation mark.
Congenital	Friendly.
Constipation	Endangered feces.
D & C	Where Washington is located.
Dilate	To live long.
Ear	Where you are now.
Elixir	What a dog gives to his owner when she gives him a bone.
Enema	Not a friend; as in "a guy like that is his own worst enema."
Fester	Quicker.
Fibrillate	To tell a small lie.
Genital	Non-Jew.
G.I. series	Military ball game.
Hangnail	Coat hook.
Hemorrhoid	Transportation given to a third person; as, "He didn't have his car so I offered hemorrhoid."

Hernia .... Referring to a female's knee.

Humerus .... Tell us what we want to hear.

Impotent .... Distinguished, well-known.

Inbred .... The best way to eat peanut butter.

Inguinal .... A new type of Italian noodle.

Intubate .... What a fisherman is.

Kidney .... Part of a child's leg.

Labor pain .... Injured at work.

Medical staff .... A doctor's cane.

Migraine .... What a Russian farmer now says about his harvest.

Minor operation .... Coal digging.

Morbid .... A higher offer.

Nitrates .... Cheaper than day rates.

Node .... Was aware of.

Organic .... Church musician.

Outpatient .... A person who has fainted.

Ova .... Finished; done with.

Pap smear .... Fatherhood test; or to slander your father.

Pelvis .... Cousin to Elvis.

Penis .... Someone who plays the piano.

Protein .... In favor of young people.

Post-operative .... A letter carrier.

Recovery room .... A place to do upholstery.

Rectum .... Dang near killed 'em.

Sacrum .... Holy.

Secretion .... Hiding anything.

Seizure .... Roman emperor.

Serology .... A study of English knighthood.

Serum .... What you do when you barbecue steaks.

Sperm .... To reject.

Tablet .... A small table.

Terminal illness .... Getting sick at the airport.

Tumor .... An extra pair.

Urine .... Opposite of you're out.

Urticaria .... Insisting to be manually transported; as, "The only reason that child is screaming at his mother is that he wants urticaria."

Varicose .... Nearby.

Vein .... Conceited.

Vitamin .... What you do when friends stop by for a visit.

REFERENCE MATERIAL

The dictionaries, texts, and magazines listed below are materials that I have found helpful in teaching my medical terminology classes. I recommend them to you and your students as sources for study of the medical language as well as related concepts in anatomy and physiology.

Dictionaries

Dorland's Illustrated Medical Dictionary, 30th edition. Philadelphia, W.B. Saunders, 2003.

Dorland's Pocket Medical Dictionary with CD-ROM, 27th edition. Philadelphia, W.B. Saunders, 2004.

Miller-Keane, O'Toole MT (editor): Miller-Keane Encyclopedia and Dictionary of Medicine, Nursing & Allied Health—Revised Reprint, 7th edition. Philadelphia, W.B. Saunders, 2005.

Mosby's Dental Dictionary, St Louis, Mosby, 2004.

Mosby's Dictionary of Medicine, Nursing & Health Professions, 7th edition. St. Louis, Mosby, 2005.

Texts

Barkauskas VH, Baumann LC, Darling-Fisher CS: Health and Physical Assessment, 3rd edition, St. Louis Mosby, 2002.

Beers MH, Porter RS, Jones TV: Merck Manual of Diagnosis and Therapy, 18th edition. Hoboken, NJ, John Wiley & Sons, 2006.
(Good reference for looking up answers to the questions you couldn't answer in class.)

Black JM, Hawks J: Medical-Surgical Nursing: Clinical Management for Positive Outcomes, 7th edition. Philadelphia, W.B. Saunders, 2005.

Boston Women's Health Book Collective: Our Bodies, Ourselves: A New Edition for a New Era. New York, Touchstone Books, 2005.
(Paperback full of readable, accurate information for women and men about many aspects of female health and physiology. Chapters include anatomy and physiology of reproduction and sexuality, venereal disease, birth control, abortion, rape and self-defense, childbearing, menopause, and many others.)

Callen JP, Greer KE, Paller AS, Swinyer LJ: Color Atlas of Dermatology, 2nd edition, Philadelphia, W.B. Saunders, 2000.

Damjanov I: Pathology for the Health Professions, 3rd edition. Philadelphia, W.B. Saunders, 2006.

Frazier MS, Drzymkowski J: Essentials of Human Disease and Conditions, 3rd Edition, Philadelphia, W.B. Saunders, 2004.

Goldman L, Ausiello DA (editors): Cecil Textbook of Medicine, 22nd edition. Philadelphia, W.B. Saunders, 2004.
(Valuable reference source for information about disease processes related to internal medicine.)

Gould BE: Pathophysiology for the Health Professions, 3rd edition. Philadelphia, W.B. Saunders, 2006.

Guyton AC: Textbook of Medical Physiology, 11th edition. Philadelphia, W.B. Saunders, 2006.
(*Excellent basic physiology text.*)

Haubrich WS (editor): Medical Meanings, A Glossary of Word Origins, 2nd edition. Philadelphia, American College of Physicians, 2003.
(*Interesting explanations of medical etymology.*)

Herlihy B: The Human Body in Health and Illness, 3rd edition, Philadelphia, W.B. Saunders, 2007.

Ignatavicius DD, Workman ML: Medical-Surgical Nursing: Critical Thinking for Collaborative Care, 5th edition. Philadelphia, W.B. Saunders, 2006.

Jarvis C: Physical Examination and Health Assessment, 4th edition. Philadelphia, W.B. Saunders, 2004.

Kumar V, Cotran RS, Robbins SL: Robbins Basic Pathology Updated Edition, 7th edition. Philadelphia, W.B. Saunders, 2005.
(*Easy to read pathology text.*)

Lewis SM, Heitkemper MM, Dirksen SR: Medical-Surgical Nursing: Assessment and Management of Clinical Problems, 6th edition. St. Louis, Mosby, 2004.

Moore KL, Persaud TVN: Before We Are Born, 6th edition. Philadelphia, W.B. Saunders, 2003.
(*Basic embryology and birth defects.*)

Sheldon H: Boyd's Introduction to the Study of Disease, 11th edition. Philadelphia, Lippincott, Williams & Wilkins, 1992.
(*Good source of information about diseases, written in nontechnical language.*)

Siedel HM et al: Mosby's Guide to Physical Examination, 6th edition. St. Louis, Mosby, 2006.

Silverman, HM: The Pill Book: The Illustrated Guide to the Most Prescribed Drugs in the United States, 12th edition. New York, Bantam Books, 2006.
(*Basic information on prescription drugs.*)

Solomon EP: Introduction to Human Anatomy and Physiology, 2nd edition, Philadelphia, W.B. Saunders, 2003.

Solomon EP, Phillips GA: Understanding Human Anatomy and Physiology. Philadelphia, W.B. Saunders, 1987.
(*Easy to read, excellent illustrations.*)

Swartz MH: Textbook of Physical Diagnosis: History and Examination with STUDENT CONSULT Access, 5th edition. Philadelphia, W.B. Saunders, 2006.
(*Explanations and diagrams of procedures related to patient care.*)

Thibodeau GA, Patton KT: Anatomy & Physiology, 6th edition, St. Louis, Mosby, 2006.

Thibodeau GA, Patton KT: Structure & Function of the Body, 12th edition., St. Louis, Mosby, 2004.
(*Simplified anatomy and physiology for the student with little or no background in science.*)

Tkachuk DC, Hirschmann JV, McArthur JR: Atlas of Clinical Hematology, Philadelphia, W.B. Saunders, 2002.

Townsend CM (et al) (editors): Sabiston Textbook of Surgery, 17th edition. Philadelphia, W.B. Saunders, 2004.
(*Helpful in describing surgical procedures and related diseases.*)

Magazines

The following is a list of magazines that I have found helpful in understanding many disease processes. I clip articles, file them by subject, and bring them into class for students to read. Although the articles are written for family practitioners and internists, they are written in simple, nontechnical, medical language and often include excellent diagrams and illustrations.

American Family Physician. American Academy of Family Physicians, Lisle, Illinois, http://www.aafp.org.

CA—A Cancer Journal for Clinicians. Lippincott Williams & Wilkins, New York, http://www.lww.com.

Emergency Medicine. Quadrant HealthCom, Chatham, New Jersey, http://www.emedmag.com.

Patient Care. Medical Economics Co., Montvale, New Jersey, http://www.patientcareonline.com/patcare.

Resident and Staff Physician. Ascend Media LLC, Princeton, New Jersey, http://www.residentandstaff.com.

Publications by R.N. Medical Economics Co., Montvale, New Jersey, 313-761-4700.

RESOURCES*

Sources for Patient Education Materials

Abbott Laboratories
100 Abbott Park Road
Abbott Park, IL 60064-3500
847-937-6100
www.abbott.com

AGC/United Learning
1560 Sherman Ave., Suite 100
Evanston, IL 60201
888-892-3484
www.unitedlearning.com

Alfred Higgins Productions, Inc.
15500 Hamner Drive
Los Angeles, CA 90077
800-766-5353
www.alfredhigginsprod.com

American Cancer Society
1599 Clifton Rd., NE
Atlanta, GA 30329
800-ACS-2345
www.cancer.org

American Dental Association
211 E. Chicago Ave.
17th Floor
Chicago, IL 60611
312-440-2500
www.ada.org

American Diabetes Association
National Center
1701 N. Beauregard St.
Alexandria, VA 22311
800-342-2383
www.diabetes.org

American Dietetic Association
120 South Riverside Plaza, Suite 2000
Chicago, IL 60606-6995
800-877-1600
www.eatright.org

American Liver Foundation
75 Maiden Lane, Suite 603
New York, NY 10038
800-465-4837
www.liverfoundation.org

American Lung Association
61 Broadway, 6th floor
New York, NY 10006
212-315-8700
www.lungusa.org

American Red Cross
2025 E Street, NW
Washington, DC 20006
202-303-4498
www.redcross.org

Arthritis Foundation
2970 Peachtree Road NW
Suite 200
Atlanta, GA 30305
404-872-7100
www.arthritis.org

Channing Bete Company
One Community Place
South Deerfield, MA 01373-0200
800-477-4776
www.channing-bete.com

*Adapted from O'Toole, M (ed): Miller-Keane Encyclopedia & Dictionary of Medicine, Nursing & Allied Health. 7th ed. Philadelphia, W.B. Saunders, 2005. Please visit our website, http://evolve.elsevier.com/chabner/language/ for updates of this information.

Cystic Fibrosis Foundation
6931 Arlington Rd
Bethesda, MD 20814
1-800-344-4823
www.cff.org

Eli Lilly and Company
Lilly Corporate Center
Indianapolis, IN 46285
317-276-2000
www.lilly.com

Elsevier/Mosby
11830 Westline Industrial Drive
St. Louis, MO 63146
800-325-4177
www.elsevier.com

Elsevier/WB Saunders
1600 John F. Kennedy Boulevard,
Suite 1800
Philadelphia, PA 19103-2899
215-239-3900
www.elsevier.com

Glaxo SmithKline
One Franklin Plaza
P.O. Box 7929
Philadelphia, PA 19101
888-825-5249
www.gsk.com

Johnson and Johnson
One Johnson and Johnson Plaza
New Brunswick, NJ 08903
732-524-0400
www.jnj.com

Juvenile Diabetes Foundation International
120 Wall Street
New York, NY 10005
800-533-2873
www.jdfcure.org

March of Dimes Birth Defect Foundation
1275 Mamaroneck Ave.
White Plains, NY 10605
914-997-4488
www.modimes.org

Maternity Center Association
281 Park Avenue South, 5th floor
New York, NY 10010
212-777-5000
www.maternity.org

McNeil Laboratories
Consumer Affairs Department
7050 Camp Hill Rd.
Ft. Washington, PA 19034-2292
215-233-7171
www.mcneilcampusrecruiting.com

Merck & Co., Inc.
One Merck Drive
P.O. Box 100
Whitehouse Station, NJ 08889-0100
908-423-1000
www.merck.com

National Autism Association
1330 W. Schatz Lane
Nixa, MO 65714
877-622-2884
www.nationalautismassociation.org

National Council on Alcoholism and Drug
  Dependence, Inc.
22 Cortlandt Street, Suite 801
New York, NY 10007-3128
212-269-7797
www.ncadd.org

National Healthy Mothers, Healthy Babies
  Coalition
2000 N. Beauregard Street
6th Floor
Alexandria, VA 22311
703-836-6110
www.hmhb.org

National Hydrocephalus Foundation
12413 Centralia Road
Lakewood, CA 90715-1623
562-402-3523
www.nhfonline.org

National Institute on Drug Abuse (NIDA)
6001 Executive Blvd., Room 5213
Bethesda, MD 20892
301-443-1124
www.drugabuse.gov

National Kidney Foundation
30 E. 33rd St.
New York, NY 10016
800-622-9010
www.kidney.org

National Mental Health Association
2000 N. Beauregard Street, 6th Floor
Alexandria, VA 22311
800-969-6642
www.nmha.org

National Multiple Sclerosis Society
733 Third Ave.
New York, NY 10017-3288
1-800-344-4867
www.nmss.org

National Safety Council
1121 Spring Lake Drive
Itasca, IL 60143
800-621-7619
www.nsc.org

National Scoliosis Foundation
5 Cabot Place
Stoughton, MA 02072
800-673-6922
www.scoliosis.org

National Tay-Sachs and Allied Diseases
   Association, Inc.
2001 Beacon St., Suite 204
Brighton, MA 02135
800-906-8723
www.ntsad.org

National Women's Health Network
514 10th St., NW, Suite 400
Washington, DC 20004
202-347-1140
www.womenshealthnetwork.org

Novartis Institutes for BioMedical
   Research, Inc.
250 Massachusetts Avenue
Cambridge, MA 02139
617-871-8000
www.novartis.com

Novo Nordisk Pharmaceuticals
Novo Nordisk Inc.
100 College Road West
Princeton, NJ 08540
800-727-6500
www.novo-nordisk.com

Organon Corporation
56 Livingston Ave
Roseland, NJ 07068
800-241-8812
973-325- 4500
www.organon-usa.com

Ortho Pharmaceutical Corporation
1000 Route 202 South
Raritan, NJ 08869-0602
800-526-7736
www.ortho-mcneil.com

Pfizer Laboratories
Pfizer, Inc.
235 E. 42nd St.
New York, NY 10017
212-733-2323
www.pfizer.com

Planned Parenthood Federation of America
434 West 33rd Street
New York, NY 10001
212-541-7800
www.plannedparenthood.org

Roche Diagnostics Corporation
9115 Hague Road
PO Box 50457
Indianapolis, IN 46256
317-521-2000
www.roche-diagnostics.com

Ross Laboratories
Consumer Relations
625 Cleveland Ave.
Columbus, OH 43215
800-986-8510
www.rosslabs.com

SAMHSA's National Clearinghouse for
   Alcohol and Drug Information
P.O. Box 2345
Rockville, MD 20847-2345
800-729-6686
www.health.org

Skin Cancer Foundation
245 Fifth Ave., Suite 1403
New York, NJ 10016
800-SKIN-490
www.skincancer.org

Spina Bifida Association of America
4590 MacArthur Blvd., NW
Suite 250
Washington, DC 20007
800-621-3141
202-944-3285
www.sbaa.org

United Ostomy Association of America, Inc.
P.O. Box 66
Fairview, TN 37062-0066
800-826-0826
www.uoaa.org

Voluntary Health and Welfare Agencies and Associations

Administration on Aging
Washington, DC 20201
202-619-0724
www.aoa.gov

Alcoholics Anonymous World Service Office
475 Riverside Drive, Suite 832
New York, NY 10115
212-870-3400
www.alcoholics-anonymous.org

Alzheimer's Association
225 N. Michigan Ave., Floor 1700
Chicago, IL 60601
800-272-3900
www.alz.org

American Academy of Allergy, Asthma,
   and Immunology
555 East Wells Street
Suite 1100
Milwaukee, WI 53202-3823
800-822-2762
414-272-6071
www.aaaai.org

American Anorexia Bulimia Association
418 E. 76th Street
New York, New York 10021
212-734-1114
www.aabainc.org

American Association of Kidney Patients
3505 E Frontage Rd, Suite 315
Tampa, FL 33607
800-749-2257
813-636-8100
www.aakp.org

American Association on Mental Retardation
444 N. Capitol Street, NW
Suite 846
Washington, DC 20001-1512
800-424-3688
202-387-1968
www.aamr.org

American Association of Retired
   Persons (AARP)
601 E Street, NW
Washington, DC 20049
888-687-2277
www.aarp.org

American Cancer Society
1599 Clifton Rd., NE
Atlanta, GA 30329
800-ACS-2345
www.cancer.org

American Dental Association
211 E. Chicago Ave.
17th Floor
Chicago, IL 60611
312-440-2500
www.ada.org

American Diabetes Association
National Center
1701 N. Beauregard St.
Alexandria, VA 22311
800-342-2383
www.diabetes.org

American Foundation for the Blind
11 Penn Plaza, Suite 300
New York, NY 10001
212-502-7600
www.afb.org

American Liver Foundation
75 Maiden Lane, Suite 603
New York, NY 10038
800-465-4837
www.liverfoundation.org

American Lung Association
61 Broadway, 6th floor
New York, NY 10006
212-315-8700
www.lungusa.org

American Pain Society
4700 West Lake Ave.
Glenview, IL 60025
847-375-4715
www.ampainsoc.org

American Parkinson Disease Association, Inc.
135 Parkinson Avenue
Staten Island, NY 10305
800-223-2732
718-981-8001
www.apdaparkinson.org

American Speech-Language-Hearing
  Association
10801 Rockville Pike
Rockville, MD 20852
800-638-8255
www.asha.org

American Tinnitus Association
PO Box 5
Portland, OR 97207
800-634-8978
www.ata.org

ARC of the United States
Association for Retarded Citizens
1010 Wayne Ave.
Suite 650
Silver Spring, MD 20910
301-565-3842
www.TheArc.org

Arthritis Foundation
2970 Peachtree Road NW
Suite 200
Atlanta, GA 30305
404-872-7100
www.arthritis.org

Asthma and Allergy Foundation of America
1233 20th St., NW
Suite 402
Washington, DC 20036
800-727-8462
www.aafa.org

Centers for Disease Control & Prevention
Department of Health and Human Services
U.S. Public Health Service
1600 Clifton Road
Atlanta, GA 30333
800-311-3435
www.cdc.gov

Crohn's and Colitis Foundation of America
386 Park Ave. South
17th Floor
New York, NY 10016-8804
800-932-2423
www.ccfa.org

Cystic Fibrosis Foundation
6931 Arlington Rd
Bethesda, MD 20814
1-800-344-4823
www.cff.org

Epilepsy Foundation
8301 Professional Place
Landover, MD 20785-7223
800-332-1000
www.efa.org

International Dyslexia Association
Chester Building
Suite 382
8600 LaSalle Rd.
Baltimore, MD 21286-2044
800-ABCD-123
410-296-0232
www.interdys.org

La Leche League International
1400 N. Meacham Road
Schaumburg, IL 60173-4808
847-519-7730
www.lalecheleague.org

Leukemia & Lymphoma Society
1311 Mamaroneck Ave.
White Plains, NY 10605
800-955-4572
914-949-5213
www.leukemia-lymphoma.org

Muscular Dystrophy Association
3300 E. Sunrise Dr.
Tucson, AZ 85718
800-344-4863
www.mdausa.org

Myasthenia Gravis Foundation
1821 University Avenue W., Suite S256
St. Paul, MN 55104
800-541-5454
www.myasthenia.org

National Center for the American Heart
  Association
7272 Greenville Ave.
Dallas, TX 75231
800-242-8721
www.americanheart.org

National Easter Seal Society
230 W. Monroe St.
Suite 1800
Chicago, IL 60606-4802
800-221-6827
www.easter-seals.org

National Hemophilia Foundation
116 W. 32nd Street, 11th Floor
New York, NY 10001
212-328-3700
www.hemophilia.org

National Institute of Allergy and Infectious
  Diseases
NIAID Office of Communications and Public
  Liaison
6610 Rockledge Drive, MSC 6612
Bethesda, MD 20892-6612
301-496-5717
www.niaid.nih.gov

National Institutes of Arthritis and
  Musculoskeletal and Skin Diseases
Information Clearinghouse
1 AMS Circle
Bethesda, MD 20892-3675
301-495-4484
www.niams.nih.gov

National Jewish Medical & Research Center
1400 Jackson St.
Denver, CO 80206
800-222-5864
303-388-4461
www.NationalJewish.org

National Kidney Foundation
30 E. 33rd St.
New York, NY 10016
800-622-9010
www.kidney.org

National Multiple Sclerosis Society
733 Third Ave.
New York, NY 10017-3288
1-800-344-4867
www.nmss.org

National Osteoporosis Foundation
1232 22nd St., NW
Washington, DC 20037-1292
202-223-2226
www.nof.org

National Parkinson's Foundation
1501 NW 9th Ave.
Miami, FL 33136
800-327-4545
www.parkinson.org

National Psoriasis Foundation
6600 SW 92nd Ave.
Suite 300
Portland, OR 97223-7195
800-723-9166
www.psoriasis.org

National Safety Council
1121 Spring Lake Drive
Itasca, IL 60143
800-621-7619
www.nsc.org

National Spinal Cord Injury Association
6701 Democracy Blvd, Suite 300-9
Silver Spring, MD 20817
800-962-9629
www.spinalcord.org

Paget's Foundation for Paget's Disease of Bone
& Related Disorders
120 Wall St.
Suite 1602
New York, NY 10005
800-23-PAGET
www.paget.org

Parkinson Disease Foundation
1359 Broadway, Suite 1509
New York, NY 10018
800-457-6676
www.pdf.org

Phoenix Society (assistance following burn
injuries)
1835 R W Berends Dr. SW
Grand Rapids, MI 49519-4955
800-888-2876
www.phoenix-society.org

Prevent Blindness America
211 West Wacker Drive
Suite 1700
Chicago, IL 60606
800-331-2020
www.preventblindness.org

Self Help for Hard of Hearing People (SHHH)
7910 Woodmont Ave.
Suite 1200
Bethesda, MD 20814
301-657-2248
www.shhh.org

Sexuality Information and Education Council
of the United States (SIECUS)
130 W. 42nd St., Suite 350
New York, NY 10036
212-819-9770
www.siecus.org

Sickle Cell Disease Association of America
231 East Baltimore St., Suite 800
Baltimore, MD 21202
800-421-8453
410-528-1555
www.SickleCellDisease.org

SIDS Alliance, Inc.
1314 Bedford Ave.
Suite 210
Baltimore, MD 21208
800-221-SIDS
www.sidsalliance.org

United Cerebral Palsy Association (UCPA)
1660 L St., NW
Suite 700
Washington, DC 20036
800-872-5827
www.ucpa.org

United Network for Organ Sharing
PO Box 2484
Richmond, VA 23218
888-894-6361
www.unos.org

1-800 Telephone Numbers for Health Care Information, Products, and Services

Alzheimer's Disease and Related Disorders Association 800-272-3900
American Academy of Allergy, Asthma, and Immunology 800-822-2762
American Cancer Society 800-ACS-2345
American Council of the Blind 800-424-8666
American Diabetes Association 800-342-2383
American Dietetic Association 800-877-1600
American Kidney Fund 800-638-8299
American Liver Foundation 800-465-4837
Lupus Foundation Information Line 800-558-0121
American Nurses Association 800-274-4ANA
Asthma and Allergy Foundation of America 800-727-8462
Cystic Fibrosis Foundation 800-344-4823
Drug Abuse Hotline 800-662-HELP
Epilepsy Foundation's National Information Center 800-332-1000
FDA Hotline (for drugs, biologics, and medical devices) 888-463-6332
National Safety Council 800-621-7619
Hearing Impaired AIDS Hotline 800-243-7889
Human Growth Foundation (growth disorders) 800-451-6434
Institute for Limb Preservation @ Presbyterian/St. Luke's Medical Center 800-262-5462
Juvenile Diabetes Foundation International 800-533-2873
Invacare 800-333-6900
The Living Bank International (organ donation) 800-528-2971
Graham Field Inc. 800-347-5678
Medco Instruments .... 800-626-3326 ext. 10
MedicAlert 888-633-4298
Medical Express (traveling health professionals) 800-544-7255
Medicare 800-MEDICARE
CDC National AIDS Hotline 800-HIV-0440
CDC TB & STD Prevention Information Network 800-458-5231
National Cancer Institute, Public Inquiries Office 800-4-CANCER
National Clearinghouse for Alcohol and Drug Information 800-729-6686
National Down Syndrome Society 800-221-4602
National Down Syndrome Congress 800-232-6372
National Health Careers Information Hotline 800-999-4248
Lung Line at National Jewish Medical and Research Center 800-222-LUNG
National Rehabilitation Information Center 800-34-NARIC
National Safety Council Call Center 800-621-7619
CDC Sexually Transmitted Diseases Hotline 800-227-8922
National SIDS Alliance 800-221-SIDS
National Spinal Cord Injury Association Resource Center 800-962-9629
Information Request Line for International Dyslexia Association 800-ABCD-123
Phoenix Society for Burn Survivors 800-888-BURN
Quality Line Health Education Videos 800-356-0986

Simon Foundation for Continence 800-237-4666
SmithKline Glaxo 888-825-5249
Spanish AIDS and STD Hotline 800-344-7432
Spina Bifida Association of America 800-621-3141
United Cerebral Palsy Foundation 800-872-5827
United Ostomy Association 800-826-0826

Professional Organizations, Associations, and Academies

American Academy of Nurse Practitioners
PO Box 12846
Austin TX 78711
512-442-4262
www.aanp.org

American Academy of Nursing
555 East Wells Street
Suite 1100
Milwaukee, WI 53202-3823
414-287-0289
www.nursingworld.org/aan

American Association for the History of
    Nursing, Inc.
PO Box 175
Lanoka Harbor, NJ 08734
609-693-7250
www.aahn.org

American Association for Medical
    Transcription
100 Sycamore Avenue
Modesto, CA 95354
800-982-2182
209-527-9620
www.aamt.org

American Association for Respiratory Care
9425 N. MacArthur Blvd., Suite 100
Irving, TX 75063
972-243-2272
www.aarc.org

American Association of Blood Banks
8101 Glenbrook Rd.
Bethesda, MD 20814-2749
301-907-6977
www.aabb.org

American Association of Critical-Care Nurses
101 Columbia
Aliso Viejo, CA 92656
800-899-2226
949-362-2000
www.aacn.org

American Association of Medical Assistants
20 N. Wacker Drive, Suite 1575
Chicago, IL 60606
312-899-1500
www.aama-ntl.org

American Association of Neuroscience Nurses
4700 W. Lake Ave.
Glenview, IL 60025
888-557-2266 (US only)
847-375-4733
www.aann.org

American Association of Nurse Anesthetists
222 S. Prospect Ave.
Park Ridge, IL 60068-4001
847-692-7050
www.aana.com

American Association of Nurse Attorneys
P.O. Box 515
Columbus, OH 43216-0515
877-538-2262
www.taana.org

American Association of Occupational Health
    Nurses
2920 Brandywine Rd., Suite 100
Atlanta, GA 30341
770-455-7757
www.aaohn.org

American Association of Office Nurses
109 Kinderkamack Rd.
Montvale, NJ 07645
201-391-2600
www.healthresource.org/HRP/proorgs.
asp?orgid=127

American Association of Spinal Cord Injury
   Nurses
75-20 Astoria Blvd.
Jackson Heights, NY 11370-1177
718-803-3782
www.aascin.org

American Clinical Laboratory Association
1250 H Street, NW
Suite 880
Washington, DC 20005
202-637-9466
www.clinical-labs.org

American College of Healthcare Executives
1 North Franklin St., Suite 1700
Chicago, IL 60606-3491
312-424-2800
www.ache.org

American College of Nurse Midwives
8403 Colesville Rd.
Suite 1550
Silver Spring MD 20910
240-485-1800
www.midwife.org

American Dental Association
211 E. Chicago Ave.
17th Floor
Chicago, IL 60611
312-440-2500
www.ada.org

American Dental Hygienists' Association
444 N Michigan Avenue, Suite 3400
Chicago, IL 60611
312-440-8900
www.adha.org

American Dietetic Association
120 South Riverside Plaza, Suite 2000
Chicago, IL 60606-6995
800-877-1600
www.eatright.org

American Health Care Association
1201 L St. NW
Washington, DC 20005-4015
202-842-4444
www.ahca.org

American Health Information Management
   Association
233 N Michigan Avenue, 21st Floor
Chicago, IL 60601
312-233-1100
www.ahima.org

American Holistic Nurses' Association
PO Box 2130
Flagstaff, AZ 86003-2130
800-278-2462
www.ahna.org

American Lung Association
61 Broadway, 6th floor
New York, NY 10006
212-315-8700
www.lungusa.org

American Massage Therapy Association
500 Davis Street
Evanston, IL 60201
877-905-2700
847-864-0123
www.amtamassage.org

American Medical Association
515 N. State St.
Chicago, IL 60610
800-621-8335
www.ama-assn.org

American Nephrology Nurses' Association
East Holly Ave.
Box 56
Pitman, NJ 08071-0056
888-600-ANNA
856-256-2320
www.annanurse.org

American Nurses Association
8515 Georgia Avenue
Suite 400
Silver Spring, MD 20910
301-628-5000
800-274-4ANA
www.nursingworld.org

American Nurses Foundation
8515 Georgia Ave.
Suite 400 West
Silver Spring, MD 20910
301-628-5227
www.nursingworld.org/anf

American Occupational Therapy Association
4720 Montgomery Lane
PO Box 31220
Bethesda, MD 20824-1220
301-652-2682
www.aota.org

American Organization of Nurse Executives
Liberty Place
325 Seventh Street, NW
Washington, DC 20004
202-626-2240
www.aone.org

American Pharmacists Association
1100 15th Street NW, Suite 400
Washington, DC 20005-1707
800-237-APHA
202-628-4410
www.aphanet.org

American Physical Therapy Association
1111 N. Fairfax St.
Alexandria, VA 22314-1488
800-999-2782
703-684-2782
www.apta.org

American Psychiatric Nurses Association
1555 Wilson Blvd, Suite 602
Arlington, VA 22209
866-243-2443
www.apna.org

American Public Health Association
800 I Street, NW
Washington, DC 20001
202-777-2742
www.apha.org

American Radiological Nurses Association
7794 Grow Drive
Pensacola, FL 32514
866-486-2762
850-474-7292
www.arna.net

American Registry of Radiologic Technologists
1255 Northland Dr.
St. Paul, MN 55120
651-687-0048
www.arrt.org

American Society for Clinical Laboratory
   Science
6701 Democracy Blvd, Suite 300
Bethesda, MD 20817
301-657-2768
www.ascls.org

American Society of Health-System
   Pharmacists
7272 Wisconsin Ave.
Bethesda, MD 20814
301-657-3000
www.ashp.org

American Speech-Language-Hearing
   Association
10801 Rockville Pike
Rockville, MD 20852
800-638-8255
www.asha.org

Association for the Care of Children's Health
19 Mantua Rd.
Mt. Royal, NJ 08061
609-224-1742
www.eparent.com/resources/associations/
   childrenshealthassoc.htm

Association of Mental Health Administrators
60 Revere Drive, Suite 500
Northbrook, IL 60062
708-480-9626

Association of Nurses in AIDS Care
3538 Ridgewood Road
Akron, OH 44333
800-260-6780
www.anacnet.org

Association of Pediatric Oncology Nurses
4700 West Lake Ave.
Glenview, IL 60025
847-375-4724
www.apon.org

Association of Peri-Operative Registered Nurses
2170 South Parker Rd.
Suite 300
Denver, CO 80231
800-755-2676
www.aorn.org

Association of Rehabilitation Nurses
4700 W. Lake Rd.
Glenview, IL 60025-1485
800-229-7530
www.rehabnurse.org

Association of Women's Health, Obstetric and
    Neonatal Nurses
2000 L Street, NW
Suite 740
Washington, DC 20036
800-673-8499 (toll free U.S.)
800-245-0231 (toll free Canada)
www.awhonn.org

Commission on Graduates of Foreign Nursing
    Schools (CGFNS)
3600 Market St., Suite 400
Philadelphia, PA 19104
215-349-8767
www.cgfns.org

Dental Assisting National Board
444 N. Michigan Avenue, Suite 900
Chicago, IL 60611
312-642-3368
www.dentalassisting.com

Development Disabilities Nurses Association
1685 H St. PMB 1214
Blaine, WA 98230
800-888-6733
www.ddna.org

Emergency Nurses Association
915 Lee St.
Des Plaines, IL 60016-6569
800-900-9659
www.ena.org

Hospice & Palliative Nurses Association
One Penn Center West, Suite 229
Pittsburgh, PA 15276
412-787-9301
www.hpna.org

Infusion Nurses Society
220 Norwood Park South
Norwood, MA 02062
781-440-9408
www.ins1.org

National Association of Hispanic Nurses
1501 16th St., NW
Washington, DC 20036
202-387-2477
www.thehispanicnurses.org

National Association of Home Care (NAHC)
228 Seventh Street, SE
Washington, DC 20003
202-547-7424
www.nahc.org

National Association of Nurse Practitioners in
    Women's Health
505 C Street, N.E.
Washington, DC 20002
202-543-9693
www.npwh.org

National Association of Pediatric Nurse
    Associates and Practitioners
20 Brace Road
Suite 200
Cherry Hill, NJ 08034-2634
856-857-9700
www.napnap.org

National Association of School Nurses, Inc.
8484 Georgia Avenue, Suite 420
Silver Spring, MD 20910
240-821-1130
www.nasn.org

National Athletic Trainers' Association
2952 Stemmons Freeway, #200
Dallas, TX 75247
214-637-6282
www.nata.org

National Black Nurses Association
8630 Fenton St.
Suite 330
Silver Spring, MD 20910
800-575-6298
301-589-3200
www.nbna.org

National Board for Respiratory Care
8310 Nieman Rd.
Lenexa, KS 66214
913-599-4200
www.nbrc.org

National Cancer Institute
NCI Public Inquiries Office
6116 Executive Boulevard
Room 3036A
Bethesda, MD 20892-8322
800-4-CANCER
www.cancer.gov
www.nci.nih.gov

National Gerontological Nursing Association
7794 Grow Dr.
Pensacola, FL 32514-7072
850-473-1174
www.ngna.org

National League for Nursing
61 Broadway, 33rd Floor
New York, NY 10006
212-363-5555
www.nln.org

National Nurses in Business Association
(NNBA)
PO Box 561081
Rockledge, FL 32956
877-353-8888
www.nnba.net

International Nurses Society on Addictions
PO Box 10752
Raleigh, NC 27605
919-821-1292
http://intnsa.org

National Student Nurses' Association
45 Main Street, Suite 606
Brooklyn, NY 11201
718-210-0705
www.nsna.org

North American Nursing Diagnosis
Association
100 N. 20th Street, 4th Floor
Philadelphia, PA 19103
215-545-8105
800-647-9002
www.nanda.org

Oncology Nursing Society
125 Enterprise Drive
Pittsburgh, PA 15275
866-257-4ONS
412-859-6100
www.ons.org

Sigma Theta Tau International Honor Society
of Nursing
550 W. North St.
Indianapolis, IN 46202
888-634-7575
317-634-8171
www.nursingsociety.org

Society for Vascular Nursing
7794 Grow Dr.
Pensacola, FL 32514
888-536-4786
www.svnnet.org

Society of Gastroenterology Nurses and
Associates, Inc.
401 N. Michigan Ave.
Chicago, IL 60611
312-321-5165
800-245-7462 (hotline)
www.sgna.org

Society of Otorhinolaryngology and Head/Neck
Nurses
116 Canal St.
Suite A
New Smyrna Beach, FL 32168
386-428-1695
www.sohnnurse.com

Transcultural Nursing Society
Madonna University
College of Nursing and Health
36600 Schoolcraft Road
Livonia, MI 48150-1173
888-432-5470 (from within the United States)
734-432-5470 (international)
www.tcns.org